Positive Psychology Interventions in Practice

Carmel Proctor
Editor

Positive Psychology Interventions in Practice

Springer

Editor
Carmel Proctor
Positive Psychology Research Centre Ltd
Guernsey, UK

ISBN 978-3-319-51785-8 ISBN 978-3-319-51787-2 (eBook)
DOI 10.1007/978-3-319-51787-2

Library of Congress Control Number: 2017930961

Printed on acid-free paper

This Springer imprint is published by Springer Nature
The registered company is Springer International Publishing AG
The registered company address is: Gewerbestrasse 11, 6330 Cham, Switzerland

I dedicate this volume to Piers my husband, Morgan my son, and Doreen my friend for their patience, love, and support and for you Danny.

Foreword

A decade ago, colleagues and I posed the question '*Does positive psychology have a future*?' In doing so, we were setting out to explore what we saw as three potential avenues for the future evolution of positive psychology. First, that it disappeared, because all psychology subsumed the positive. Second, that it continued as an independent discipline, while in parallel becoming more broadly absorbed by psychology as a whole. Or third, that it became increasingly marginalised as a specialist subdiscipline (see Linley et al. 2006).

The advent of this book is a striking testament to the fact that over this intervening decade, positive psychology has followed the middle course. It has become ever more embedded within psychology as a whole while still maintaining its own vibrant ecosystem of research and practice. I suspect a better outcome for positive psychology—and most importantly, its beneficial impact on the people of the world—we could not have hoped for.

The chapters of this book show how much has changed in relation to the applications of positive psychology, together with our ability to document and evidence the positive influence that positive psychology can have on people's lives. Earlier writings on positive psychology applications and interventions tended to be speculative and theoretical. In *Positive Psychology Interventions in Practice*, we see these applications and interventions brought to life with evidence and data. Targeted insight and understanding allow us to develop more nuanced perspectives on what works for whom and why, when, and where.

Throughout these chapters, we see positive psychology being integrated within a wider literature of research and practice, across myriad areas of practice and intervention. These perspectives start with the self—as any viable intervention always must then blossom out to consider targeted interventions for desired outcomes, before embarking on the exploration and enabling of human flourishing in specific environments—through relationships with others, at school, or in the workplace.

Embracing the challenge and opportunity of the modern world, the chapters then embrace the positive potential of technologies and design, before concluding with an invitation and instructions for effective engagement on the development and implementation of positive policy—our ability to impact the greatest number in the most positive ways, through leveraging positive psychology interventions against the fulcrum of government legislation and practice.

In everything throughout, the emphasis is on practice. To change, we must act. To improve, we must strive. To serve others, we must step forward. *Positive Psychology Interventions in Practice* provides us with the evidence, the frameworks, and the practical steps we need to take to have a positive impact on our world.

We should all seize the opportunity that is before us and do so.

Capp & Co Ltd, The Venture Centre,
University of Warwick Science Park
Sir William Lyons Road, Coventry,
CV4 7EZ, UK
alex.linley@capp.co

Alex Linley

Reference

Linley, P. A., Joseph, S., Harrington, S., & Wood, A. M. (2006). Positive psychology: Past, present and (possible) future. *Journal of Positive Psychology, 1*(1), 3–16.

Contents

List of Contributors

Fredrike Bannink Bannink Therapy, Training, Coaching and Mediation Practice, Amsterdam, The Netherlands

Rosa Maria Banos Department of Personality, Evaluation and Psychological Treatment, University of Valencia, Valencia, Spain

Cristina Botella Department of Basic Psychology, Clinical and Psychobiology, Jaume I University, Castellon, Spain

Kim Cameron Ross School of Education, University of Michigan, Ann Arbor, MI, USA

Natalia Carro INIBIOMA (CONICET-University of Comahue), Bariloche, Argentina

Ron Chu University of Toronto Scarborough, Toronto, ON, Canada

Lucian Gideon Conway III Department of Psychology, University of Montana, Missoula, MT, USA

Andrea Czar AWE, Buenos Aires, Argentina

University of Palermo, Buenos Aires, Argentina

Paola D'Adamo INIBIOMA (CONICET-University of Comahue), Bariloche, Argentina

AWE, Buenos Aires, Argentina

Madeline Dobrin Department of Psychology, Kwantlen Polytechnic University, Surrey, BC, Canada

Olivia Evans The Career Guide, Melbourne, Australia

Jenny Fox Eades Edge Hill University, Ormskirk, Lancashire, UK

Judith Gray Frodingham Infant School, Scunthorpe, North Lincolnshire, UK

Suzy Green The Positivity Institute, Sydney, NSW, Australia

Veronica Guillen Department of Personality, Evaluation and Psychological Treatment, University of Valencia, Valencia, Spain

Centro Clínico Previ, Valencia, Spain

Irfan Hakim University of Toronto Scarborough, Toronto, ON, Canada

Jenny Hofmann Abteilung für Persönlichkeitspsychologie und Diagnostik, Psychologisches Institut, Zürich, Switzerland

Marcela Kapelmayer AWE, CABA, Argentina

Jandi Kelly Ross School of Education, University of Michigan, Ann Arbor, MI, USA

Viviana Kelmanowicz AWE, Buenos Aires, Argentina

University of Belgrano, Buenos Aires, Argentina

University of Palermo, Buenos Aires, Argentina

Bruce Kidd University of Toronto Scarborough, Toronto, ON, Canada

Thomas J. Lottman Children, Inc., Covington, KY, USA

Ruth Louden University of Toronto Scarborough, Toronto, ON, Canada

Mariana Lozada INIBIOMA (CONICET-University of Comahue), Bariloche, Argentina

Aryel Maharaj University of Toronto Scarborough, Toronto, ON, Canada

Eric Mah Department of Psychology, Kwantlen Polytechnic University, Surrey, BC, Canada

Ryan Niemiec VIA Institute on Character, Cincinnati, OH, USA

Rachel Van Poele Department of Psychology, Kwantlen Polytechnic University, Surrey, BC, Canada

Anna E. Pohlmeyer Department of Industrial Design, Delft University of Technology, Delft, The Netherlands

Denise M. Quinlan Māori Hill, Dunedin, New Zealand

Tayyab Rashid University of Toronto Scarborough, Toronto, ON, Canada

Sue Roffey School of Education, Western Sydney University, Penrith, NSW, Australia

Vera Roos Optentia Research Focus Area, North-West University, Vanderbijlpark, South Africa

Willibald Ruch Abteilung für Persönlichkeitspsychologie und Diagnostik, Psychologisches Institut, Zürich, Switzerland

Roger G. Tweed Department of Psychology, Kwantlen Polytechnic University, Surrey, BC, Canada

Danielle Uy University of Toronto Scarborough, Toronto, ON, Canada

Belinda Williams The Whole Being Group, Sydney, Australia

Piers Worth The Faculty of Society and Health, School of Social Sciences and Education, Buckinghamshire New University, Buckinghamshire, UK

Laurie Wright University of Toronto Scarborough, Toronto, ON, Canada

Ronette Zaaiman Optentia Research Focus Area, North-West University, Vanderbijlpark, South Africa

Sarah Zawaly Children, Inc., Covington, KY, USA

The original version of this book was revised. An erratum to this book can be found at DOI 10.1007/978-3-319-51787-2_16

Chapter 1
Positive Psychology Interventions: The First Intervention Is Our Self

Piers Worth

Abstract This book is focused on positive psychology interventions (PPIs) in practice. This chapter advocates that we pause ahead of looking at PPI themselves and consider that any positive psychology practitioner seeking to facilitate an intervention with others, should recognise that the first intervention they bring is their own self—the qualities of attention, openness, and presence along with a willingness to suspend personal prior experiences. If, in turn, they can acknowledge what Carl Rogers (1961) described as the 'actualising tendency', they are trusting and accepting of the unique unfolding that may occur within individuals and groups, and potentially offering Rogers' core conditions for growth. The chapter takes a provocative step in suggesting that the kind of behaviours this may involve, are a reflection of Fredrickson's (2013) research and writing on love. The chapter concludes with a proposal that this perspective is a central reflection of the professionalism and professional practice of any positive psychology practitioner.

Abbreviation

PPI Positive psychology intervention

Introduction

For those of us introducing and facilitating a positive psychology intervention (PPI) for others, my proposal is that who you are as a person, what you live and bring, will affect everything that you do, and are as important as learning an intervention. My

P. Worth (✉)
The Faculty of Society and Health, School of Social Sciences and Education,
Buckinghamshire New University, Buckinghamshire, UK
e-mail: piers.worth@bucks.ac.uk

C. Proctor (ed.), *Positive Psychology Interventions in Practice*,
DOI 10.1007/978-3-319-51787-2_1

motive in writing this chapter is to illustrate a small number of the perspectives and insights that may be involved in the 'self-as-instrument' (Cheung-Judge 2001). We see individuals entering the discipline and work of positive psychology from many educational and professional backgrounds. Motivated by a commitment to personal and professional practice and development in the discipline (Schon 1991), and profession of 'intervening' with others, this chapter offers psychologically-related theoretical and research insights (e.g., Ryan and Deci 2000; Joseph 2015) to help individuals to bring themselves to the positive psychology intervention in a perceptually open and resourceful way.

In the chapter we will reflect upon the perceptions and habits that shape your reactions to the work you undertake. Reflecting our discipline, we will in turn anticipate the positive in you that will influence and shape what you bring to positive psychology interventions. The chapter will explore the presence and the influence of Carl Rogers' concept of the actualising tendency (Rogers 1961; Glassman and Hadad 2009) and its capacity to shape your beliefs and expectations within the practice of positive psychology. The chapter will conclude with a consideration of the reflective and reflexive impact of the perspectives on our practise of positive psychology.

Our Busy 'Auto Pilot' World

We see and encounter our world through habits of perception. As sense-making beings, we seek commonly and compulsively to understand, anticipate, and predict causation within the world we live in (Martin et al. 2007). All our experience shapes how we believe the world to be. We analyse, categorise, and label the world we encounter. By doing this, by judging, naming, labelling, and predicting our world, we feel safer and potentially more in control (Hogg and Vaughan 2008). Our work and professional responses also become shaped by these habits, and in turn they become how we explain experiences to ourselves (Martin et al. 2007; Seligman 2006).

To complicate matters further, we live in a digitally frantic world. Our computers, telephones, and tablets, all create a flood of information and demands on us that may, in reality, be at best cognitively distracting from the world around us and at worst impossible to deal with. This level of information and stimulation floods us with demands to do or act—requiring a response primarily from our rationality rather than our being or heart. Coping with these demands may push or force us to live out of habit, on 'autopilot', or by automatic reactions, rather than meeting our experiences in their fullness, in each moment.

This life context and style runs the risk that we become, at the same time, potentially disconnected from our 'being' while flooded with demands on our 'doing'. We want to review, within this book, positive psychology interventions in practice. Yet, what I propose within this chapter is that the first and primary intervention with others comes from being, our self, as the primary vehicle for connecting with and influencing others. It is in the finding and understanding of our self that we become prepared and resources to 'intervene' with others. The purpose of this chapter is to review what, in practise, this might mean, and how we may develop and access its characteristics.

What Do You Bring to the PPI Interaction?

As we enter and start to encounter and deal with any situation, we bring all of our experiences to date with us. These shaping and guiding memories or internal schemas are our expectations of how the world around us works and how we would wish it to work (Maltby et al. 2010; Martin et al. 2007; Hogg and Vaughan 2008). If you were to summarise your story, its big themes or patterns, what would they be? These are a combination of expectations and beliefs. They form both what we see and expect. They are, in turn, habits of perception. When we originally had an experience that shaped our views of the world, our perception and reaction were occurring within our awareness. Over time, in what we come to believe is their predictability, they become habits of perception, and something we do outside awareness or unconsciously.

For those of us drawn to and engaged in positive psychology these may also be beliefs about the positive in life, the balance of the positive and the negative, or challenging experiences in our world, and what kind of outcomes we may seek via a positive psychology intervention. These beliefs will also include expectations around helping others, their need for helping, and why you *must* help. If we must help, then we actually *need* those who require help. Perhaps, bizarrely, we are dependent on them. Help may actually represent a measure of your personal value. The ability to help others change may in turn represent your personal success.

If you offer help, an intervention, to others, you may *need* them to accept and respond as a mark of your own value. Their reaction and your success becomes a form of pressure from you on or direction towards them.

To explore these ideas further, please consider what your habits of perception are? What are your beliefs or expectations? What do you expect to see and find in the world around you, particularly your work? How might these habits of perception shape the direction of work you undertake, such as a positive psychology intervention? Do any of these habits or perceptions have the qualities of 'should' or 'must'? What should you be doing? What must you be doing? What story has brought you to this point? How, in turn, do these direct or drive the work you undertake? How much of your mental awareness is either processing the events or experiences, or is rehearsing how you believe you will respond? How much do you *really* see? Even if you only explore and answer a proportion of these questions, please consider what influence your insights may have on your approach to facilitating or creating a positive psychology intervention?

Our Individuation: Our Actualising Tendency

Joseph and Linley (2006) made a profound step within the practice of our discipline, by asserting and assuming one of Carl Rogers (1961) tenets, the actualising tendency, as a 'central foundation stone' of positive psychology. Given the power of this assertion in its own right and, if accepted, the potential influence on the education of individuals entering the discipline, this section seeks to articulate and define these ideas.

The actualising tendency is a theory that proposes all biological life, including human beings, will grow towards its inherent best given the necessary conditions for growth (Glassman and Hadad 2009). This implies, whatever our circumstances, age, or context, there is some part of us that will be drawing us towards our best. If we combine this perspective with that of Carl Jung, and what he termed 'individuation', the view would become that not only do we seek to grow towards our best, but also we seek to grow towards our own wholeness (Levinson et al. 1978). Glassman and Hadad (2009) write as if this is a literal biological process, which the descriptions appear to imply. Thorne (2002), however, presents this more as metaphor and symbolism of something that occurs within us all. Joseph (2015) acknowledges that the concept of the actualising tendency remains unusual if not challenging even in modern time. As professionals and practitioners the idea creates the invitation and need to reflect on how our behaviour and work might change if we accept its presence.

Living and Working with the Belief of the Actualising Tendency?

If we hold a belief that individually we will grow towards our best given the supportive conditions, then what we propose is this changes everything in the relationship we might hold with those we facilitate in a positive psychology intervention.

We may know the shape an intervention may have and the direction it may draw individuals. We know, within the context of the theory of our discipline, that some interventions fit us, or elicit our motivation, in ways that others will not (Lyubomirksy 2007). However, if we believe that the experiences and the outcome of an intervention will be unique to an individual and an expression of their individual, personal unfolding, then in turn we need to hold an openness, a willingness to let the unexpected happen, not to judge, push, or shape an outcome with *our* expectations. Whichever view we take or accept, if we assume a move towards our best, and wholeness, then it has an implication of openness and acceptance to the reaction of those on or towards whom we are intervening.

If you were to accept the presence of the actualising tendency, how do you feel this would shape or change your habits of perception or attention? How would it change your relationship with those you are working with as a positive psychology practitioner?

Bringing About, Eliciting the Actualising Tendency in Others

Rogers (1961) proposed three core conditions for growth, which, if offered to an individual, received or found by them, facilitate the actualising tendency, and subsequent personal growth is probably inevitable. He found this from years of clinical practice, and subsequently applied this in an education environment (Rogers et al. 2014). The first was offering 'unconditional positive regard' which is where we prize another individual for being human and for their humanity, even if we may have questions, for example, with their behaviour. The second was experiencing empathy for another individual, the ability to have a sense of their experiences and their perspectives, and to communicate this via our attention or words. The final condition is the capacity for what was called 'congruence', an acceptance of ourselves, in the moment, and overall, and being willing to work from this, and to let others see us doing so. In simple terms, congruence is living from the position of giving ourselves unconditional positive regard, and an ongoing empathy for our own experiences and letting others see us in our humanity, modelling, living, what we might wish to offer them (Glassman and Hadad 2009).

In our humanity, this offering of core conditions is always an effort or potentially incomplete, but Rogers (1961) believed the attempt was more important than necessarily this being 'right' (Glassman and Hadad 2009). Rogers' views on the core conditions for growth, which in turn elicit and support the actualising tendency, arguably become a 'loop'. If we offer the core conditions to others, we support the development of their actualising tendency. If we bring about the actualising tendency, in turn we may bring about further expressions of the core conditions for growth from others to us, and those in their context. While this is a theory and a practise described in its own right, the willingness to relate to it describes what would, in turn, imply a mindful approach, and a willingness to engage with the moment-by-moment 'life' and change present in a positive psychology intervention (Kabat-Zinn 2004; Segal et al. 2002). Consider exploring the implications of practising and experiencing the core conditions? Do you believe you experience these now? Where? From whom? Which of these core conditions do you offer now? Which of them is harder for you to offer? Why? Is there a way in which you might develop this perspective and skill?

How Do the Ideas and Assumptions of the Actualising Tendency Link to Other Areas of Positive Psychology?

I believe what I am suggesting in bringing this approach to a PPI is a reflection of theories proposed by Barbara Fredrickson (2013) on love. The aliveness, openness to, and acceptance of others in this approach of offering the core conditions for growth to facilitate a PPI is potentially a reflection of the interconnectedness Fredrickson sees as fundamental to micro moments of love. The behaviours we offer to others have the potential to broaden-and-build their emotional experiences in the openness they create in those experiencing the PPI (e.g., Fredrickson and Joiner 2002). Fredrickson implies they may turn full circle and become an openness we give ourselves. However, I believe we can go further in proposing this is a reflection of love, by linking her ideas to Fromm's (1957) psychotherapeutic exploration of what he termed the 'art of loving' considered in the next paragraph.

This quality of attention to others involves an openness, a capacity for listening and attention, and a stillness to respond creatively and a potential vulnerability that represents a functioning at a peak of our own strengths and emotional capacity. Fromm (1957) asserts this quality of 'giving' is an experience of our strength, power, vitality, and potency. It involves or creates an aliveness and joyousness. This form of giving may be an attention to those we are with, but the openness is a reflection of ourselves, our aliveness, and our life. Perhaps, in turn, the quality of focus and attention may also create the characteristics of flow (e.g., Csikszentmihalyi 1992). In a manner that preceded and reflected the ideas of Fredrickson (2013), Fromm saw this quality as an act of respect that was in turn a reflection of love. This is a respect in which we are willing to see an individual or others as they are, in their uniqueness and individuality, with a concern for and an openness towards the growth of those we love (Fromm 1957).

Again, as a forerunner to the positive psychology ideas put forward by Fredrickson (2013), Fromm (1957) saw love as an attitude, a way of behaving that shaped his or her relatedness towards the world. Love is an action and an activity, not solely bound up with a person or focus of our love. The characteristics, nature, or quality of our action and activity involve not simply looking *at* the surface of others, but involves looking *in*. A surface will portray differences, whereas insight, 'in-sight' towards another will involve our relatedness and connection. Fromm argues that this form of love can only take place between equals. Through this we move beyond seeing others as those that need help—we experience and relate to the compassion we share with others. If we accept these perspectives they have a profound influence and challenge to our professional practice in positive psychology.

Quietening Inside in Order to See and Hear Openly, Rather than Through Habit

Given what I described earlier about our habits of perception, as you commence working in a positive psychology intervention, a question you face is how much of what you see and hear in front of you, will you actually perceive? Can you quieten or stop the inner processing, interpretation, and labelling of what you encounter to allow yourself to see what is in front of you (Davies 2012)?

A simple fact and reality of our cognitive psychology is the more we are engaged in interpreting what we see, let alone rehearsing internally how we will respond and act, the less we actually have available to us to perceive. The act of processing removes or takes up cognitive capacity, and reduces our capacity to perceive. Can we allow ourselves to *just* see, to perceive, to take in, before we actually have to act? Can we allow ourselves time and opportunity to fully perceive, encounter, and accept what we see, before choosing its meaning and deciding to act (Davies 2012)? Davies proposes that this form of attention has a meditative or mindful quality. This gives us the time to communicate our attention towards those we work with, to witness and accept what we encounter, before rushing into interpretation and action. The quiet and gentleness on our perception before the action, arguably is one way to offer the core conditions for growth. Are we able and willing to perceive, to not fully know, and to be surprised? If so, we may perceive more than we had expected or believed possible.

Listening and Mirroring in Depth

As we allow ourselves the time to perceive, to be with, to be surprised and to be present with those we seek to help, we can listen in depth. What might the words, the tone of the words, and the bodies of those who speak tell us about their experience or what they need? For example, is voice tone at variance with the words spoken? Do the words say *yes*, but the tone say *uncertainty*? As positive psychology professionals, do we allow ourselves to explore these experiences, and what we perceive, without the rush to label or categorise. Our experience, our struggle to understand, may mirror that of the person or people we are working with. When we free ourselves to perceive openly, rather than to 'do', we give ourselves the opportunity to relate in the intervention we are supporting. We have the chance to notice what the possibility of change is really bringing about for those we work with (Machon 2010).

Surfing the Edge of Awareness

A pivotal experience of my own, in allowing myself to listen and perceive in depth, is what I have come to describe as 'surfing the edge' of awareness. A gift of being deaf is the amount of effort I have to put in to ensure I hear those I work with. I know, most of the time, I do well. Yet one afternoon a decade ago, I began to notice particularly the last 5–10 s of what individuals said to me. Their voice tone became uncertain, their words were hesitant, and it was as if they were asking an incomplete question, not of me, but of themselves. I simply mirrored to them their own half-formed question, which they in turn, then, answered. I had noticed, heard, the process of what these individuals were working out for themselves, perhaps without them realising what was emerging or happening. This edge of awareness proved an area of priority for the individual because it was the point at which some new part of themselves appeared to be taking shape, growing, and being born. While I will always listen to all words spoken, I now place a major priority on the final, uncertain, and half-formed words, which is a question the individual is asking of themselves. When the individual in turn asks their question to himself or herself, in awareness, they then have the ability to act.

Attempt your own listening to others. Do not think or rehearse what to say until they have finished speaking. Allow them to *see* the extent of your listening, and your own working out, finding words for what you in turn need to say to them.

Creating Form and Shape for Moving Forward

When we perceive, feel, and listen in this way as positive psychology practitioners do we, in turn, become a 'mirror of hope' for the individual or group? If we work in this way, whatever the coming PPI, I propose we are reflecting the self or selves in the process of becoming (Machon 2010). Drawing on the structure of Snyder's (1994, 2000) model of hope, we may hear their goals, 'will power' and 'way power'. Working in this way allows us to conversationally give form and shape to the emerging hope within the PPI.

Using Snyder's (1994, 2000) model, do you hear a 'goal', will power and way power evident in conversation, in what individuals may describe to you? Which of the two may be lacking in form or precision to support an individual's action? What questions may gently support an individual or a group becoming more exact about a goal, will power, or way power?

The Professional Implications of This Perspective

If as positive psychology practitioners, we accept perspectives like the actualising tendency we are in a journey of 'process' rather than 'ending' (Joseph and Linley 2006; Machon 2010; Joseph 2015). For example, how we unfold towards the best in us will change with time and age. An unfolding in our 30s will be different to one in our 40s or 50s (Levinson et al. 1978; Levinson 1986; Vaillant 1977, 2002). We are challenged therefore, in ourselves and in our work with others, to accept they are in the process of becoming, rather than ever reaching an end-point. We bring to those we work with that authentic acceptance of our own process of becoming, and of theirs, and in turn the attentiveness to what this might be (Machon 2010). If, as facilitators and practitioners, we can accept this is happening for those we work with, our role changes to one of observation and stillness, that in turn witnesses and supports the unfolding of others (Machon 2010).

Further, the related discipline of appreciative inquiry proposes that this depth of attention and listening offers others the majority of what are termed 'the six freedoms' which are believed to release a personal and/or organisational power when experienced. These 'freedoms' are described as being known in relationship, to be heard, to be positive, to act with support, to dream in community, and to contribute to the world around them (Whitney and Trosten-Bloom 2010). I believe as positive psychology practitioners we would infer a positive psychology intervention provides most if not all of these freedoms to those we seek to support. Offering the rarity of attention and belief to others in the way implied in this chapter initiates a capacity to relate and respond to the creative growth that may emerge in a positive psychology intervention.

Worth (2015) implies that the willingness to work openly with the uncertainty of what may occur in those we facilitate is in turn an acceptance of the fundamental qualities of creation occurring in life, and our lives. This acceptance of uncertainty and creativity is part of what is described as the 'hero's journey' (Worth 2015).

If we can accept that the attitude we bring to a PPI is a reflection of actions and behaviours of love, we will be accepting and honouring the human qualities of those we are with (Fromm 1957). Yet Fromm challenges us deeply: he asserts to love in this way must also involve our own self-acceptance and self-love. Through this a PPI, in turn, becomes a paradox, a part of our own positive psychology practice towards ourselves.

To work in this manner is an act of love, art, and creation. The skill it involves includes discipline, patience, concentration, and reflection, as part of our journey of development as positive psychology practitioners (Fromm 1957). While I have not, to date, seen these types of ideas in positive psychology writing, I know they exist in other disciplines, such as social work, organisation development, and coaching (Cheung-Judge 2001; Curran et al. 1995; Heydt and Sherman 2005). This chapter is a description and an advocacy of what these writers would call 'self-as-an-instrument'. A positive psychology practitioner facilitating an intervention becomes an 'instrument of the profession'. He or she, in a helping relationship, is guiding a process of change (Heydt and Sherman 2005). The relationship is the vehicle and medium through which a practitioner facilitates change, even if this is part of a positive psychology intervention. Whether advocating system-level change, facilitating group or individual change, Heydt and Sherman (2005) use the striking musical image of the practitioner being both player and conductor in this process.

In earlier writing from the perspective of organisation development, Curran et al. (1995) highlight that a professional's capacity to use him or herself in this way relies on self-awareness, presence, and influence. They offer a detailed and insightful diagrammatic representation of what the self-as-instrument of change may involve which makes this reference particularly valuable to locate for readers. This diagram, illustrates factors, such as communication skills, a living out of personal values, worldview beliefs, and a capacity to monitor our own reactions and feelings, which are all characteristics that may be found within positive psychology interventions. This argues and illustrates what Peterson (2006) proposed and advocated: positive psychology is not a spectator sport. Facilitating others in these processes needs from a practitioner their own experience and practice, a willingness to live what they offer to others. Cheung-Judge (2001) summarises these demands graphically. She says the willingness to draw on the 'self-as-an-instrument' involves commitment, time, and energy to knowing who we are now and who we will be as we unfold in time. Cheung-Judge also asserts that an unwillingness to engage in the activities we advocate will come at a cost to ourselves in a strain or implied lack of authenticity in our work with others.

Geller and Greenberg's (2002) work takes an additional step, again from the perspective of person-centred counselling. The combination of what is advocated here involves a self-awareness and living what we offer to others, while at the same time being willing to be in relationship with others, openly work to their experiences while suspending or letting go of our own assumptions, bias, and habits of labelling. If we can find a confidence in our own self-awareness, a capacity to rely upon it, it creates an opportunity to let go, and be in a deeper presence with those we facilitate and lead. This has all the characteristics described earlier of Rogers' (1961) core conditions for growth, but goes further. Geller and Greenberg (2002) imply that in this type of relationship we 'blend' with the other. The receptivity and immersion they describe appear to have the characteristics of flow (e.g., Csikszentmihalyi 1992) we know well from within the discipline of positive psychology.

This is the paradox: by a willingness to acknowledge ourselves as an instrument in the work with others, to live the discipline we advocate, we in turn may find an openness and a capacity to be available with others that has the qualities of love described by Fromm (1957) and Fredrickson (2013).

The characteristics and possibilities that occur in this level of connection appear also to reflect the descriptions of 'presence' being described by Senge et al. (2005), as a creative and profoundly interpersonal space in which exceptional change may occur between individuals, in groups, and organisations.

Positive psychology as a discipline is drawing from many backgrounds beyond mainstream psychology or the social sciences. The perspectives of this chapter might be considered reflections of the personal development, professionalism, professional practice, and ethical awareness for those who are practitioners. This practice of interpersonal awareness, both of what we bring to the interaction and what we see and expect within it, is the reflective and reflexive skill expected in many professions. This chapter advocates that positive psychology interventions in practice is an environment and place in which they must be seen for the healthy unfolding of our discipline.

References

Cheung-Judge, M.-Y. (2001). The self as an instrument—A cornerstone for the future of OD. *The OD Practitioner, 33*(3), 11–16.

Csikszentmihalyi, M. (1992). *Flow: The psychology of happiness*. London: Rider Books.

Curran, K. M., Seashore, C. N., & Welp, M. G. (1995, November 17). *Use of the self as an instrument of change*. Paper presented at the ODN National Conference, Seattle, WA.

Davies, J. (2012). *Too busy to live your life: Take another look and walk with joy*. London: Aldgate Press.

Fredrickson, B. (2013). *Love 2.0*. New York: Hudson Street Press.

Fredrickson, B., & Joiner, T. (2002). Positive emotions trigger upward spirals toward emotional well-being. *Psychological Science, 13*(2), 172–175.

Fromm, E. (1957). *The art of loving*. London: Thorsons.

Geller, S. M., & Greenberg, L. (2002). Therapeutic presence: Therapists' experience of presence in the psychotherapy encounter. *Person-Centred and Experiential Psychotherapies, 1*(1–2), 71–86.

Glassman, W. E., & Hadad, M. (2009). *Approaches to psychology* (5th ed.). London: McGraw Hill.

Heydt, M. J., & Sherman, N. E. (2005). Conscious use of self: Tuning the instrument of social work practice with cultural competence. *The Journal of Baccalaureate Social Work, 10*(2), 25–40.

Hogg, M. A., & Vaughan, G. M. (2008). *Social psychology* (5th ed.). London: Pearson Education.

Joseph, S. (2015). *Positive therapy: Building bridges between positive psychology and person-centred psychotherapy* (2nd ed.). London: Routledge.

Joseph, S., & Linley, P. A. (2006). *Positive therapy: A meta-theory for positive psychology practice*. London: Routledge.

Kabat-Zinn, J. (2004). *Full catastrophe living: How to cope with stress, pain and illness using mindfulness meditation* (15th Anniversary ed.). New York: Dell.

Levinson, D. (1986). *Seasons of a woman's life*. New York: Alfred Knopf.

Levinson, D., Darrow, C. N., Klein, E. B., Levinson, M. H., & McKee, B. (1978). *Seasons of a man's life*. New York: Balantine Books.

Lyubomirksy, S. (2007). *The how of happiness: A scientific approach to getting the life you want*. New York: Penguin Press.

Machon, A. (2010). *The coaching secret: How to be and exceptional coach*. London: Prentice Hall Business.

Maltby, J., Day, L., & Macaskill, A. (2010). *Personality, individual differences and intelligence* (2nd ed.). London: Pearson Education.

Martin, G. N., Carlson, N. R., & Buskist, W. (2007). *Psychology* (3rd ed.). London: Pearson Education.

Peterson, C. (2006). *Positive psychology: A primer*. Oxford: Oxford University Press.

Rogers, C. R. (1961). *On becoming a person: A therapist's view of psychotherapy*. London: Constable.

Rogers, C. R., Lyon, H. C., & Tausch, R. (2014). *On becoming an effective teacher*. London: Routledge.
Ryan, R. M., & Deci, E. L. (2000). Self-determination theory and the facilitation of intrinsic motivation, social development and well-being. *American Psychologist, 5*(1), 68–78.
Schon, D. A. (1991). *The reflective practitioner: How professionals think in action*. Aldershot: Ashgate.
Segal, V., Williams, J. M. G., & Teasdale, J. D. (2002). *Mindfulness-based cognitive therapy for depression*. London: Guildford Press.
Seligman, M. E. P. (2006). *Learned optimism*. New York: Vintage Books.
Senge, P., Scharmer, C. O., Jaworski, J., & Flowers, B. S. (2005). *Presence: Exploring profound change in people, organizations and society*. London: Nicholas Brealey.
Snyder, C. R. (1994). *The psychology of hope*. London: Free Press.
Snyder, C. R. (Ed.). (2000). *Handbook of hope: Theory, measures and application*. London: Academic Press.
Thorne, B. (2002). *The mystical power of person-centred therapy*. London: Whurr.
Vaillant, G. (1977). *Adaptation to life*. Cambridge: Harvard University Press.
Vaillant, G. (2002). *Ageing well*. Boston: Little Brown.
Whitney, D., & Trosten-Bloom, A. (2010). *The power of appreciative inquiry: A practical guide to positive change* (2nd ed.). San Francisco: Berrett-Koehler.
Worth, P. (2015). The hero's quest. In I. Ivtzan, T. Lomas, K. Hefferon, & P. Worth (Eds.), *Second wave positive psychology: Embracing the dark side of life*. London: Routledge.

Part I
Clinical and Focused Interventions

Chapter 2
Positive CBT in Practice

Fredrike Bannink

Abstract Recent decades have witnessed the development of competency-based, collaborative approaches to working with clients. This article reveals how cognitive behavioural therapy (CBT) becomes positive CBT, with a shift in the focus of therapy from what is wrong with clients to what is right with them, and from what is not working to what is. The concept of positive CBT, which can be seen as Fourth Wave CBT, aimed at improving the well-being of clients and their therapists, draws on research and applications from positive psychology and solution-focused brief therapy. A functional behaviour analysis of exceptions to the problem and the 'upward arrow' instead of the 'downward arrow' technique are two of the many practical applications of positive CBT, described in this chapter.

Abbreviations

CBT	Cognitive behaviour therapy
FBA	Functional behaviour analysis
SFBT	Solution-focused brief therapy

Introduction

Cognitive behavioural therapy (CBT) has evolved to address a broad array of client presentations and an impressive body of evidence attests to its efficacy. Yet outcomes, and particularly longer-term outcomes, leave a substantial margin for improvement. What will it take to help more clients benefit more substantively from therapy? What more can therapists do to support their clients to develop longer-term resilience and well-being? How can therapists use the least demanding interventions on their clients? How can therapists increase clients' self-efficacy and

F. Bannink (✉)
Bannink Therapy, Training, Coaching and Mediation Practice, Amsterdam, The Netherlands
e-mail: solutions@fredrikebannink.com

C. Proctor (ed.), *Positive Psychology Interventions in Practice*,
DOI 10.1007/978-3-319-51787-2_2

self-esteem? What will it take to make CBT better and faster and therefore more cost-effective? And last but not least: How can CBT be more kind to its therapists? *Positive CBT* (Bannink 2012) emerged from the desire to find a new way forward in the application of traditional CBT. It aims to provide answers to the above questions.

CBT has been strongly influenced by the medical model of diagnosis and treatment. The structure of problem-solving—determining the nature of the problem and then intervening—influences the content of interaction between therapists and clients: they focus on pathology and on what is wrong with clients. Assessments focus on problems, limitations, and deficiencies and mention few or no client strengths and abilities. It is, however, the clients' strengths, abilities, and resources that are most important in helping to bring about change. Seligman (2011), cofounder of the positive psychology movement, states that if we want to flourish and have well-being, we must minimise our misery; but in addition, we must have positive emotion, meaning, accomplishment, and positive relationships.

Positive CBT draws on research and applications from positive psychology and solution-focused brief therapy. *Positive psychology* is the academic study of what makes life worth living and what enables individuals and communities to thrive. It is also the study of the conditions and processes that lead to optimal functioning in individuals, relations, and work. *Solution-focused brief therapy* (SFBT) is the pragmatic application of a set of principles and tools, best described as finding the direct route to 'what works' for this client, at this moment, in this context. The emphasis is on constructing solutions as a counterweight to the traditional emphasis on the analysis of problems. It is an approach to change, which invites conversations about what is wanted, what is working, and what might constitute progress (Bannink and Jackson 2011).

This chapter provides a condensed description of positive CBT, with information regarding the same cognitive behavioural process as used in traditional CBT. This process includes enhancing the therapeutic alliance, followed by doing an assessment (although in positive CBT assessment is first and foremost about strengths, resources, what works, and goals), including making functional behaviour analyses. The next part of the treatment is inviting clients to change: changing their viewing, doing, and feeling. Homework tasks and the evaluation of the treatment are described, as well as the changing role of the positive CBT therapist.

From a theoretical point of view positive CBT is different from traditional CBT. Traditional CBT uses a logical positivist view (the foundations of science remain in objectively quantifiable observations), whereas positive CBT—as does SFBT—uses a social constructivist view (the individual's notion of what is real—including his sense of the nature of problems, abilities, and solutions—is constructed in daily life in communication with others). This also means a shift in the language used in therapy: instead of terms like 'learning' and 'unlearning' following learning principles (CBT), positive CBT uses the term 'becoming better at', because there are always exceptions to the problem (Wittgenstein 1968).

Positive CBT

If there is a *positive* CBT, is there also a *negative* CBT, one may wonder. I don't believe that there is a negative form of CBT, since all forms of psychotherapy—including *traditional* problem-focused CBT—have as their main goal to help clients bring about desired changes in their lives. In the past 30 years however, there has been a paradigm shift with the development of competency-based, more collaborative approaches to working with clients. Positive psychology and SFBT are amongst these approaches directed toward clients' strengths and their preferred futures, instead of their past or present deficits and problems.

Mental health is more than the absence of mental illness. The focus of positive CBT is not on mental illness and pathology, on what is wrong with clients and on repairing what is worst, but on mental health and strengths, what is right with them and on creating what is best. In this quest, positive CBT does not have to be constructed from the ground up, but it does involve a change of focus from reducing problems to a focus on building on clients' strengths and on what works. Positive CBT can be seen as being the other side of the 'CBT coin' and can be easily combined with traditional CBT. This positive focus has helped SFBT to become shorter in time than other psychotherapies (Franklin et al. 2012; Gingerich and Peterson 2013). The same may be true for positive CBT, because it uses the same positive focus. Many professionals working in the fields of positive psychology and SFBT claim that conversations with their clients are more light-hearted, which results in less burnout (Medina and Beyebach 2014).

A *strengths-based approach* with its roots in positive psychology is a philosophical perspective in which people are seen as capable and as having abilities and resources within themselves and their social systems. When activated and integrated with new experiences, understandings, and skills, strengths offer people pathways to reduce pain and suffering, resolve concerns and conflicts, and more effectively cope with life stressors. The outcome is an improved sense of well-being and quality of life and higher degrees of interpersonal and social functioning.

Saleebey (2007) describes the *strengths perspective* in psychotherapy. Despite life's struggles, all persons possess strengths that can be marshalled to improve the qualities of their lives. Therapists should respect these strengths and the directions in which clients wish to apply them. Client motivation is increased by a consistent emphasis on strengths, as the client defines them. Discovering these strengths requires a process of cooperative exploration between clients and therapists; therapists do not have the last word on what clients need to improve in their lives. Focusing on strengths turns therapists away from the temptation to judge or blame clients for their difficulties and toward discovering how clients have managed to survive, even in the most difficult circumstances. All environments—even the most bleak—contain resources.

Kuyken et al. (2009) state that in the CBT literature there has been a much greater emphasis on identifying precipitating, predisposing, and perpetuating factors for problems than on identifying strengths. They advocate the inclusion of strengths whenever possible during case conceptualisation.

Furthermore, a *solutions-based approach*, focusing on what works for this client in this context and in this moment, with its roots in SFBT (Bannink 2007, 2010a, b, 2014, 2015a, b) adds to the well-being of clients by inviting them to describe their preferred future (instead of their problems or their feared future) and finding strengths and solutions to reach their goal.

Research shows that successful therapists focus on clients' strengths, abilities, and available support, from the very start of a therapy session. They create an environment in which clients feel they are perceived as well-functioning persons. Successful therapists also make sure they end sessions by returning to their clients' strengths (Gassman and Grawe 2006), enhancing a good therapeutic alliance along the way.

The Therapeutic Alliance

Therapeutic alliance has been defined in many ways and despite of this diversity of definitions, the consensus is that the alliance represents a positive attachment between therapist and client, as well as an active and collaborative engagement in therapeutic tasks designed to help the client. Therapists make explicit efforts to facilitate the creation of a positive alliance and systematically monitor the alliance with the now available instruments, rather than relying on clinical impression. It is important to keep in mind that the client's view of the alliance (and not the therapist's) is the best-known predictor of outcome (Duncan 2010).

Positive CBT starts with *building rapport*. The therapist makes a positive start by asking questions about the daily life of the client: *'What kind of work do you do?'*, *'What grade are you in?'* (when the client is a child), followed by questions as: *'What do you like about your work?'*, *'What are you good at?'*, *'What hobbies do you have?'*, *'What is your best subject in school?'*, *'Who is your favourite teacher?'*. These questions can be seen as icebreakers, but are also the start for uncovering useful information about strengths and solutions already present in the client's life. They set the tone for a more light-hearted conversation than the client may have been expecting.

Many clients like to have the opportunity to talk about problems, not least because they think that that is the intent of the therapy. Positive CBT therapists listen respectfully to their stories and offer acknowledgment, but do not ask for details of the problem. With the question: *'How is this a problem for you?'*, clients can often begin to talk about the problem in a different way. It may be helpful to provide information about positive CBT with its focus on possibilities instead of impossibilities and strengths instead of weaknesses. When clients insist on talking about their problems, therapists may ask: *'How many sessions do you think you need to talk about problems and what is wrong with you before we can start looking at your preferred future and what is right with you?'*.

Assessment

Positive CBT is more interested in what clients want to change in their lives rather than exploring their problems and more interested in what is right with clients than in what is wrong with them. Therefore, the first challenge positive CBT therapists encounter is inviting clients to shift from *problem talk* to *strengths and solutions talk* at the point at which they have had enough time to describe their problems to feel heard (10–15 min is often enough). Assessing what clients want to be different (their goals), strengths and resources (exceptions to the problem and their competences), motivation to change, progression, hope, and confidence are all part of the assessment and *case conceptualisation* in positive CBT.

Kuyken et al. (2009) propose that psychotherapy has two overarching goals: to alleviate distress and to build resilience. Most current CBT approaches are concerned either exclusively or largely with clients' problems, vulnerabilities, and history of adversity. A strengths focus is often more engaging for clients and offers the advantages of harnessing client strengths in the change process to pave a way to lasting recovery. Clients are often not aware of the coping strategies they use to be resilient and highlighting these increases the likelihood clients will consider their use during future challenges. Noticing the strategies a person employs to manage adversity is often a first step toward conceptualising resilience. These strategies may be behavioural (e.g., persisting in efforts), cognitive (e.g., problem solving, acceptance), emotional (e.g., humour, reassurance), social (e.g., seeking help), spiritual (e.g., finding meaning in suffering), or physical (e.g., sleeping and eating well).

Setting goals emphasises the possibility of change, and begins to focus clients on future possibilities rather than on problems. It reinforces the notion that clients' are an active member of the therapeutic relationship, and that full involvement is required: they will not be 'done' to. Hawton et al. (1995) state that defined goals help to impose structure on treatment. It also prepares clients for discharge: making explicit that therapy will be terminated when goals are achieved, or that therapy will be discontinued if there is little progress. This is not to say that goals cannot be renegotiated during treatment, but that this should be done explicitly together with clients, thus reducing the risk that clients and therapist are pursuing different agendas. Finally, setting goals provides the opportunity for an evaluation of outcome related to the clients' problems.

Goals can be stated as increasing strengths or positive values (approach goal: e.g., be more considerate) as well as reducing distress (avoidance goal: e.g., feel less anxious). *'What will be the best outcome of you coming to see me?'* is a good way to start this part of the session, or *'When can we stop meeting like this?'*, or *'What are your best hopes?'*, followed by *'What difference will it make when your best hopes are met?'*.

Positive CBT is not *problem-phobic*. Clients are given an opportunity to describe their problems, to which therapists listen respectfully. But no details about the nature and severity of the problem are asked and causes are not analysed. By asking about exceptions to the problem—a form of differential diagnosis—may reveal that some disorders can be eliminated (e.g., when asked about exceptions, a child who would otherwise be diagnosed with ADHD, appears to be able to sit still in the classroom).

Another way of conducting positive CBT, granting due acknowledgement, is to first collect all symptoms, complaints, and constraints and then to 'translate' all problem-descriptions into goals: *'What would you like to see instead?'* and then discard the problems collection by tearing it up or just ignoring it when working with what clients want different in their lives. Another useful question is: *'Suppose these problems would not be there, how will you or your life/relationship/work be different?'*.

Bakker et al. (2010) state that therapists may choose to commence treatment immediately and if necessary pay attention to diagnostics at a later stage. Severe psychiatric disorders or a suspicion thereof justify the decision to conduct a thorough diagnosis, since the tracing of the underlying organic pathology has direct therapeutic consequences. Ambulant intakes in primary or secondary health care are suitable for a positive CBT approach. During the first and follow-up conversations it will become clear whether an advanced diagnosis is necessary, for example if there is a deterioration in the client's condition or if the treatment fails to give positive results. Analogous to *stepped care* one could think of *stepped diagnosis*.

In traditional CBT, *self-monitoring* of problems is used to gain an accurate description of behaviours (rather than relying on recall) to help adept the intervention in relation to client progress and to provide clients with feedback about their progress. Self-monitoring is often integrated into therapy, both in the sessions and as part of homework assignments. In positive CBT self-monitoring is not about clients' problems or symptoms, but about clients' strengths and about exceptions to the problems. When clients use this form of *positive self-monitoring* they often feel more competent and can choose to do more of what works to change their situation for the better.

Functional analysis methodology identifies variables that influence the occurrence of problem behaviour and has become a hallmark of behavioural assessment. Behavioural research demonstrates that behaviours can be learned and unlearned on the basis of patterns of association, reward, and punishment. Functional behaviour analysis (FBA) looks beyond the behaviour itself: the focus is on identifying significant factors associated with the (non) occurrence of specific behaviours. In FBA each problem is analysed in terms of A-B-Cs: antecedents, behaviours and beliefs, and consequences. Each of these factors increase or decrease the probability that the behaviour will occur. In traditional CBT a FBA is made of the ABCs of problem behaviour, whereas in positive CBT (see below) a FBA is made of desired behaviour and/or exceptions of the problem behaviour. CBT therapists may also choose to use both traditional and positive FBAs.

Positive FBA interview in three questions:

1. Suppose tonight while you are sleeping, a miracle happens and your problems are all solved. But because you are asleep, you don't know that this miracle happens. What will be the first thing you notice tomorrow morning that will tell you

that this miracle has happened? What will be the first thing you notice yourself doing differently that will let you know that this miracle occurred? What else? What else? What do you expect to see and find in the world around you, particularly your work?
2. Tell me about some recent times when you were doing somewhat better or (part of) the miracle was happening, even just a little bit.
3. When things are going somewhat better for you, what have you noticed that you or others do differently then? What other consequences have you noticed?

In Positive CBT clients do more of what works: there is not need to try something different, because solutions are already present. Clients' reports on the helpfulness of the intervention and collect further observations by self-monitoring, and the cycle of FBA repeats itself. By identifying strengths and exceptions, intervention plans focus on increasing the use of appropriate skills clients already possess rather than relying on manipulating antecedents and consequences to reduce negative behaviours. Questions are: *'What is better (since the last time we met)?'*, *'What is different (since the last time we met)?'*, *'What has been helpful (even just a little bit)?'*.

Changing the Viewing

O'Hanlon (2000) states that when people are not happy or are not getting the results they want, they should do something different. Clients have to change either the viewing or the doing of the problem, or both. This will almost certainly result in a change in the feeling of the problem.

In *changing the viewing* of the problem the focus is on changing how clients think and what they pay attention to as a way to change their situation for the better. This can involve five interventions. The first intervention is to acknowledge feelings and the past without letting them determine what clients can do. They are invited to create more compassionate and helpful stories and find a kinder, gentler view of themselves, others, and/or the situation (Gilbert 2010).

The second intervention is to invite clients to change what they are paying attention to in a problem situation. The point of departure is that a problem does not always manifest itself to the same degree. Directing attention to the clients' past or present successes instead of their failures generates a positive expectation: clients begin to see themselves and/or the situation in a more positive light.

The third intervention is to focus on what clients want in the future rather than on what they do not like in the present or the past. Setting goals about what clients want to be different in the future emphasises the possibility of change and begins to focus clients on future possibilities rather than on their symptoms and problems.

The fourth intervention is to challenge unhelpful beliefs about themself and their situation. Traditional CBT assists clients to identify and reality-test unhelpful cognitions, which underlie repeated negative patterns of emotion and behaviour, whereas positive CBT assists clients to find adaptive helpful cognitions that give rise to a more positive experience of the self, others, and the world. These (more) adaptive cognitions do not have to be developed, because they are already present (exceptions to the problem) and may be used again.

The fifth and last intervention is to use a spiritual perspective to help clients transcend their troubles and to draw on resources beyond their usual abilities. O'Hanlon (2000) describes the three Cs of spirituality as sources of resilience. *Connection* means moving beyond your little, isolated ego, or personality into connection with something bigger, within or outside yourself. *Compassion* means softening your attitude towards yourself or others by 'feeling with' rather than being against yourself, others, or the world. And *contribution* means being of unselfish service to others or the world.

Upward Arrow Technique

As an example of how positive CBT differs from traditional CBT, which uses the *downward arrow technique*, I introduced the *upward arrow technique,* with a focus on positive reactions to a given situation, or to exceptions to the problem. So-called *core beliefs* are central, absolute beliefs about self, others, and the world. People develop both positive and negative beliefs. The automatic thoughts and underlying assumptions lead therapist and clients toward relevant core beliefs. The problem-focused *downward arrow technique* is one of the ways to identify beliefs that underpin negative reactions to a given situation. Questions are: *'What does that matter?'*, *'What is so bad about…?'*, *'What is the 'worst case scenario?'*. These questions are repeated in response to each answer clients provide.

Questions using the *upward arrow technique* are: *'How will you like the situation/yourself/others to be different?'*, *'What will be the best outcome?'*, *'What will be the "best case" scenario?'*, *'Suppose that happens, what difference will that make (for yourself, for others)?'*. These questions are also repeated in response to each answer clients provide.

Changing the Doing

One way to solve a problem is not to analyse why the problem arose, but to change what clients are doing to solve it. The way to do that is to determine how they keep acting in the same way over and over again (the problem pattern), and begin to experiment with doing something different (breaking the pattern). In changing the *doing of the problem* the focus is on concrete actions clients can take to make these changes. The first intervention is to invite clients to *pay attention to repetitive patterns* that they are caught up in or that others are caught up in with them and change anything possible about these patterns. Clients may change the doing of the problem by changing any part they can of their regularly repeated actions in the situation. By using paradox clients are invited to go with the problem or try to make it worse (more intense or more frequent) or try to deliberately make the problem happen. Invite clients to stop avoiding the problem or try to fix the problem, and instead embrace it and allow it to happen. In linking new actions to the problem pattern clients are invited to find something they can do every time they have the problem, something that is good for them, usually something burdensome. Or ask them to do this avoided action first, every time they feel the urge to 'do' the problem.

The second intervention is to notice what clients are doing when things are going better, and invite them to do more of that. Ask clients: *'When didn't you experience the problem after you expected you would?'*. Find a time that is an exception to the usual problem pattern and look for changes clients can make by deliberately repeating whatever action worked. Invite clients to notice what happens as the problem ends or starts to end. Then invite clients to deliberately do some of the helpful actions they did then, but earlier in the problem situation. Or import solution patterns from other situations in which clients feel competent. Examine patterns at work, in hobbies, with friends, and in other contexts to find something clients can use effectively in the problem situation. Ask clients: *'Why isn't the problem worse?'*. Use their own natural abilities to limit the severity of the problem they have been using without noticing. Most of the time clients know very well—often better than therapists do—what works and what doesn't work, but for a change they have to do something different from what they are currently doing.

In traditional CBT the *modification procedures* (like self-control procedures or behavioural experiments) are usually advised by the therapist, whose role is that of the expert. In positive CBT the modification procedures are already available: clients, coexperts on what works, are competent to make changes and have made changes before. Also there are always exceptions to the problem. The modification procedures may be the same as advised by traditional CBT therapists, with the difference that in positive CBT clients come up with modification procedures, which have helped before, are therefore 'evidence-based' and may be repeated.

Changing the Feeling

Traditional CBT aims to obtain a clear picture of situations which are distressing to clients, by helping them to clearly differentiate thoughts from emotions, it empathises with their emotions throughout the process and helps them to evaluate the dysfunctional thinking which has influenced their mood. The therapist's job is to minimise negative effect: by dispensing drugs or in instigating psychological interventions, thereby rendering people less anxious, angry, or depressed. Seligman (2011), however, described some disappointing results with this approach of making miserable people less miserable. He found that as a therapist, he would help a client get rid of his anger, anxiety, or sadness. He thought he would then get a happy patient, but he never did. He got an empty patient, because the skills of flourishing are something over and above the skills of minimising suffering.

As an example of how reducing negative affect does not automatically increase positive affect, research in a coaching context done by Grant and O'Connor (2010) showed that problem-focused questions reduce negative affect and increase self-efficacy, but do not increase understanding of the nature of the problem or enhance positive affect. Solution-focused questions increase positive affect, decrease negative affect, increase self-efficacy, as well as increase participants' insight and understanding of the nature of the problem.

In positive CBT the focus is on positive emotions: *'How will you feel when your best hopes are met?'*, *'What will you be feeling differently when you notice that the steps you take are in the right direction?'*. Also bringing back the best from the past by asking questions about previous successes and competences triggers positive emotions.

The *broaden-and-build theory of positive emotions* (Fredrickson 2009) suggests that negative emotions narrow our thought-action repertoires, whereas positive emotions broaden our awareness and encourage novel, varied, and exploratory thoughts and actions. The power of asking open questions, focused on what clients do want (*'How will you know this session has been useful?'*, *'How will you know the problem has been solved?'*, *'What has been working well?'*, *'What is better?'*), all serve to widen the array of thoughts and actions. Using imagination (for example using the *miracle question*) also creates positive emotions and has a powerful impact on the capacity to expand ideas and activities. The use of compliments and competence questions (*'How did you manage to do that?'*, *'How did you decide to do that?'*) also elicit positive emotions. The focus of positive CBT therapists is on noticing skills and resources of their clients and to compliment or play those resources back to them.

Homework Tasks

In traditional CBT homework is considered important, because learning and unlearning are required following learning principles and it is assumed that change takes place especially between therapy sessions. For example, *self-monitoring* is the most widely used adjunct to CBT, and is almost invariably used both at the initial assessment stage and to monitor subsequent change. Another widely used adjunct are *behavioural experiments*. There are three types of experiments in CBT (Bennett-Levy et al. 2004). One type is *experimental manipulation of the environment*. This necessitates doing something, which is different to what the client usually does in a particular situation. For example, the client may try to answer the question: *'If I go the supermarket alone and do not take my usual precautions, will I actually faint (as my existing belief would predict) or will I just feel anxious (the prediction of an alternative theory)'*.

Another type constitutes of *observational experiments*, in that it is either not possible or not necessary to manipulate key variables. Instead clients set out to observe and gather evidence, which is relevant to their specific negative thoughts or beliefs. For example, a client may try to answer the question: *'Will people think I am stupid or abnormal if I sweat in social situations?'*.

The third type constitutes of *discovery-oriented experiments*, when clients have little or no idea what will happen when they undertake a behavioural experiment and need to collect data systematically in order to 'build a theory'. For example, a client may try to answer the question: *'What would happen if I acted "as if" I was valued by others?'*. Or the client may be encouraged to try out different ways of behaving in order to collect those data (*'How might a valued person act in these circumstances?'*).

Positive CBT employs the same types of behavioural experiments, but again with a positive focus. Experimental manipulation of the environment: clients are invited to explore exceptions to the problem: what has the client done—even slightly—differently before? How has that been helpful? Does the client think it might be a good idea to use this solution again? Observational experiments: clients are invited to observe and gather evidence, which is relevant to their specific *positive* thoughts and beliefs. For example, the client may answer the question: *'Will people think I am likeable if I go to this party?'*. When they pay attention to their positive thoughts or beliefs, chances are that clients will find evidence for these positive ones, whereas when they pay attention to negative thoughts or beliefs, chances are that clients will find evidence for the negative ones too. Discovery-oriented experiments: clients are invited to act as if their preferred future has already arrived or are one or two points higher on the scale of progress. During the session clients may be invited to pretend things are going better and show the therapist (for some minutes) how their life/relationships will be different and how this will appear.

In positive CBT homework tasks are only important if clients think it is useful. The solution-focused idea in positive CBT is that when clients change their construction, which is assumed to take place during and between therapy sessions, behaviour change follows naturally.

Homework is intended to direct clients' attention to those aspects of their experiences and situations that are most useful in reaching their goals. Presenting homework or tasks as an 'experiment' or even a 'small experiment' may make it easier for clients, because it alleviates the pressure to be successful at accomplishing the task. Before coming up with suggestions, it is useful to ask whether clients want to do homework anyway. If they say that they don't have any need for them, they will probably have a good reason: perhaps they don't consider it useful, or maybe they don't have time. In those instances, therapists needn't come up with suggestions or may ask clients what they would consider to be useful. When clients are feeling somewhat hesitant about change, invite them to observe rather than to do something.

Solution-focused therapists Walter and Peller (1992) mention four basic homework tasks. The first task is to observe for positives: *'Between now and the next time, notice what is going on in your life (marriage, family, work, etc.) that you would like to see continue'*. The second task is to do more of the positives or exceptions when these are perceived as deliberate and within clients' control: *'Keep up what you are doing that is helpful and take notice of what you are doing that is helpful so that you can tell me about it next time'*.

The third task is to find out how spontaneous exceptions happen: *'On the odd-numbered days of the week you pretend to feel different and see what happens. I know that you might not always feel that way, in fact, you might feel the same old way. However, I think there is some potential in how you act and think differently when you do. So, every other day, pretend to feel different and on the even-numbered days just do as you normally do. Observe what differences you notice'*. The fourth task is to do some small piece of a hypothetical solution (*'Suppose a miracle happened and your problems are gone'*): *'You might want to experiment with this new idea. You might want to do just a small piece of it to try it on for size'*.

Evaluation

In *subsequent sessions* clients and therapist carefully explore what is better. Therapists ask for a detailed explanation of positive exceptions, give compliments, and emphasise clients' input in finding solutions. At the end of every session clients are asked whether they think another meeting is useful, and if so, when they like to return. In fact, in many cases clients think it is not necessary to return or schedule an appointment further into the future than is typical in other forms of psychotherapy. The goal of subsequent sessions is further described in Bannink (2010a, b, 2012). At the end of every session clients are invited to give feedback about the relationship with the therapist, whether the goals and topics were discussed that they wanted to talk about and whether the method or approach was a good fit for them (e.g., Session Rating Scale; Duncan 2010).

Role of the Positive CBT Therapist

In Positive CBT the role of the therapist is different from the role in traditional CBT. From being the only expert in the room, who explores and analyses the problem and then gives advise to clients on how to solve their problems, the role changes to one where the therapist does not need to push or pull. Positive CBT therapists are 'not-knowing' (they ask questions) and are 'leading from one step behind'. In this therapists, metaphorically speaking, stand behind their clients and tap them on the shoulder with solution-focused questions, inviting them to look at their preferred future and, in order to achieve their goal, to envisage a wide horizon of personal possibilities.

Clients are seen as coexperts and therapists invite them—by asking solution-focused questions—to share their expertise to reach the preferred future. Therapists also change their focus of attention by using learning principles during the therapy sessions: positive reinforcement of *strengths and solutions-talk* (paying attention to conversations about goals, exceptions, possibilities, strengths, and resources) and negative punishment of *problem-talk* (not paying attention to conversations about problems, causes, impossibilities, and weaknesses).

Conclusion

Positive CBT offers the best constructive vision to date of what cognitive behaviour therapy looks like when joined with positive psychology and solution focused brief therapy. Positive CBT shifts the focus of therapy from what is wrong with clients to what is right with them, and from what is not working to what is. This transition represents a paradigm shift from problem analysis to goal analysis, from a focus on deficits and weaknesses to one that builds on resources and strengths, and from reducing distress to building success. Positive CBT recently emerged from the desire to find a new way forward in the application of traditional CBT. Research is currently being done at the Maastricht University in the Netherlands to find out how positive CBT is distinct from, or may be even superior to traditional CBT.

References

Bakker, J. M., Bannink, F. P., & Macdonald, A. (2010). Solution-focused psychiatry. *The Psychiatrist, 34*, 297–300.

Bannink, F. P. (2007). Solution-focused brief therapy. *Journal of Contemporary Psychotherapy, 37*(2), 87–94.

Bannink, F. P. (2010a). *1001 Solution-focused questions. Handbook for solution-focused interviewing*. New York: Norton.

Bannink, F. P. (2010b). *Handbook of solution focused conflict management*. Cambridge, MA: Hogrefe.

Bannink, F. P. (2012). *Practicing positive CBT. From reducing distress to building success*. Oxford: Wiley.

Bannink, F. P. (2014). *Post traumatic success*. New York: Norton.

Bannink, F. P. (2015a). *Handbook of positive supervision*. Cambrigde, MA: Hogrefe.

Bannink, F. P. (2015b). *101 Solution-focused questions for help with anxiety/depression/trauma* (3 Vols.). New York: Norton.

Bannink, F. P., & Jackson, P. Z. (2011). Positive psychology and solution focus—Looking at similarities and differences. *InterAction. The Journal of Solution Focus in Organisations, 3*(1), 8–20.

Bennett-Levy, J., Butler, G., Fennell, M., Hackman, A., Mueller, M., & Westbrook, D. (2004). *Oxford guide to behavioural experiments in cognitive therapy*. New York: Oxford University Press.

Duncan, B. L. (2010). *On becoming a better therapist*. Washington, DC: American Psychological Association.

Franklin, C., Trepper, T. S., Gingerich, W. J., & McCollum, E. E. (Eds.). (2012). *Solution-focused brief therapy: A handbook of evidence-based practice*. New York: Oxford University Press.

Fredrickson, B. L. (2009). *Positivity*. New York: Crown.

Gassman, D., & Grawe, K. (2006). General change mechanisms: The relation between problem activation and resource activation in successful and unsuccessful therapeutic interactions. *Clinical Psychology and Psychotherapy, 13*, 1–11.

Gilbert, P. (2010). *Compassion focused therapy. The CBT distinctive features series*. New York: Routledge.

Gingerich, W. J., & Peterson, L. T. (2013). Effectiveness of solution-focused brief therapy: A systematic qualitative review of controlled outcome studies. *Research on Social Work Practice, 23*, 266–283. doi:10.1177/1049731512470859.

Grant, A. M., & O'Connor, S. A. (2010). The differential effects of solution-focused and problem-focused coaching questions: A pilot study with implications for practice. *Industrial and Commercial Training, 42*(4), 102–111.

Hawton, K., Salkovskis, P. M., Kirk, J., & Clark, D. M. (1995). *Cognitive behaviour therapy for psychiatric problems: A practical guide*. Oxford: Oxford University Press.

Kuyken, W., Padesky, C. A., & Dudley, R. (2009). *Collaborative case conceptualization*. New York: Guilford.

Medina, A., & Beyebach, M. (2014). The impact of solution-focused training on professionals' beliefs, practices and burnout of child protection workers in Tenerife Island. *Child Care in Practice, 20*(1), 7–36.

O'Hanlon, B. (2000). *Do one thing different*. New York: Harper Collins.

Saleebey, D. (Ed.). (2007). *The strengths perspective in social work practice*. Boston: Allyn & Bacon.

Seligman, M. E. P. (2011). *Flourish*. New York: Free Press.

Walter, J. L., & Peller, J. E. (1992). *Becoming solution-focused in brief therapy*. New York: Brunner/Mazel.

Wittgenstein, L. (1968). *Philosophical investigations* (G. E. M. Anscombe, Trans., 3rd ed.). New York: Macmillan.

Chapter 3
Flourish: A Strengths-Based Approach to Building Student Resilience

Tayyab Rashid, Ruth Louden, Laurie Wright, Ron Chu, Aryel Maharaj, Irfan Hakim, Danielle Uy, and Bruce Kidd

Abstract Flourish is a strengths-based collaborative project bringing together four student services departments on a post-secondary campus with the aim of building resilience of students in college and university settings. Its overarching mission is to help students grow intellectually, socially, and emotionally and to teach them concrete skills so that they can translate this growth into action, habit, and purpose. Broadly based on theories of positive psychology and student development, the programme aims to help all students in post-secondary educational settings, but first year students in particular, acquire concrete skills that build their emotional, academic, and physical resilience. The premise is that these components of resilience, in turn, will facilitate emotional, intellectual, and social growth of students towards flourishing. The programme starts with a comprehensive online assessment, which helps determine whether the student is flourishing, languishing, or functioning somewhere between these two states. The assessment includes a comprehensive feedback report and a rich repository of online and campus-wide resources to support their resilience. With staff from four student services departments and student leaders, students in the programme can participate in a range of interventions that support their resilience. This chapter describes Flourish, as a strengths-based assessment and intervention for young adults, in post-secondary settings. It describes the theoretical background of the Flourish assessment battery, programme interventions and initial results. The chapter concludes with a brief discussion about the future direction of the programme.

T. Rashid (✉) • R. Louden • L. Wright • R. Chu • A. Maharaj
I. Hakim • D. Uy • B. Kidd
University of Toronto Scarborough, 1265 Military Trail, Toronto, ON, Canada, M1C 1A4
e-mail: trashid@utsc.utoronto.ca; louden@utsc.utoronto.ca; lwright@utsc.utoronto.ca; ron.chu@mail.utoronto.ca; aryel.lutchmie.maharaj@mail.utoronto.ca; irfan.hakim@mail.utoronto.ca; danielle.uy@mail.utoronto.ca; bruce.kidd@utsc.utoronto.ca

C. Proctor (ed.), *Positive Psychology Interventions in Practice*,
DOI 10.1007/978-3-319-51787-2_3

Abbreviations

FI	Flourishing Inventory
GPA	Grade point average
MHC-SF	Mental Health Continuum-Short Form
OQ-45	Outcome Questionnaire
PERMA	Positive emotion, engagement, relationships, meaning, accomplishment
PRP	Penn Resilience Project
SEI	Student Engagement Inventory
SSQ-72	Signature Strengths Questionnaire

Introduction

Post-secondary educational settings offer students numerous opportunities for growth. With these opportunities come challenges, mental health concerns being perhaps the most significant barrier to student flourishing on post-secondary campuses (MacKean 2011; Kettmann et al. 2007; Sharkin and Coulter 2005; Schwartz 2006; Erdur-Baker et al. 2006; Gallagher 2010; Blanco et al. 2008). Mental illness is also the most common medical condition to emerge during adolescence, with half of all mental disorders having their onset by age 14, and three-quarters having their onset by age 24 (Kessler et al. 2005). In Canada, where this present study is being conducted, about 18% of Canadian adolescents (ages 15–24) report a mental illness or substance abuse problem (Kirby and Keon 2006). This is consistent with trends reported on other North American campuses (National College Health Survey 2016). Overall, statistics indicate that mental health concerns on post-secondary campuses are increasing. Further, the research studies conclude that it is not just a result of increased awareness or sophisticated assessment techniques (Pedrelli et al. 2015; Much and Swanson 2010; Conway et al. 2006). That is, the increase in prevalence, chronicity, and severity appears to be real. Further complicating this reality, are stigma associated with seeking mental health treatment and the remedial approach to student problems that characterise a post-secondary setting. Given substantial transition challenges of first-year students, new models exploring strengths-based approaches provide promise of a more complete approach to supporting their mental health and wellbeing.

Stigma Against Seeking Mental Health Treatment

Mental health concerns pose a significant barrier to student success. Yet, one of the most enduring challenges in post-secondary settings, documented by numerous studies, is the striking number of students who need treatment, but refuse to seek it.

This is true even when the student may have significant pathology and potential risk (Drum et al. 2009; Eisenberg et al. 2011). Many students do not seek much-needed counselling services due to lack of knowledge about mental health problems, services, stigma, or denial of the severity of the problem. Left unrecognised and untreated, mental health problems may lead to otherwise capable students dropping out of or failing in university, attempting or committing suicide, or engaging in other risky behaviours that may result in serious injury, disability, or death (Cook 2007). Corey Keyes and colleagues, in their Healthy Minds Study of 5589 students, found that students who reported having mental illness, are at a greater risk of suicidal behaviour and academic impairment (Keyes et al. 2012).

Remedial Approach

Historically, post-secondary institutions have approached the above noted concerns by a remedial approach. Academic units consider salient markers of student success to be grade point average, registration, and graduation status. In support of these academic targets, student support services focus on remediating deficits. For example, counselling services offer counselling to manage symptoms of stress and motivation. Disability services focus on providing accommodations, while academic advising focuses on specific ways to improve academic abilities, such as time management and study skills. As a result, post-secondary institutions have evaluated effectiveness by measuring the extent to which students utilise remedial services (e.g., number of students utilising academic or counselling services or number of students accommodated).

However, over the last two decades, it has become increasingly clear that remedial effectiveness, grade point average, and graduation are not the only determinants of student success (Lounsbury et al. 2009; Karris 2007). Remediation only corrects for weaknesses, and academic achievement only accounts for 22–25% of student success among full-time students enrolled in 4-year university programmes (Zwick and Schlemer 2004). Remedial focus also poses another serious challenge. Take psychological counselling for instance. Many students from diverse cultural backgrounds find largely euro-centric diagnostic psychological labels irrelevant to their cultural experiences (Loya et al. 2010; Mitchell et al. 2007; Nilsson et al. 2004). Furthermore, signs of stress may differ from culture to culture. They may hesitate to register with 'accessibility' services because for most part, these services require documentation that the student has a psychological disorder. Similarly, students on probation tend to receive more academic advising and more focused services. Remedial services for students who need them are critical to ensure their success. However, we argue that student services may benefit by expanding their focus on remediation to include building resilience.

Transitional Challenges

Building resilience is especially important for students transitioning from secondary to post-secondary settings. As the research shows, the first year of university is the most challenging phase of the post-secondary educational experience (Ishitani 2003; Lee et al. 2009). Along with questioning their identity, first year students have to cope with the stress of transitioning to a new institution, separating from family and friends, meeting new people, and managing academic challenges. Often they have to face the discrepancy between expectations and reality. If already languishing, these challenges can evolve into serious academic concerns ranging from academic probation to breaches of academic integrity and suspension. Depression, anxiety, difficulties with emotional regulation, alcohol and drug abuse can ensue, along with lethargy, lack of concentration, sleeping difficulties, and unhealthy eating patterns.

Complete Mental Health

A college or university campus is a fertile ground for students to grow intellectually, emotionally, and socially. According to Corey Keyes' model of mental health, the absence of symptoms is not the presence of mental health. The presence of mental health, according to Keyes, can be termed as flourishing. Flourishing university students have healthy mental functions, fulfilling relationships, engaging meaningful and productive activities, and are resilient, that is, they bounce back from setbacks quickly (Keyes 2007; Ouweneel et al. 2011; Russo-Netzer and Ben-Shahar 2011). The absence of flourishing is a condition described as *languishing*. Although not clinically depressed, languishing students experience few positive emotions, feel academically and socially disengaged, and lack a sense of meaning or purpose in their lives. Languishers are neither mentally ill nor mentally well adjusted. They describe their lives as hollow or empty (Keyes et al. 2011).

From Remediation to Resilience

Most post-secondary institutions do not systematically facilitate or foster student flourishing (Lopez and Louis 2009). Instead, as discussed above, they correct for weaknesses that are mostly cognitive (Lounsbury et al. 2009; Karris 2007). However, they are becoming increasingly mindful that in a globalised knowledge-based economy, a remedial approach alone will not help students to accomplish their intellectual, social, and personal goals (Oades et al. 2011; Lopez and Edwards 2008; McGovern and Miller 2008). Furthermore, in our ever-increasing diverse campuses, strengths, not weaknesses, especially among students from diverse cultural backgrounds, can build trust. Students will approach various services if they feel that instead of being labelled as depressed, emotionally dysregulated, and learning disabled, they will be understood as holistic human beings who have challenges but also potential, risks but also resources, liabilities but also abilities. They will be more likely to take advantage of services that engage and understand them, not just assess and label them. A remedial approach gives an implicit message that students with challenges are a burden on campus whereas a strengths-based approach could offer students a feeling of *mattering*—a feeling that others (e.g., faculty, staff, administrators) are interested in them and that they matter to the institution (Rayle and Chung 2007). Similarly, on- and off-campus civic engagement of students serves as a buffer against mental health problems (Mitchell et al. 2016).

Compared to stressors, strengths are more ubiquitous and do not carry a negative connotation. Therefore, incorporating strengths in student services can likely encourage students to seek help. Finally, strengths can tap into the 'communal potential' of students in ways symptoms, stressors and problems cannot.

Resilience Programming in Post-secondary Settings

Models of student success have started underscoring the importance of incorporating strengths in student services in order to build student resilience and well-being (Louis 2011; Clifton et al. 2006; Lounsbury et al. 2009; Karris 2007). Leading models of university student development have also started echoing the importance of strengths in student development (Chickering and Reisser 1993; Tinto 2004). There are a few successful illustrations where these models have and are being applied in creating learning environments that maximise student potential by building resilience and well-being (e.g., Seligman et al. 2006). Some of these illustrations are:

1. **Penn Resilience Project:** Perhaps the most widely researched and applied programme in this regard is the *Penn Resilience Project* (PRP; Brunwasser et al. 2009), which has been in place for more than 20 years, from the University of Pennsylvania. PRP teaches students resilience, optimism, and citizenship. Validated through more than 21 controlled, mostly randomised studies, this programme teaches students resilience, optimism, and interpersonal skills, thereby enhancing their flourishing (Seligman et al. 2007).
2. **Bounce Back:** Designed in 2004, the *Bounce Back* programme was created at the University of San Diego. The overarching goal of the programme was to increase resilience of students, especially those most vulnerable to dropout from the university (Hanger et al. 2007). The programme has demonstrated its effectiveness in terms of academic outcomes including probation removal, probation continued, disqualification, retention, credits earned, and grade point average (Hanger et al. 2011).
3. **What Makes Life Worth Living:** More recently, a comprehensive campus-wide initiative called *What Makes Life Worth Living* at University of Michigan,

Ann Arbor, has been introduced. This programme engages university students and community groups to create events centring on the theme of flourishing in art, dance, music, film, play, toys, foods, religion, and service to others. To date, no empirical data is available on the programme. However, anecdotal reports suggest that the program is well received by students and community members. http://wmlwl.com.

Integrating these lines of research, we conceived of the *Flourish* programme and posited that understanding and building student strengths will enhance their emotional, academic, and physical resilience, which in turn, will enhance students' flourishing.

Flourish: Project Goals

The overarching goal of the Flourish project at the University of Toronto Scarborough is to build resilience of students entering the post-secondary educational setting, particularly those who are considered at a greater risk for developing mental illness or of struggling with transition. This goal is operationalised through the following specific exploratory questions:

1. What is the well-being profile of incoming students in relation to their states of flourishing or languishing?
2. What changes in the well-being profile of students from semester to semester and year to year will correspond with changes in their academic performance? In particular, will those who no longer score in the flourishing range show changes in their academic performance?
3. Which specific character strengths predict flourishing and languishing and which strengths predict academic performance?
4. Can resilience and well-being be increased by a systematic strengths-based intervention?
5. Are students who attend the full-day Flourish workshop more likely to report higher well-being compared to their counterparts who do not?

Project Execution

The research on the project has been approved by the University of Toronto's Research Ethics Board. We invited students to participate in the Flourish programme by completing an online assessment. Participating students receive a profile that includes their scores presented graphically (see Appendix) and accompanying explanatory text. The profile provides feedback on the following measures:

- *Signature Strengths Questionnaire* (SSQ-72; Rashid et al. 2013): A 72-item questionnaire which measures 24 core character strengths according to the *Values-In-Action* (VIA) model of character strengths (Peterson and Seligman 2004).
- *Flourishing Inventory* (FI; Rashid 2016): This inventory assesses students' well-being in terms of their positive emotions, engagement, relationships, meaning, and accomplishment.
- *Student Engagement Inventory* (SEI; Rashid and Louden 2014): This 40-item inventory assesses students' academic habits. It has six subscales: assignments, examinations, academic motivation, academic resilience, campus engagement and campus adjustment.
- *Outcome Questionnaire* (OQ-45; Lambert et al. 1996): This well-established 45-item measure assesses symptoms of mental distress in three domains: (a) symptomatic distress, (b) interpersonal relations, and (c) social roles.
- *Cumulative GPA*: Grade point averages from semester to semester are tracked, as long as students continue to participate in the Flourish programme by completing the assessment. The assessment can be completed once every academic term.

Theoretical Underpinning

As discussed, Flourish is based on Corey Keyes' model (Keyes 2007; Keyes et al. 2011). Keyes has examined flourishing and languishing across numerous samples using the Mental Health Continuum-Short Form (MHC-SF; Keyes 2009). The MHC-SF consists of 14 items that measure the degree of emotional well-being, as defined in terms of happiness, satisfaction, and interest in life; social well-being in terms of social acceptance, social actualisation, social contribution, social coherence, and social integration; and psychological well-being in terms of autonomy, environmental mastery, personal growth, positive relations with others, purpose in life, and self-acceptance. Using this measure with a sample of 5698 college students, Keyes found that approximately 49.3% of students were flourishing and did not screen positive for a mental health disorder. Those who were not flourishing and screened positive for a mental disorder had impaired academics and also experienced suicidal ideation.

Modified Criteria of Flourishing

Our university also included MHC-SF along with the National College Health Assessment (ACHA 2016). Based on data of 631 students from our university who completed MHC-SF, 53% of students reported flourishing, less than 2% reported languishing, and the rest reported functioning in the moderately healthy range. Given the escalating rates of psychopathology on campuses, reported above, we found these rates higher than expected and inconsistent with rates previously reported by Keyes (2002). Instead of using MHC-SF, we opted to use two

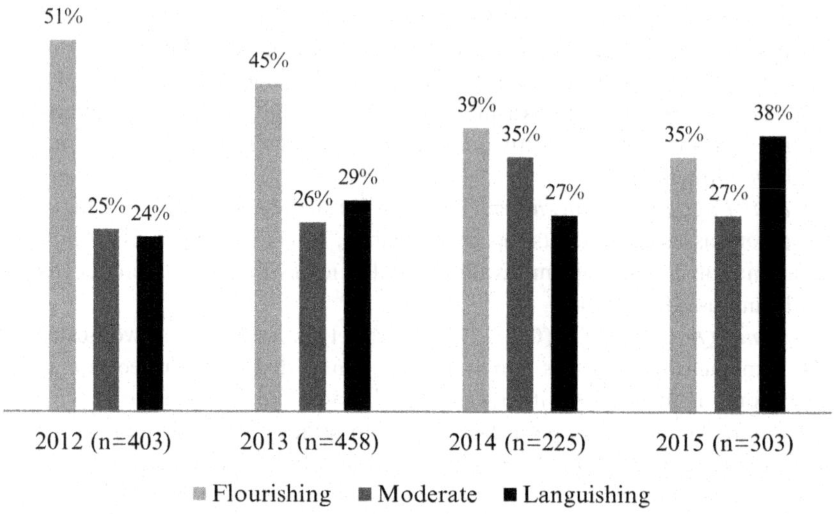

Fig. 3.1 Percentage of students flourishing, languishing, and moderately functioning based on stress and well-being scores, 2012–2015

independent measures, one measuring psychopathology and one well-being. As noted in the measures section above, psychiatric stress was measured by OQ-45, a well-established measure of overall psychiatric distress. We measured well-being with the 25-item FI, which measures five aspects of well-being including: (a) Positive emotion, (b) Engagement, (c) Relationships, (d) Meaning, and (e) Accomplishment (PERMA; Seligman 2011).

We opted to categorise students as *flourishing* if their scores were within the non-clinical range on OQ-45 (<63), and within the upper quartiles of the FI. We categorised them as *languishing* if their scores fell within the clinical range on OQ-45 (>63) and fell below the mean on the well-being measure (<97). Students not belonging to either of these categories are considered to be moderately mentally healthy.

Figure 3.1 presents four first year cohorts (2012–2015), a total of 1289 students (70.6% females; age 21.12 years, *SD 2.5* who completed their flourish assessment within the first month of their school year.

To date, more than 2000 students have participated in the programme. The data in Fig. 3.1 includes only Canadian residents, excluding international students. We invited incoming students through two orientation programmes. Participating students are eligible to enter a draw (e.g., $100 credit deposited on their student identity cards). Students receive an online link via email, presenting an overview of the project and outlining expectations for their participation. The online assessment and profiles are housed on a secure site; individual profiles are accessible only to the participating student. The consent procedure details potential risks and benefits. For example, students who endorse two critical items on the symptom measure receive a list of support resources. Participants are reassured that they can leave the project voluntarily at any time without academic or financial penalty and that their individual academic records will not be shared with anyone including faculty, staff of student services, or administration without their explicit consent.

Students are provided comprehensive feedback and a rich repository of online and campus-wide resources to support their flourishing (see Appendix for a sample). The programme, in collaboration with peer leaders and professional staff, offered day-long experiential workshops to struggling students focusing on building their psychological, physical, and academic well-being and resilience.

Flourish Intervention: Workshop: The Becoming

The primary intervention of the program is a full-day workshop titled *The Becoming*. The programme team has designed this full-day workshop around three components of resilience: emotional, physical, and academic. Each component includes an experiential activity facilitated by professional staff members from Health and Wellness, Athletics and Recreation, and the Academic Advising and Career Centre. After focusing on three components of resilience, students are encouraged to set up a personal goal that uses their signature strengths towards adaptive problem solving or towards becoming the sort of person they aspire to. The programme also offers a 2-h follow-up session, approximately 6 weeks later, where students discuss their progress and learn about additional resources. This session also offers students opportunities to get involved with the programme as a peer leader to help with facilitating future full-day workshops or other programme activities. Students who participate in our full-day workshops are invited to participate in research to assess the potential impact of the workshop and subsequent Flourish involvement. To date, 27 students have attended a full-day workshop and completed the Flourish assessment more than twice. We tested change in participants' level of understanding before and after each activity. Figure 3.2 presents changes. Significant changes were found in all four activities in terms of participant levels of learning before and after. We also assessed the overall effectiveness of the full-day workshops. Figure 3.3 presents a summary of anonymous feedback provided by participants (Table 3.1).

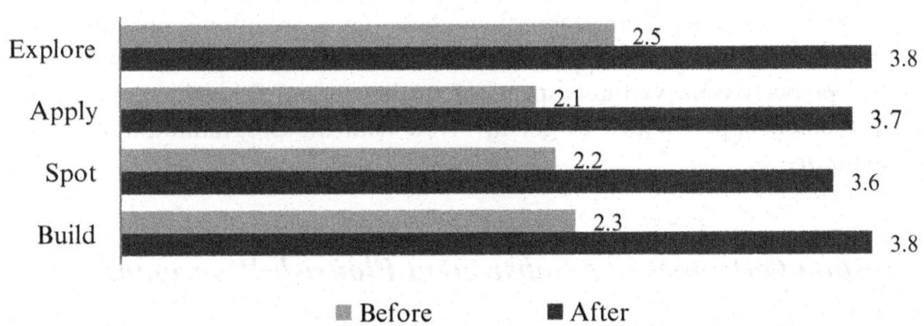

Fig. 3.2 Flourish full-day workshop: changes in level of knowledge before and after resilience activities. Changes in level of knowledge reported by participants ($n = 33$) before and after participating in the following four experiential activities: (1) Exploring one's character strengths from affective and intellectual perspectives; (2) Applying character strengths to resolve tough academic challenges; (3) Spotting other's character strengths through a team-building physical activity; (4) Building one's character strengths by pursuing a goal-setting activity

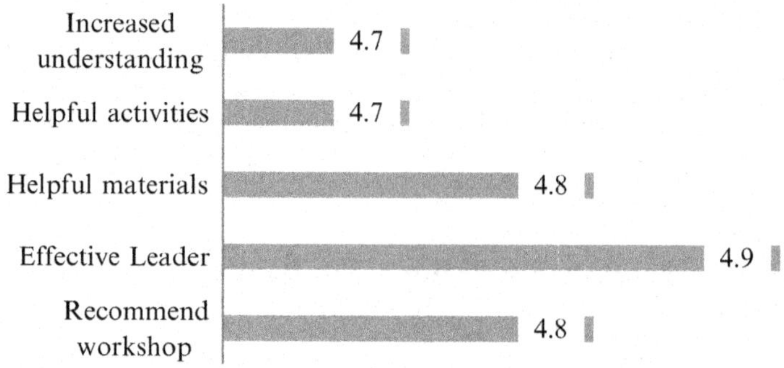

Fig. 3.3 Flourish full-day workshops: feedback from participants. Summary of feedback from students (n = 21) who attended our full-day Flourish workshops in Fall 2015 and Winter 2016. Participants rated various aspects of the workshop on a 5-point Likert Scale (5 = Strongly Agree; 4 = Agree; 3 = Neutral; 2 = Disagree; 1 = Strongly Disagree): (1) The workshop increased my understanding of my strengths; (2) Having done the activities today has helped me to better understand about various sources of my well-being and resilience; (3) The workshop materials (hand out, video clips, slides) were helpful to support my learning; (4) The leaders were effective in guiding the sessions; (5) I would recommend that this workshop be given to every UTSC student, especially first-years

Table 3.1 Changes in scores on measures of well-being, stress, and student engagement for students (n = 12) who attended full-day Flourish workshops in 2015

	Pre	Post		
Activity	Mean *(sd)*	Mean *(sd)*	*df*	*t*
Explore your strengths	2.54 *(0.93)*	3.75 *(0.60)*	31	*7.61***
Spot strengths in others	2.14 *(0.84)*	3.66 *(0.69)*	30	*9.49***
Apply your strengths	2.22 *(0.94)*	3.63 *(0.65)*	31	*8.49***
Build your strengths	2.25 *(0.84)*	3.75 *(0.62)*	31	*9.64***

**p<.001

We host a 2-h follow-up session, approximately 6 weeks after each workshop, where students discuss their progress and learn about additional resources. These sessions also offer students opportunities to discuss their progress and hear about others' perspective on various aspects of resilience and flourishing. Students are also presented opportunities to get involved with the programme as a *Flourish Ambassador*.

Workshop Outcomes and Subsequent Flourish Programme

All students who participated in the Flourish assessment received invitations to a full-day Flourish workshop, *The Becoming*, offered once every academic term, usually during a mid-semester break where there are no classes. Students who participate in our full-day workshops are then invited to participate in research to assess

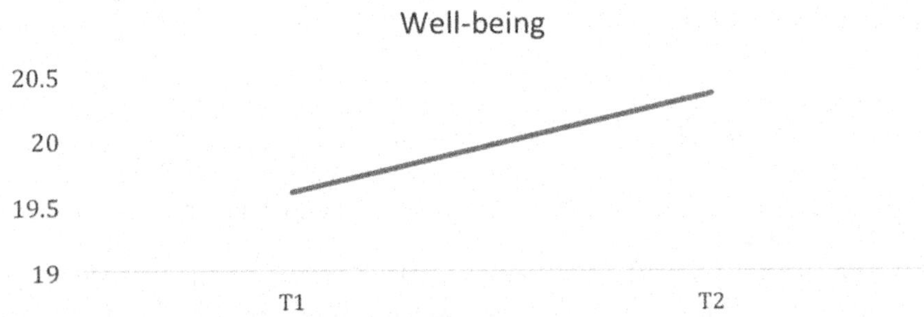

Fig. 3.4 Changes in scores of well-being for participants who engaged with the Flourish programme consistently

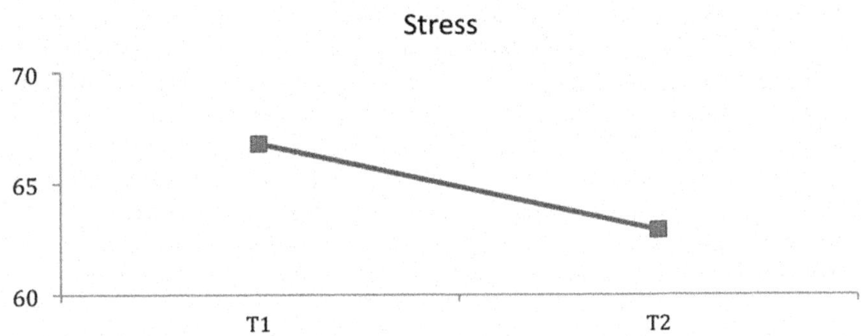

Fig. 3.5 Changes in scores of stress for participants who engaged with the Flourish programme consistently

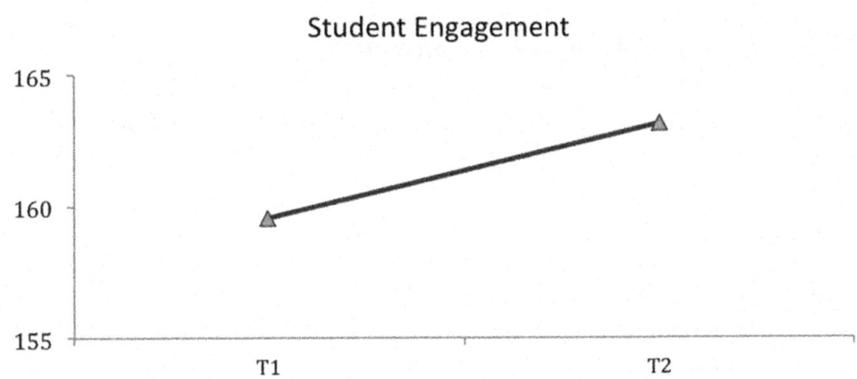

Fig. 3.6 Changes in scores of student engagement for participants who engaged with the Flourish programme consistently

the potential impact of the workshop and subsequent Flourish involvement. Generally, students who participated in a Flourish full-day workshop reported decreased stress, increased well-being, and increased student engagement. However, this data is preliminary and based on 12 ambassadors who completed the assessment at least twice (Figs. 3.4, 3.5 and 3.6).

Future Directions

1. **Longitudinal Analysis:** We continue to analyse succeeding cohorts to explore patterns of flourishing, including well-being, stress, and student engagement. Our longitudinal analyses will offer valuable insights about factors to better understand the malleability of various aspects of flourishing, resilience and well-being of young adults.
2. **Service Utilisation:** We also plan to conduct analysis regarding participants' utilisation of various student services, which will help us differentiate how students who are flourishing or languishing utilise student services. For example, are languishing students more likely to utilise counselling services, or students in the moderate range more likely to access academic advising services?
3. **Flourish Ambassador Program:** Currently we are also working with student leaders who have completed the Flourish assessment and subsequently participated in flourish interventions. These ambassadors will help in co-facilitating flourish workshops and also share their experience of participation. In addition, a group of Flourish ambassadors is working on curating stories of resilience from first year students, which can serve as exemplars for other students. We are developing a peer-training program that will train future ambassadors.
4. **Dissemination:** We are currently preparing a web-based assessment portal which will enable audiences across the world to assess their flourishing.

Acknowledgment This project, in part, was supported through the Mental Health Innovation Fund (MHIF) from the Ministry of Advanced Education and Skills Development.

Appendix: Flourish Profile (Feedback)

Signature Strengths (Based on Your Responses on November 2, 2015)

- **Curiosity**: You find yourself interested in exploring new things. When things are not clear, you strive to explore them further. You are fascinated by new topics and constantly ask questions to discover more about them. You are able to focus sharply on acquiring new information about a specific topic. Also, you are open to experiencing new and different things.
- **Kindness**: You are a kind and generous person who loves doing favours and good deeds for others, even for those you don't know well. You are never too busy to do a favour for a friend or family member; in fact, you enjoy doing that. You are always more inclined to give than to receive. Your acts of kindness are in the best interest of the other person, not to fulfil your own needs and wishes.
- **Love of Learning**: You love to learn new things—in school or on your own. You make very good use of opportunities where you can gain knowledge about skills, concept, ideas, and facts. You have always enjoyed school and reading. When it

comes to learning, you are persistent; even if you get frustrated or distracted, you refocus and don't give up until you have mastered the topic or skill.

- **Gratitude**: You never take things for granted and appreciate the good things in your life. When someone does a good thing for you, you just don't say 'thank you', but also take time to express your heartfelt thanks through words and action. You recognise that it is important to sit down and regularly count your blessings. Therefore, you savour looking at the pictures and other memorabilia of the pleasant memories of the past. You share your joys and pleasant experiences with others with enthusiasm.
- **Modesty and Humility**: You always let your accomplishments speak for themselves and do not seek the spotlight. You do not regard yourself as a special person, nor do you insist on being treated specially. You usually do not use status symbols (e.g., brand-name clothes or products) to impress others. Also, if you excel at something, you do not make others feel bad who may not be good at that. You are aware of your shortcomings and do not hesitate to admit them. Others recognise you as a humble or modest person.

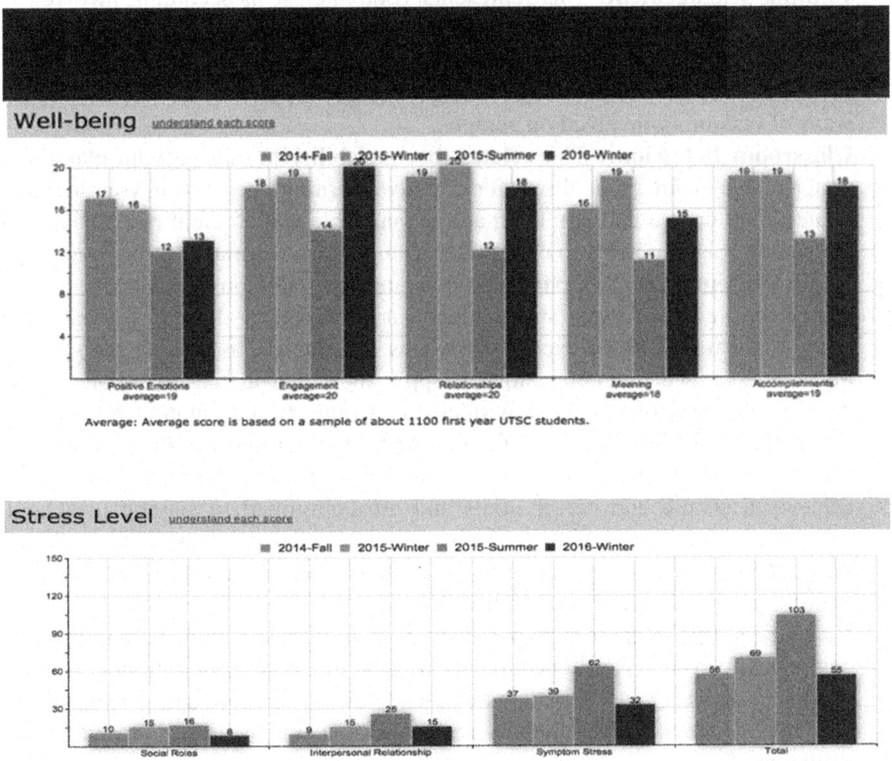

Your latest scores fall into following ranges:

	Social Roles	Interpersonal Relationship	Symptom Stress	Total
Normal Range	0-11	0-14	0-35	0-62
Moderate Range	12-18	15-20	36-50	63-78
High Range	19-36	21-44	51-100	79-180

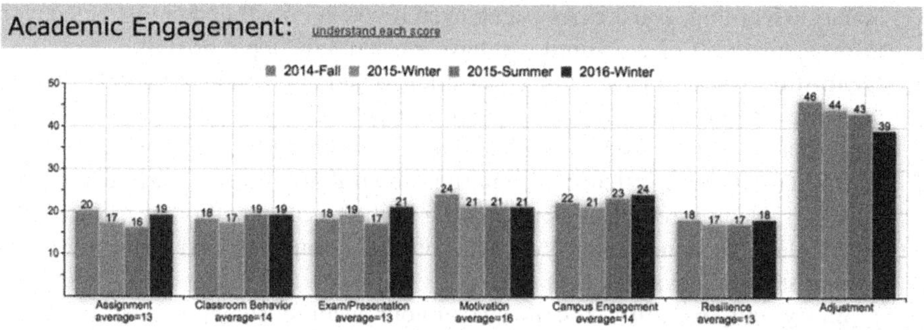

Resources

- **Assignment**: This relates to your ability to organise your personal time to ensure that you are able complete assignments in a timely and effective manner. Fostering strategies for managing assignments is essential to academic success.
- **Campus Engagement**: This represents your interest in becoming involved in university activities. Students engaged on campus take on leadership roles, join university clubs and organizations, and participate in extracurricular activities. Campus engagement is a strong predictor of student persistence. There are many ways of becoming involved on campus.
- **Classroom Behaviour**: This relates to your ability to engage with classroom material in a manner that allows for effective learning. Structuring your learning strategies to ensure that you learn at a manageable and efficient rate throughout the semester is important to effective learning and performance at university.
- **Exam/Presentation Behavior**: Exams and presentations provide a unique source of stress that many students can find particularly difficult to deal with, even if they are otherwise excellent students. Fortunately, as with all skills, learning strategies and practicing how to apply them can increase confidence and decrease the anxiety associated with exam writing and presentation delivery.
- **Motivation**: This is your level of commitment to your undergraduate education. Students committed to their education understand that a degree is essential to achieve academic and career goals and are committed to staying in school. Education commitment is one of the best predictors of student persistence. Many factors contribute to student motivation and you have the power to make changes in order to improve your own motivation.
- **Resilience**: This refers to how positively you might respond to challenging academic or life events. Resilient students are able to respond appropriately to life's challenges and remain focused on their academic and career goals. By exercising your own personal and community resources, you are able to cultivate your own resiliency.

References

American College Health Association. (2016). *American College Health Association-National College Health Assessment II: Reference group executive summary*. American College Health Association.: Hanover, MD. Spring 2016.

Blanco, C., Okuda, M., Wright, C., Hasin, D. S., Grant, B. F., Liu, S., & Olfson, M. (2008). Mental health of college students and their non-college-attending peers: Results from the National Epidemiologic Study on Alcohol and Related Conditions. *Archives of General Psychiatry, 65*(12), 1429–1437.

Brunwasser, S. M., Gillham, J. E., & Kim, E. S. (2009). A meta-analytic review of the Penn resiliency program's effect on depressive symptoms. *Journal of Consulting and Clinical Psychology, 77*(6), 1042–1054.

Chickering, A. W., & Reisser, L. (1993). *Education and identity* (2nd ed.). San Francisco: Jossey-Bass.

Clifton, D. O., Anderson, C. E., & Schreiner, L. A. (2006). *StrengthsQuest: Discover and develop your strengths in academics, career, and beyond* (2nd ed.). New York: Gallup Press.

Conway, K. P., Compton, W., Stinson, F. S., & Grant, B. F. (2006). Lifetime comorbidity of DSM-IV mood and anxiety disorders and specific drug use disorders: Results from the National Epidemiologic Survey on Alcohol and Related Conditions. *Journal of Clinical Psychiatry, 67*, 247–257.

Cook, L. J. (2007). Striving to help college students with mental health issues. *Journal of Psychosocial Nursing Mental Health Services, 45*, 40–44.

Drum, D. J., Brownson, C., Burton Denmark, A., & Smith, S. (2009). New data on the nature of suicidal crises in college students: Shifting the paradigm. *Professional Psychology: Research and Practice, 3*, 213–222.

Eisenberg, D., Hunt, J., Speer, N., & Zivin, K. (2011). Mental health service utilization among college Students in the United States. *Journal of Nervous and Mental Disease, 199*, 301–308.

Erdur-Baker, O., Aberson, C. L., Barrow, J. C., & Draper, M. R. (2006). Nature and severity of college students' psychological concerns: A comparison of clinical and nonclinical national samples. *Professional Psychology: Research and Practice, 37*, 317–323.

Gallagher, R. (2010). *National survey of counseling centre directors*. The International Association of Counseling Services. Monograph Series Number 85. Retrieved September 11, 2011, from http://www.iacsinc.org/

Hanger, M. A., Goldenson, J., Weinberg, M., Schmitz-Sciborski, A., & Monzon, R. (2011). The bounce back retention program: One-year follow-up study. *Journal of College Student Retention, 13*(2), 205–227.

Hanger, M., Schmitz-Sciborski, A., & Weinberg, M. (2007). *Bounce back retention program: Facilitator and coach manual*. San Diego, CA: Montezuma Publishing.

Ishitani, T. T. (2003). A longitudinal approach to assessing attrition behavior among first generation students: Time-varying effects of pre-college characteristics. *Research in Higher Education, 44*, 433–449.

Karris, M. A. (2007). *Character strengths and well-being in a college sample*. ProQuest Dissertations and Theses, University of Colorado at Boulder. Retrieved April 24, 2012, from http://search.proquest.com/docview/304889523?accountid=14771

Kessler, R. C., Chiu, W. T., Demler, O., & Walters, E. E. (2005). Prevalence, severity, and comorbidity of twelve-month DSM-IV disorders in the National Comorbidity Survey Replication (NCS-R). *Archives of General Psychiatry, 62*, 617–627.

Kettmann, J. D. J., Schoen, E. G., Moel, J. E., Cochran, S. V., Greenberg, S. T., & Corkery, J. M. (2007). Increasing severity of psychopathology at counseling centers: A new look. *Professional Psychology: Research and Practice, 38*, 523–529.

Keyes, C. L. M. (2002). The mental health continuum: From languishing to flourishing in life. *Journal of Health and Social Behavior, 43*(2), 207–222. Retrieved from http://www.ncbi.nlm.nih.gov/pubmed/12096700

Keyes, C. L. M. (2007). Promoting and protecting mental health as flourishing: A complementary strategy for improving national mental health. *American Psychologist, 62*, 95–108.

Keyes, C. L. M., Eisenberg, D., Perry, G. S., Dube, S. R., Kroenke, K., & Dhingra, S. S. (2011). The relationship of level of positive mental health with current mental disorders in predicting suicidal behavior and academic impairment in college students. *Journal of American College Health, 60*, 126–133.

Kirby, M. J. L., & Keon, W. J. (2006). *Out of the shadows at last: Transforming mental health, mental illness and addiction services in Canada. The Standing Senate Committee on Social Affairs, Science and Technology*. Ottawa: Senate Canada.

Lambert, M. J., Burlingame, G. M., Umphress, V., Hansen, N. B., Vermeersch, D. A., Clouse, G. C., & Yanchar, S. C. (1996). The reliability and validity of the Outcome Questionnaire. *Clinical Psychology and Psychotherapy, 3*, 249–258.

Lee, D., Olson, E. A., Locke, B., Michelson, S. T., & Odes, E. (2009). The effects of college counselling services on academic performance and retention. *Journal of College Student Development, 50*, 305–319.

Lopez, S. J., & Edwards, L. M. (2008). The interface of counseling psychology and positive psychology: Assessing and promoting strengths. In S. Brown & R. Lent (Eds.), *Handbook of counseling psychology* (4th ed., pp. 86–99). Hoboken, NJ: Wiley.

Lopez, S. J., & Louis, M. C. (2009). The principles of strengths-based education. *Journal of College and Character, 10*, 1–8.

Louis, M. C. (2011). Strengths interventions in higher education: The effect of identification versus development approaches on implicit self-theory. *The Journal of Positive Psychology, 6*, 204–215.

Lounsbury, J. W., Fisher, L. A., Levy, J. J., & Welsh, D. P. (2009). An investigation of character strengths in relation to the academic success of college students. *Individual Differences Research, 7*, 52–69.

Loya, F., Reddy, R., & Hinshaw, P. (2010). Mental illness stigma as a mediator of differences in Caucasian and South Asian college students' attitudes toward psychological counseling. *Journal of Counseling Psychology, 57*, 484–490.

MacKean, G. (2011). *Mental health and well-being in postsecondary education settings: A literature and environmental scan to support planning and action in Canada.* Canadian Association of University and College Student Services. Retrieved September 11, 2011, from https://www.cacuss.ca/en/news/CACUSSnews/MentalHealth_report.htm

McGovern, T. V., & Miller, S. L. (2008). Integrating teacher behaviors with character strengths and virtues for faculty development. *Teaching of Psychology, 35*, 278.

Mitchell, S. L., Greenwood, A. K., & Guglielmi, M. C. (2007). Utilization of counseling services: Comparing international students and U.S. college students. *Journal of College Counseling, 10*, 117–129.

Mitchell, J. J., Reason, R. D., Hemer, K. M., & Finley, A. (2016). Perceptions of campus climates for civic learning as predictors of college students' mental health. *Journal of College and Character, 17*(1), 40.

Much, K., & Swanson, A. L. (2010). The debate about increasing college student psychopathology: Are college students really getting "sicker?". *Journal of College Student Psychotherapy, 24*, 86–97.

Nilsson, J. E., Berkel, L. A., Flores, L. Y., & Lucas, M. S. (2004). Utilization rate and presenting concerns of international students at a university counseling center. *Journal of College Student Psychotherapy, 19*, 49–59.

Oades, L. G., Robinson, P., Green, S., & Spence, G. B. (2011). Towards a positive university. *The Journal of Positive Psychology, 6*, 432–439.

Ouweneel, E., Le Blanc, P. M., & Schaufeli, W. B. (2011). Flourishing students: A longitudinal study on positive emotions, personal resources, and study engagement. *The Journal of Positive Psychology, 6*(2), 142–153.

Pedrelli, P., Nyer, M., Yeung, A., Zulauf, C., & Wilens, T. (2015). College students: Mental health problems and treatment considerations. *Academic Psychiatry, 39*(5), 503–511.

Peterson, C., & Seligman, M. E. P. P. (2004). *Character strengths and virtues: A handbook and classification (First)*. New York: Oxford University Press.

Rashid, T. (2016). *Flourishing inventory*. Unpublished Data, University of Toronto Scarborough.

Rashid, T., & Loudan, R. (2014). *Student engagement inventory*. Unpublished data, University of Toronto Scarborough.

Rashid, T., Anjum, A., Lennex, C., Quinlin, D., Niemiec, R., Mayerson, D., & Kazemi, F. (2013). Assessment of positive traits in children and adolescents. In C. Proctor & P. A. Linley (Eds.), *Research, applications, and interventions for children and adolescents: A positive psychology perspective* (pp. 81–114). The Netherlands: Springer.

Rayle, A. D., & Chung, K. Y. (2007). Revisiting first-year college students' mattering: Social support, academic stress, and the mattering experience. *Journal of Student Retention, 9*, 21–37.

Russo-Netzer, P., & Ben-Shahar, T. (2011). Learning from success: A close look at a popular positive psychology course. *The Journal of Positive Psychology, 6*, 468–476.

Schwartz, A. J. (2006). Are college students more disturbed today? Stability in the acuity and qualitative character of psychopathology of college counseling center clients: 1992–1993 through 2001–2002. *Journal of American College Health, 54*, 327–337.

Seligman, M. E. P. (2011). *Flourish: A visionary new understanding of happiness and well-being*. New York: Free Press.

Seligman, M. E. P., Rashid, T., & Parks, A. C. (2006). Positive psychotherapy. *American Psychologist, 61*, 774–788.

Seligman, M. E. P., Schulman, P., & Tryon, A. (2007). Group prevention of depression and anxiety symptoms. *Behaviour Research and Therapy, 45*, 1111–1126.

Sharkin, B. S., & Coulter, L. P. (2005). Empirically supporting the increasing severity of college counseling center client problems: Why is it so challenging? *Journal of College Counseling, 8*, 165–172.

Tinto, V. (2004). Linking learning and leaving: Exploring the role of the college classroom in student departure. In J. M. Braxton (Ed.), *Reworking the student departure puzzle* (pp. 81–94). Nashville, TN: Vanderbilt University Press.

Zwick, R., & Schlemer, L. (2004). SAT validity for linguistic minorities at the University of California, Santa Barbara. *Educational Measurement: Issues and Practice, 25*, 6–16.

Chapter 4
Active Ageing as Positive Intervention: Some Unintended Consequences

Vera Roos and Ronette Zaaiman

Abstract The aim of this chapter is twofold: first, to access the subjective experiences of older residents in an urban residential facility which has adopted an active ageing approach; and second, to indicate how active ageing enables growth goals, but also produces unintended consequences. Data were obtained (from 16 Afrikaans- and English-speaking, White males and females, ranging in age from 65 to 84) by means of the Mmogo-method®, a projective visual data-collection method (Roos 2012). Textual data were analysed thematically and visual data were analysed by using the Roos and Redelinghuys's (2016) six-step method of analysis. Even though the active environment enabled growth goals (autonomy, independence, and interrelatedness), it provoked some unintended consequences, including: exclusion of some residents due to ill health or limited financial resources; a feeling of obligation to participate; increased emphasis on self- and relational-regulation; and unmet emotional needs. Suggestions are proposed to deal with the unintended consequences of active ageing in an attempt to optimise it as a positive intervention.

Background and Introduction

Contextualised against the backdrop of the observed and projected global ageing of populations, this chapter has a two-pronged aim: (1) to obtain older people's subjective expressions of their experiences in an active ageing environment, and (2) to highlight some of the unintended consequences of adopting an active ageing approach.

It has become common knowledge that the proportion of people aged 60 and over is globally growing faster than that of any other age group (ILC 2015; World

V. Roos (✉) • R. Zaaiman
Optentia Research Focus Area, North-West University, Vanderbijlpark, South Africa
e-mail: Vera.Roos@nwu.ac.za; ronettezaaiman@gmail.com

C. Proctor (ed.), *Positive Psychology Interventions in Practice*,
DOI 10.1007/978-3-319-51787-2_4

Health Organization 2015). The current world population (including older people) had already exceeded seven billion people by the end of 2011 (ILC 2015), and it is estimated that people aged 60 years and older will outnumber children under the age of 15 by 2050 (ILC 2015). Although still an overwhelmingly young country, South Africa follows a similar trend. The World Population Data Sheet (Population Reference Bureau 2014) identified South Africa, with almost 5% of 58.7 million people over the age of 60, as having one of the most rapidly ageing populations compared with other populations in Sub-Sahara Africa.

Reasons for the increase of older people may be ascribed to many factors, such as: the temporary increase in the birth rate following the Second World War, known as the 'baby-boom'; lowered fertility and mortality rates; improved life expectancy, as a direct consequence of the impact of progressive medical developments; and migration (Apt 2012; ILC 2015; Powell and Taylor 2015; Velkoff and Kowal 2007). There is general agreement that how people age is a product of: the particular socio-cultural context in which they live; their unique genetic, biological disposition, psychological constellation that has developed over their total lifespan; their unique responses to life-changing events; the development of habits; and the adoption of a particular lifestyle (Fernández-Ballesteros et al. 2013; ILC 2015; Nolan and Scott 2009).

Ageing, in the South African context, should also be contextualised against the legacy of apartheid. Pre-1994, job opportunities, health, and social services were reserved for a minority group of Whites, while the majority of Blacks, who are now elderly, found themselves living in communities with limited infrastructure, unfavourable and age-unfriendly physical environments, and with limited support for their health and social needs (Lombard and Kruger 2009; Krout 2014; Roos et al. 2014a, b). Even though a lifespan approach, by which ageing is understood as a process that starts from birth, is acknowledged, for the purpose of this chapter individuals who are 60 years and older will be discussed.

Active Ageing

Definitions of active ageing vary and cover a wide spectrum of concepts. For example, concepts such as successful ageing, healthy ageing, robust ageing, productive ageing, positive ageing, and optimal ageing (Cosco et al. 2013) are used as synonyms for active ageing. However, these constructs are embedded in particular theoretical frameworks or are used to inform practice or to test hypotheses. For example, successful ageing is used as a probable variable that is associated with good health, low probability of illness, high physical and mental functioning, and high social participation (Fernandez-Ballesteros et al. 2013). In line with the reasoning of Paoletti (2015) the use of these indicators may imply that older people who are frail and experience illness are aging unsuccessfully. For the purpose of this chapter, *active ageing* was chosen as an operational term (ILC 2015).

Active ageing was introduced as: part of a broad global positive intervention for the management of ageing populations (Stenner et al. 2011), to reduce expenses associated with increasing age-declining health (Paoletti 2015), to bring about a change in society's views and prejudices regarding ageing and older people (Stenner et al. 2011), and to promote the social inclusion of older people in all life domains. The ideology underlying active ageing was the introduction of a different discourse about ageing and older people and it found expression in the development of active ageing programmes and campaigns to encourage individuals to change their behaviour to ensure their own personal well-being and life quality as they age (Van Dyk et al. 2013).

To deal with the number of older growing people there was also a shift from a primarily medical approach that viewed older people in terms of their incapacities or illnesses, to the maintenance and improvement of people's functional abilities during their life course in order to raise the quality of their lives when they are old (Department of Social Development 2010). Even though this would appear to be a 'win-win' situation, the onus of ageing actively falls on individuals' making use of the available opportunities and on remaining actively involved (Van Dyk et al. 2013). Accordingly, the aim of this study was to obtain data from the personal experiences of older individuals who find themselves in an environment that adopts an active ageing approach. This motivation resonates with Van Dyk et al.'s (2013) view that even though there is a political discourse about active ageing and interventions to manage older growing populations, very little empirical evidence has been obtained from the older people themselves. Moreover, research has been conducted mostly on older people who are frail, vulnerable, or disabled and have specific physical care needs (Buswell 2011; Persoon et al. 2010). Therefore, the following question guided this chapter: What do functional older people experience in an active ageing environment?

Contextualising the Discussion

The director of a private residential facility in Johannesburg, Gauteng Province (an urban area), in South Africa, who also manages other facilities caring for older people, invited researchers to explore residents' lifestyle experiences in the residential facility because he wanted to enhance the services provided at their facilities. As this particular facility adopts an active ageing approach, its residents were regarded as being competent to provide detailed data of their subjective experiences.

The residents in this particular setting were mainly White Afrikaans-speaking people (although there were also some English-speaking residents) between the ages of 50 and 95 years. The residential facility had approximately 350 residents and a support staff of 35 care workers, 90 volunteers, seven permanent nurses, a lifestyle consultant, and a centre manager. The lifestyle consultant and the centre manager were responsible for the day-to-day planning and implementation of the activities. The lifestyle consultant developed specific programmes for every day of the week, with time slots allocated for different activities in which she encouraged the older people to participate. The activities included snooker, bingo, line-dancing, bridge, Scrabble, choir singing, and brisk walks. They filled the day, usually from 9:00 a.m. until 4:00 p.m. Each resident could choose if he or she wanted to participate at all, or in which activity to participate, and when.

It is important to note that this example is not representative of all older people in South Africa, because residential facilities for older people in South Africa were available exclusively for White people until Apartheid ended in 1994. It was only in post-Apartheid South Africa that these facilities were opened up to all South Africans, regardless of race or colour (Department of Social Development 2010). However, the placement of these residential facilities were geographically determined by Apartheid policies in force at the time and are therefore still concentrated within wealthier provinces and in areas with a large proportion of White older people (Bekhet et al. 2009; Donaldson and Goldhaber 2012). For the most part, older South Africans do not have access to residential facilities, but spend their last years in community settings that are age-unfriendly with limited infrastructure (Keating et al. 2013; Mayosi et al. 2009).

A residential facility is a building used primarily to provide accommodation and 24-h care to older people (South Africa 2006). In South Africa, the Older Persons Act makes provision for three categories of residential facilities: Category A—independent living, Category B—assisted living, and Category C—frail care. In Category C, the focus is mainly on the physical care of older people. This study focuses on the first two categories—on functional older people who, despite the challenges that accompany ageing, can still look after themselves, get about on their own, and are still actively engaged in their environment (Aiken 1995; Papalia et al. 2009).

In collaboration with the staff of the residential facility, independently-living older people who were willing to and capable of participating in the data-gathering process were invited to participate in the research. A group of 16 Afrikaans- and English-speaking White individuals, consisting of 13 female and 3 male participants ranging in age from 65 to 84, was recruited. By implication this group of residents may be in any case those who are already pursuing active ageing and therefore agreed to participate. Nevertheless, they are regarded as being capable of providing detailed information about their experiences.

To elicit rich and deep data about lifestyle experiences from the participants, the data-gathering method which was chosen for this study was the Mmogo-method®, a projective visual data-collection method (Roos 2008, 2012, 2016a). The Mmogo-method® involves obtaining personal and group experiences by requesting participants to use unstructured materials to make visual representations of their experiences in a group setting. Before engaging in the task, a context of optimal participation is created by means of explaining in detail what the research entails and by requesting participants to treat information shared in the group as confidential.

In applying the method, participants were requested to divide themselves into two similar-sized groups of eight and to be seated in a circle. They were provided with unstructured materials: a lump of clay, colourful beads, and sticks of different lengths, and asked: *'Please make a visual representation with the materials provided that can tell us more about how you experience your life here at the residential facility'*.

After the visual representations had been completed, photos were taken and served as visual data. The visual representations became the stimulus material for each participant to present his or her perspective and for the group to discuss shared experiences, which could thus lead to the social construction of the meaning attached to shared experiences (Roos 2008, 2012, 2016a). The explanations and discussions, transcribed verbatim, produced the textual data.

The textual data were analysed using thematic analysis (Clarke and Braun 2013), and the visual data were analysed using Roos and Redelinghuys's (2016) proposed steps: (1) the research production context was described, (2) researchers assumed an empathic position towards data, (3) the literal observations of visual elements were described, (4) the symbolic meanings attributed by participants to the elements in their visual representations were described, (5) if applicable, the contexts that participants introduced spontaneously were described, and (6) an interpretative analysis based on the previous steps was conducted to identify transferrable knowledge. In this research an onto-epistemological approach was used: first, there is a focus on the subjective experiences of people (relativism), and next, in the analysis and interpretation of data, researchers assume a realist perspective, viewing participants' visual representations and the discussions as the participants' social constructions in relation to a social reality (Roos and Baart 2016).

Active Ageing: Growth Goals

The discussion of participants' subjective experiences will be supported with theories and literature.

An Optimal Environment Promotes Active Ageing

Not surprisingly, a safe environment was mentioned by many participants as an optimal environment; this was expressed as a sense of physical and organisational safety. Following Barker's (1968) behaviour setting theory, which holds that the setting in which people function is a significant determinant of human behaviour, the subjective experiences of participants should be understood against the South African context, which is regarded as a violent society that regularly targets older people as vulnerable victims (Policastro et al. 2015; Roberts 2010). Safety for these participants meant the absence of, or protection against, unmanageable, dangerous or harmful incidents. Participant 7, for example, indicated that her need for safety was one of the reasons why she and other older people chose to relocate to residential facilities: *'[It] is different from when you lived in a big house'* where you *'used to feel like you have to lock all the doors and put the alarm on'*. Now *'you can sit with your doors open until you go to bed'*.

Research by Bekhet et al. (2009) also found that older people required an optimal environment that, among other things, implies a safe environment when they relocate to a residential facility. When people feel safe it enables them to relax and to engage in living their lives fully without fearing for their physical safety: *'You are never troubled or concerned at night, you do not worry about anything...peace'* (Participant 12). Maslow's (1943) hierarchy of human needs confirms that lower (deficiency) needs must at least be partially satisfied before the higher growth goals become influential.

Interestingly, safety in this study also refers to older participants' expression of organisational safety which Baumgardner and Crothers (2010), link to an orderly and predictable world. Participant 2 explained that: *'You feel so safe, because you know it is well organised. We do not stand on our own'*. Since people's subjective experiences are embedded in the environment in which they function (Barker 1968; Nelson and Prilleltensky 2005; Roos 2016b), the finding that an organised environment, with structure, routine, and predictability is associated with a sense of safety, is also important to consider when contexts are designed to promote active ageing.

Growth Goals

Growth goals refer to what the self-determination theory calls 'growth needs' (Alderfer 1969; Deci and Ryan 2000; Dahlgaard and Dahlgaard 2003). The term 'growth goals' is preferred because 'needs' could also imply 'deficiencies' (Alderfer 1969; Dahlgaard and Dahlgaard 2003). However, what is relevant is that growth goals are regarded as innate psychological nutriments which, Deci and Ryan (2000) suggest, arouse people to purposeful, self-direction action to pursue contentment, happiness, and fulfilment. The three growth goals include: autonomy, independence, and interrelatedness.

Autonomy

Autonomy refers to people's sense that their actions are freely chosen and mastery of the environment (Covinsky et al. 2003; Deci and Ryan 2000). In the well-organised environment studied, participants expressed freedom of choice in maintaining their active lifestyle. They decide autonomously whether or not to participate in a range of physical activities that are formally organised and/or arranged by the facility (both inside and outside) or self-organised, and include: going to the gymnasium in the facility, going for walks outside the facility, playing tennis, or playing snooker. Participant 2, referring to his visual presentation of a tap as a metaphor (see Fig. 4.1), explained that he had the autonomy to decide if, where and how he would

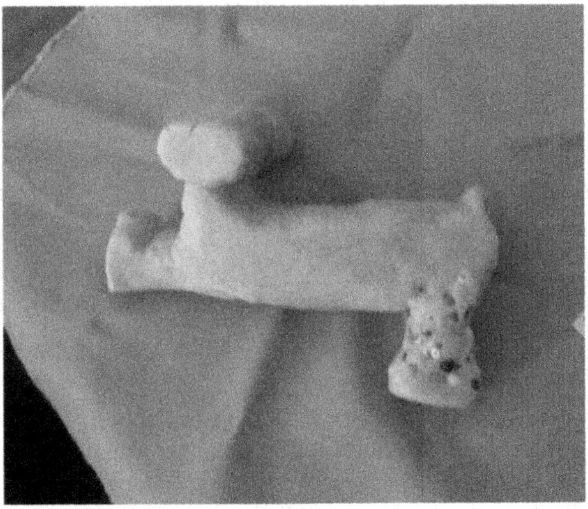

Fig. 4.1 Presentation of a tap demonstrating freedom of choice

like to participate in the active environment: *'If you open the tap, you can participate in many activities within the facility as well as outside…; that is right, you can turn it open or close it…'.*

Many participants also demonstrated mastery of the environment by pursuing the active lifestyles they were used to. They found that their busy schedules before relocating to the residential facility had been complemented by the environment and therefore appreciated now being able to take part in as many activities as they had done before: *'I'm a very active person, I can't sit still. I do everything, and I love it, I love it. As long as I can, I will do it!'* (Participant 11). This active involvement could be a consequence for some participants of having to adjust to psychosocial developmental changes, such as retirement, fewer responsibilities, and the loss of loved ones (Deci and Ryan 2000). It could also be that residents wished to experience mastery and interpersonal connection (Compton 2005). However, according to Van Dyk et al. (2013), another explanation is that the group of older people who are involved in an 'endless motion' of activities to 'simulate being busy and to imitate occupational schedules, do so in order to be recognised as active citizens' (p. 17).

Independence

Freedom to choose and the opportunity to exercise this freedom is a deep driver of people's actions to remain in control of the management of everyday life (Deci and Ryan 2000). Interestingly, in this research older people differentiated between autonomy and independence. Autonomy is expressed and confirmed in literature as the individual's sense that his or her actions are freely chosen and expressive of the true self (Deci and Ryan 2000). In contrast, independence refers to the ability to perform basic self-care activities without assistance (Covinsky et al. 2003).

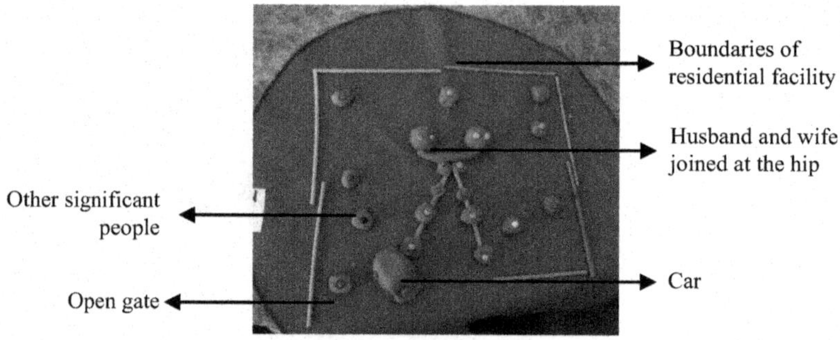

Fig. 4.2 Enclosed facility with an open gate through which car is leaving

Independency was also demonstrated by participants who come and go freely. Participant 4 described this by using her visual presentation (see Fig. 4.2): *'The gate is open for me to come and go as I please. That is why I placed the car there. Because, my husband and I often go…at least once a month to different places'*.

Interrelatedness

The need to have mutually supportive interpersonal relationships and the optimisation of this growth goal are vital for the facilitation of optimal functioning, constructive social development, and well-being (Compton 2005; Deci and Ryan 2000). Social interactions depend, however, on the subjective experience of the impact of the reciprocal processes of the relational interactions between people (Roos 2016b; Vorster 2011), and how people define the social space in their relational interactions in the interpersonal context. In this study participants described the social distance between them and other people either as a close or general social space, also confirmed by literature (Antonucci et al. 2013, 2004; Thomése et al. 2005).

Close Social Space

This space is very specifically described as relationships with close family members and friends (Antonucci et al. 2004). Most participants indicated the importance of family relations by stating that it was *'very, very important'*. In relation to close family relationships, regular and physical contact with children and grandchildren was emphasised. In fact, *'if you don't see them'*, as Participant 2 said, he wondered if they *'aren't interested anymore?'* In the close social space, a goal is to remain *'influential in the lives of [their] children and grandchildren'*. Older people may accordingly choose to invest their time and energy in a few significant relationships and selected activities which are deemed important (Van Dyk et al. 2013).

However, when family relationships and regular contact limit relational interactions in a close interpersonal space (for example when people do not have children or grandchildren or when they have migrated), participants create a sense of family between them: *'With all the activities... We are a big family'*. Literature confirmed that when circumstances such as losses interfered with the availability of close family relationships, increased interest in close friendship relationships (Thomése et al. 2005) was noted.

General Social Space

The general social space was where people engaged in various activities, such as: playing snooker with friends inside the facility, visiting friends outside the facility, sing-alongs in the facility, watching sport on television, taking photos and creating photo albums, reading books, making birthday cards, making scrapbooks, gardening, playing computer games, and going fishing.

Participants emphasised that their growth goals were achieved in this space when they received affirmation and emotional care through having conversations, sharing, and instrumental support. According to Vorster (2011) and Vorster et al. (2013), affirmation is one of the psychosocial needs that contribute to relational well-being. Affirmation was expressed by some participants. Participant 8 indicated that his snooker team had *'won the league'* for the *'last 5 years'*. Participants 2, 15, and 16 described how they *'greet everyone' by 'waving and greeting'* or *'say[ing] hello'*.

Emotional care was expressed by participants, who also provide compassion and mutual support, within the contexts of: losses experienced, health or other problems experienced, and feeling sad. Participant 12 described how when *'you have a problem or received bad news, you can always go to your friend and receive care'* which may contribute to new *'strength'* and *'enrichment'* (growth). Participant 3 described how everyone *'supported and assisted'* her *'during the time of [my] husband's illness and death'*. Emotional care in the residential setting, included sharing *'a cup of tea or coffee'* (Participants 11 and 16), which created opportunities for *'shared life experiences'*. The various shared activities also provided people with opportunities to *'have fun together'*. Participant 12 described how she and her friend *'can have so much fun dancing together'*.

Participants provided instrumental support to one another. They mentioned that their *'garden being watered'* by other residents enabled them to travel (Participant 5). Older residents, who were still able to drive cars, often provided instrumental support by offering residents without a car or who unable to drive, *'a lift'* (Participant 4). The importance of relationships in promoting older people's well-being in residential facilities has been well described in the literature (Roos and Du Toit 2014; Roos and Malan 2012; Van Biljon and Roos 2015, 2016).

Active Ageing: Some Unintended Consequences

Despite the benefits of active ageing, participants also indicated threats attached to the positive intervention of active ageing. These unintended consequences have implications for the individual's as well as the group's functioning.

Threats to Autonomy and Independence and Active Participation

Threats to the autonomy of older people may be experienced through financial difficulties or inevitably deteriorating health, making them dependent on others for assistance, as confirmed by Papalia et al. (2009). Participant 2 explained how financial problems, caused by the insufficiency of *'small pensions'* can hinder active participation, particularly if the activities have a financial implication.

A deteriorating health status was particularly linked to being unable to live independently and maintain their lives actively. The drive to live autonomous and independent was so strong that some residents kept *'on and on and on in their little old house and eventually even become unkempt'* and *'they cling to their little house where they can live independently'* (Participant 2). Participant 8 emphasised this drive to maintain independent living by stating that he would rather be *'[put] to sleep'*, than to *'suffer in frail care'*, supporting what Van Dyk et al. (2013) refer to as an attempt to try to 'prevent the nightmare of post-human advanced old age' (pp. 17–18).

Feeling Obliged to Participate

In line with the concern raised that the idealisation of active ageing can become oppressive, as proposed by Stenner et al. (2011), participants indicated that they experienced participation as a group norm which they violated if they did not want to participate.

It appeared that some of the residents who did participate in activities did not always feel free to stay in their rooms at times even if they felt they needed solitude. In this active environment, the well-intentioned encouragement to participate becomes a social norm guiding behaviour. However, participants often preferred to be alone: *'Yes it is important to be alone sometimes. [People] need their own time, their own space and that you have to accept it'* (Participant 8). Older people often want to disengage from an active environment in an attempt to adapt to the various psychosocial developmental changes that occur in late adulthood (Baltes and Baltes 1990), or to deal with losses by drawing on their remaining resources (Papalia et al. 2009), or from personal preference.

Some said that they also felt excluded from activities if their physical disabilities prevented them from participating. This supports Walker (2002), who proposed that active ageing runs the risk of marginalising certain groups if not properly applied.

Norm of Obligation Emphasises Self-Regulation

The theme of being 'too busy' recurred throughout the study, which consequently placed much emphasis on the regulatory skills of older people. The participants indicated that they wanted to have more control over their time so that they could spend it on other activities. The participants experienced their lives as being very busy, so much so that they felt they had not actually retired: *'You are really busy; we're actually more busy now because we haven't gone on retirement. I want to still one day play snooker but I haven't had a chance; I'm too busy'* (Participant 10).

Some older residents, however, seem easily to regulate their freedom of choice to *'participate in whatever (you) wish, which is very good, or stay by yourself. It is completely up to you, whether you want to do things or whether you can stay in your room and be quiet'* (Participant 11). Even if participants did not want to be involved in activities—*'I don't take part in all of them [activities]'* (Participant 1)—they were able to express their wishes.

However, some older people seemed over-committed to participating: *'I am active, I need to switch off'* (Participant 2). This raises the question: how can functional older people navigate themselves in an environment where the focus is on being actively engaged? One could also speculate whether in such a context it is assumed that all people have the same skills to regulate themselves and whether attention should not also be paid to vulnerable individuals who need support to navigate themselves in a very busy environment. As older people's age and experience change, their ways of self-regulation also change (Schunk and Zimmerman 1997). Combining this with the norms of participation, some individuals may be at risk of compensating to be able to continue to engage despite personal preferences and capabilities, resulting in a statement like this: *'I am now too busy, I can't...'*.

Norm of Obligation Emphasises Relation Regulation

Relational regulation is defined as the way in which people navigate themselves in relation to others in order to address their social goals or psychosocial needs (Steyn 2015). Experiences of residents who *'intrude into your space'* may have raised an awareness of the importance to *'guard against becoming selfish'*, to *'be sensitive'* and thoughtful in how you *'treat each individual'*. Therefore, relational regulation was deemed especially important, considering the inevitable and regular contact between residents: *'Inside the facility we have many people, in close proximity: you live in a small block'*. It is also a fallacy that relational regulation is a skill that develops naturally for all people: *'Look, you get people who are...they chatter all the time and you have to accept that'* (Participant 8). Older people may often lack *'judgement and tact'* (Participant 13) to regulate relationships.

Ineffective strategies to regulate relationships are to adopt an either or approach, as demonstrated by participants who said: *'One must either get along with others, despite inevitable differences, or avoid people you do not get along with'*. Another ineffective strategy to regulate relationships is to avoid conflict. Participant 7 stressed her *'strong dislike of fighting and conflict'*. Avoiding people or conflict resulted in the unintended consequence that participants might disengage from general social spaces and limit their opportunities to achieve their growth goals. Participant 15 said that in an attempt to prevent further conflict [she] *'stopped going to the gym'*, *'stopped popping at others' for tea'* and *'stopped walking through the complex'*. These strategies may seem to avoid conflict but could unintentionally contribute to self-designed isolation which in turn could contribute to loneliness. Relation regulation consists of assisting older people in dealing effectively when *'people intrude into your space and you don't like it. There are times where you want to be by yourself and you hear a knock at the door, and you think oh my goodness, who can that be? But you have to let them in'*. Group pressure and pressure from a well-meaning environment often dictate conforming, to the detriment of some individuals.

Unmet Needs

With the focus on active ageing, there may not be a space in which emotional needs can be expressed or dealt with. These come to the foreground especially when loss occurs. Losses in the form of the deaths of spouses and friends, health problems, physical constraints, or a shrinking social world are inevitable accompaniments of ageing, as also confirmed by Papalia et al. (2009). In Participant 3's words, *'You know, I feel as if I don't have that help and if I don't reach out to other people, people don't reach out to me'*, as well as the fact that her *'children are overseas'* may be indicative of an unsatisfied need for emotional care. Her visual presentation (Fig. 4.3), in conjunction with her words, also shows a significant gap which needs to be bridged in order to receive the necessary care from others. The consequences of unsatisfied emotional needs may be *'isolation'*, *'loneliness'* and a fear of becoming *'depressed because of what has happened'* (Participant 3).

Consequences of the unattended need for social interaction are isolation and loneliness. Participant 16 described the experience: *'There's nothing worse than loneliness. That's true. We all know that'*. Opportunities for social interaction may at times be compromised by factors outside an older person's control, such having to care for a disabled or ill spouse. The necessity of caring for an unwell partner may contribute to frustration: *'I spend a hell of a lot of time with my wife'* and *'I'm with her the whole day'* (Participant 8), which may interfere with the need for participation in activities and social interaction with friends.

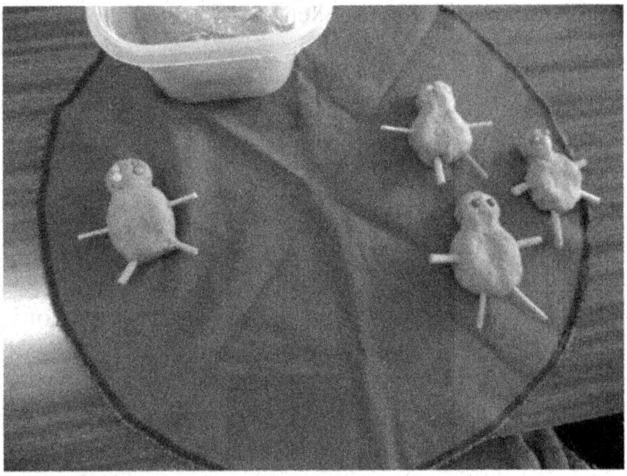

Fig. 4.3 Distance between participant and three other residents

Some Thoughts for Consideration

From our perspective, the greatest contribution of a positive intervention is that it highlights 'what works well'. In this regard, active ageing as a positive intervention has proved that it has many benefits for people: it informed policies to approach ageing differently; it changed organisations' view of older people from a medical perspective to focusing on using potential and creating optimal environments for people to engage in age-friendly environments; it stimulated strategies for assisting older people to function autonomously and independently for as long as possible; and acknowledged the importance of relational interactions in close or general social spaces (ILC 2015; Antonucci et al. 2004, 2013; Keating et al. 2013; Provencher et al. 2014).

There is no doubt that an optimal environment that promotes active ageing enhances the quality of people's lives. However, even though the development of age-friendly communities has gained much attention internationally, the reality in South Africa is that the majority of older people live in age-unfriendly and unsafe environments that limit their autonomy and independence. Even though attempts are made by local governments to address the needs of older people, not much has been achieved (Roos et al. 2014a, b).

When the focus is attuned only to promoting an optimal environment to promote growth goals, it is possible that the broader environment in which individuals' functioning is embedded is not acknowledged. For example, difficult economic circumstances may have an impact on financial resources of older people and consequently on their participation in activities and events.

We know that people age differently and that changes during the life course require the development of new lives. Therefore, a possible suggestion to support the adjustment of people in sharing their lives with others in a bounded community is to make use of group activities to introduce newcomers with an emphasis on their potential contributions to the group.

The unintended consequences of a group norm of participation that guided residents' actions highlighted the danger of exclusion. However, if a different group norm, such as respect for diversity, can be introduced it would recognise that older people as a group are not homogenous and should be treated as individuals with individual preferences.

It is also very likely that the activities in an active ageing environment could become the goal itself. By using existing opportunities for interaction, activities may be introduced so that group members can get to know one another on a deeper level. This could also provide possible avenues for addressing emotional needs and for discovering mutual interests. Positive interventions could benefit from including life coaches to assist older people with basic life skills such as time management, self- and relational-regulation, and dealing with conflict in a constructive manner.

Old age is associated with all kinds of losses and often there are no formal spaces to mourn these. In this study, emotional support was offered as part of informal group interactions and by residents' who 'became like family'. To promote the inclusion of people who have lost their mobility and therefore their autonomy and independence it could be helpful to hold group meetings in an venue that is accessible to them, provided they are given a choice of whether to participate or not. A more formalised service could provide much needed psychological help.

In essence, active ageing as a positive intervention should adopt a holistic approach to promote older people's well-being for as long as possible.

References

Aiken, L. R. (1995). *Aging: An introduction to gerontology*. Thousand Oaks, CA: Sage.

Alderfer, C. P. (1969). An empirical test of a new theory of human needs. *Organizational Behavior and Human Performance, 4*, 142–175.

Antonucci, T. C., Akiyama, H., & Takahashi, K. (2004). Attachment and close relationships across the life span. *Attachment and Human Development, 6*(4), 364–366.

Antonucci, T. C., Ajrouch, K. J., & Birditt, K. S. (2013). The convoy model: Explaining social relations from a multidisciplinary perspective. *The Gerontologist, 118*(1). doi:10.1093/geront/gnt118.

Apt, N. A. (2012). Aging in Africa: Past experiences and strategic directions. *Ageing International, 37*(1), 93–103. doi:10.1007/s12126-011-9138-8.1.

Baltes, P. B., & Baltes, M. M. (1990). *Successful ageing: Perspectives from the behavioral sciences*. New York, NY: Cambridge University Press.

Barker, R. (1968). *Ecological psychology: Concepts and methods for studying the environment of human behaviour*. Stanford, CA: Stanford University Press.

Baumgardner, S. R., & Crothers, M. K. (2010). *Positive psychology*. New Jersey, NJ: Pearson Education. doi:10.1111/j.1752-0606.1978.tb00537.x.

Bekhet, A. K., Zauszniewski, J. A., & Nakhla, W. E. (2009). Reasons for relocation to retirement communities. *Western Journal of Nursing Research, 31*(4), 462–479.

Buswell, J. (2011). Rising to the challenge and meeting the needs—Older people in critical care. *Nursing in Critical Care, 16*(6), 279–280. doi:10.1111/j.1478-5153.2011.00472.x.

Clarke, V., & Braun, V. (2013). Teaching thematic analysis: Overcoming challenges and developing strategies for effective learning. *The Psychologist, 26*(2), 120–123.

Compton, W. C. (2005). *An introduction to positive psychology*. Virginia, VA: Thomson/Wadsworth.

Cosco, T. D., Stephan, B. C. M., & Brayne, C. (2013). Letter to the editor: On the success of the successful ageing paradigm. *Journal of Applied Gerontology, 32*(3), 275–276. doi:10.1177/0733464813481562.

Covinsky, K. E., Palmer, R. M., Fortinsky, R. H., Counsell, S. R., Stewart, A. L., Kresevic, D., Burant, C. J., & Landefeld, C. S. (2003). Loss of independence in activities of daily living in older adults hospitalized with medical illnesses: Increased vulnerability with age. *Journal of the American Geriatric Society, 51*(4), 451–457.

Dahlgaard, J. J., & Dahlgaard, S. M. P. (2003). Towards a holistic understanding of human motivation: Core values—The entrance to people's commitment? *International Journal of Artificial Intelligence and Society, 17*(2), 150–180. doi:10.1007/s00146-003-0257-y.

Deci, E. L., & Ryan, R. M. (2000). The 'what' and 'why' of goal pursuits: Human needs and the self-determination of behaviour. *Psychological Inquiry, 11*(4), 227–268.

Department of Social Development. (2010). *Audit of residential facilities*. Pretoria South Africa: Government Printers.

Donaldson, R., & Goldhaber, R. (2012). Alternative reflections on the elderly's sense of place in a South African gated retirement village. *South African Review of Sociology, 34*(3), 64–80.

Fernández-Ballesteros, R., Robine, J., Walker, A., & Kalache, A. (2013). Active aging: A global goal. *Current Gerontology and Geriatrics Research, 2013*, 1–4.

International Longevity Centre Brazil. (2015). *Active aging: A policy framework in response to the longevity revolution*. Rio de Janeiro: Brazil. Retrieved from http://ilcbrazil.org/blog/2015/07/20/active-ageing-a-policy-framework-in-response-to-the-longevity-revolution/

Keating, N., Eales, J., & Phillips, J. E. (2013). Age-friendly rural communities: Conceptualizing 'best-fit'. *Canadian Journal on Aging, 32*, 319–332. doi:10.1017/S0714980813000408.

Krout, J. A. (2014). Providing services to rural older adults. In K. M. Hash, E. T. Jurkowski, & J. A. Krout (Eds.), *Aging in rural places: Policies, programs, and professional practice* (pp. 119–136). New York, NY: Springer.

Lombard, A., & Kruger, E. (2009). Older persons: The case of South Africa. *Ageing International, 34*(3), 119–135.

Maslow, A. H. (1943). A theory of human motivation. *Psychological Review, 50*(4), 370–396. doi:10.1037/h005346.

Mayosi, B. M., Flisher, A. J., Lalloo, U. G., Sitas, F., Bradshaw, D., & Tollman, S. M. (2009). The burden of non-communicable diseases in South Africa. *Lancet, 374*, 9347–9349.

Nelson, G., & Prilleltensky, I. (2005). *Community psychology: In pursuit of liberation and well-being*. London, England: Palgrave Macmillan.

Nolan, J., & Scott, J. (2009). Experiences of age and gender: Narratives of progress and decline. *International Journal of Aging and Human Development, 69*(2), 133–157.

Paoletti, I. (2015). Active aging and inclusive communities: Inter-institutional intervention in Portugal. *Ageing International, 40*(2), 165–186. doi:10.1007/s12126-014-9216-9.

Papalia, E. D., Olds, S. W., & Feldman, R. D. (2009). *Human development* (11th ed.). New York, NY: McGraw-Hill.

Persoon, A., Theunisse, L., Perry, M., & van Kempen, J. (2010). EASYcare: A standardized assessment for individual needs in health and social care. In *Proceedings from Fourth European Nursing Congress Symposium,* Rotterdam, The Netherlands.

Policastro, C., Gainey, R., & Payne, B. K. (2015). Conceptualizing crimes against older persons: Elder abuse, domestic violence, white-collar offending, or just regular 'old' crime. *Journal of Crime and Justice, 38*(1), 27–41.

Population Reference Bureau. (2014). *2014 World population data sheet*. Retrieved from http://www.prb.org/publications/datasheets/2014/2014-world-population-data-sheet.aspx

Powell, J. L., & Taylor, P. (2015). The Global South: The case of populational aging in Africa and Asia. *World Scientific News, 12*, 89–99.

Provencher, C., Keating, N., Warburton, J., & Roos, V. (2014). Ageing and community. Introduction to the special issue. *Journal of Community and Applied Social Psychology, 24*(1), 1–11. doi. 10.1002/casp.2171.

Roberts, B. (2010). Fear factor: Perceptions of safety in South Africa. In B. Roberts, M. Kivilu, & Y. D. Davids (Eds.), *South African social attitudes: 2nd report: Reflections on the age of hope (South African social attitudes survey (SASAS))* (pp. 250–275). Cape Town South Africa: HSRC Press.

Roos, V. (2008). The Mmogo-method™: Discovering symbolic community interactions. *Journal of Psychology in Africa, 18*(4), 659–668.

Roos, V. (2012). The Mmogo-Method®: An exploration of experiences through visual projections. *Qualitative Research in Psychology, 9*(3), 249–261. doi.org/10.1080/14780887.2010.500356.

Roos, V. (2016a). Conducting the Mmogo-method®. In V. Roos (Ed.), *Understanding relational and group experiences through the Mmogo-method®*. Cham, Switzerland: Springer.

Roos, V. (2016b). Theorizing from the Mmogo-method®: Self-interactional group theory (SIGT) to explain relational interactions. In V. Roos (Ed.), *Understanding relational and group experiences through the Mmogo-method®*. Cham, Switzerland: Springer.

Roos, V., & Baart, A. (2016). Theories and heuristic constructs informing the Mmogo-method®. In V. Roos (Ed.), *Understanding relational and group experiences through the Mmogo-method®*. Cham, Switzerland: Springer.

Roos, V., & Du Toit, F. (2014). Perceptions of effective relationships in an institutional care setting for older people. *South African Journal for Industrial Psychology, 40*(1), 1–9. doi.org/10.4102/sajip.v40i1.1139.

Roos, V., & Malan, L. (2012). The role of context and the interpersonal experiences of loneliness of older people in a residential care facility. *Global Health Action, 5, 18861*. doi:10.3402/gha/v10.1886.

Roos, V., & Redelinghuys, A. (2016). Analyzing visual data with text from the Mmogo-method®: Experience of meaning during the third trimester of pregnancy. In V. Roos (Ed.), *Understanding relational and group experiences through the Mmogo-method®*. Cham, Switzerland: Springer.

Roos, V., Hoffman, J. R., Ferreira, M., & Stols, A. (2014a). *Local government in South Africa and the provision of series to older persons*. Unpublished manuscript.

Roos, V., Kolobe, P. S., & Keating, N. (2014b). (Re)creating community: Experiences of older women forcibly relocated during Apartheid. *Journal of Community and Applied Social Psychology, 24*(1), 12–25. doi:10.1002/casp.2177.

Schunk, D. H., & Zimmerman, B. J. (1997). Social origins of self-regulatory competence. *Educational Psychologist, 32*, 195–208.

South Africa. (2006). *Older Persons Act, No. 13*. Retrieved from http://www.justice.gov.za/legislation/acts/2006-013_olderpersons.pdf

Stenner, P., McFarquhar, T., & Bowling, A. (2011). Older people and 'active ageing': Subjective aspects of ageing actively. *Journal of Health Psychology, 16*(3), 467–477. doi:10.1177/1359105310384298.

Steyn, S. E. (2015). *Exploring relational regulation in older persons' mobile phone use*. Unpublished master's thesis, North-West University, Potchefstroom, South Africa.

Thomése, F., Van Tilburg, T., Van Groenou, M. B., & Knipscheer, K. (2005). Network dynamics in later life. In M. L. Johnson (Ed.), *The Cambridge handbook of age and ageing* (pp. 463–467). New York, NY: Cambridge University Press.

Van Biljon, L., & Roos, V. (2015). The nature of quality of life in residential care facilities: The case of White older South Africans. *Journal of Psychology in Africa, 25*(3), 201–207. doi:10.1080/14330237.2015.1065054.

Van Biljon, L., & Roos, V. (2016). Using the Mmogo-method® to obtain quality of life contributors and inhibitors in the lives of older people in residential care facilities in South Africa. In R. Ferreira (Ed.), *Thinking innovatively about psychological assessment in a contexts of diversity*. Cape Town, South Africa: Juta.

Van Dyk, S., Lessenich, S., Denninger, T., & Richter, A. (2013). The many meanings of 'active ageing'. Confronting public discourse with older people's stories. *Recherches Sociologiques et Anthropologiques, 44*(1), 97–115.

Velkoff, V. A., & Kowal, P. R. (2007). *Population aging in Sub-Saharan Africa: Demographic dimensions 2006* (P95/07-1). Washington, DC: Government Printing Office. Retrieved from US Census Bureau, Current Population Reports. https://www.census.gov/prod/2007pubs/p95-07-1.pdf

Vorster, C. (2011). *Impact: The story of interactional therapy*. Pretoria, South Africa: Satori.

Vorster, C., Roos, V., & Beukes, M. (2013). A psycho-diagnostic tool for psychotherapy: Interactional pattern analysis (IPA). *Journal of Psychology in Africa, 23*(3), 163–169. doi:10.1080/14330237.2013.10820663#.VGC.

Walker, A. (2002). A strategy for active ageing. *International Social Security Association, 55*(1), 121–139. doi:10.1111/1468-246X.00118.

World Health Organization. (2015). *World report on ageing and health*. Retrieved from http://reliefweb.int/report/world/world-report-ageing-and-health

Chapter 5
Fostering Humour

Willibald Ruch and Jennifer Hofmann

Abstract Research on humour and humour trainings/interventions has preceded the formal foundation of positive psychology. Yet, humour in its benevolent forms [as also operationalised as one of the 24 character strengths in Peterson and Seligman's (2004) classification fits well into the realm of positive psychology and its interventions. The chapter describes current humour interventions stemming from both traditions, humour research and positive psychology. Most interventions have been designed for groups and differ in whether they are delivered in a standardised way (i.e., manuals) or more ad hoc (i.e., clinic clown interventions). Moreover, recent advances have shown the benefits of short-term online self-administered interventions. Yet, future efforts need to concentrate on the concept of humour and its measurement, as well as the development of theoretically based interventions and their evaluation of short- and long-term benefits.

Abbreviations

7HHP	7 Humor Habits Program
BENCOR	Benevolent and Corrective Humor
CLEM-29	29 Clown Emotion List
FACS	Facial Action Coding System
HBQD	Humorous Behavior Q-Sort-Deck
HSQ	Humor Styles Questionnaire
SHS	Sense of Humor Scale
STCI	State-Trait-Cheerfulness Inventory
VIA-IS	Values in Action—Inventory of Strengths

W. Ruch (✉) • J. Hofmann
Abteilung für Persönlichkeitspsychologie und Diagnostik, Psychologisches Institut, Binzmühlestrasse 14/7, 8050 Zürich, Switzerland
e-mail: w.ruch@psychologie.uzh.ch; j.hofmann@psychologie.uzh.ch

C. Proctor (ed.), *Positive Psychology Interventions in Practice*,
DOI 10.1007/978-3-319-51787-2_5

Introduction

Research on humour and positive interventions utilising humour preceded the formal foundation of positive psychology. Ruch (2010) and Ruch et al. (2010a) showed how humour fits into positive psychology: (a) the study of humour contributes to the study of positive experience, that is, amusement, hilarity, and cheerfulness (see Ruch and Hofmann 2012). Furthermore, (b) humour is a positive trait and various components of the sense of humour are seen to help individuals in a variety of ways. For example, humour assists the adaptive coping with stress, smoothens social interactions, increases creativity, and enhances life satisfaction and well-being (e.g., Kuiper and Martin 1998; Martin 2001; Martin and Lefcourt 1983; Marziali et al. 2008; Park et al. 2004; Proyer et al. 2011; Ruch et al. 1996, 2004; Ruch et al. 2010b, c). Also, higher levels of humour correspond to lower levels of depression, anxiety, and negative emotion (Deaner and McConatha 1993; Kuiper and Martin 1998; Lefcourt and Martin 1986; Moran and Massam 1999; Nezu et al. 1988; Yovetich et al. 1990). Thus, humour does not only induce positive emotions and builds personal resources, it also reduces negative emotions, and both pathways contribute to well-being. Moreover, (c) humour is a key component that may make an institution a positive institution. Indeed, the presence of humour is one factor that fosters positive experience and growth in institutions (family, schools, workplace, nations). Furthermore, studies show (d) that humour may support different virtues, but is most frequently associated with humanity and wisdom (Ruch and Proyer 2015). Finally, (e) Ruch (2010) argued that humour trainings also contribute to the field of positive interventions aimed at increasing happiness and lowering depression.

What Is Humour?

Humour (from the Latin '*umor*', i.e., liquid) originally referred to the four body fluids whose mixture (*temperare* = to mix) determines the four temperaments (choleric, sanguine, phlegmatic, melancholic). Later it acquired different meanings, and was used to refer to different qualities including mood, talents, temperament, virtue, worldview, defence mechanism. Humour is nowadays often used as an umbrella term for all forms of the comic/funny but also, and more rightfully so, in opposition to other terms, such as wit, nonsense, fun, irony, satire, sarcasm, or cynicism. In this context, humour only has positive connotations. When conceptualising humour as a character strength, Peterson and Seligman (2004) excluded the negative forms and humour in the VIA classification seems to be mostly related to humanity and wisdom (e.g., Ruch and Proyer 2015). Overall humour and virtues only have a small overlap and there are forms of humour that are morally neutral or even related to vice. Labels of assessment instruments are very diverse and include 'sense of humour', 'styles of humour/comic styles', 'humour appreciation', and 'humour creation/wit', but also more specific instruments assed the liking of various forms of jokes and cartoons and or producing or reproducing humour. Clearly, no shared conceptualisation of a sense of humour exists in the research community and this foremost goal should be achieved first.

Measurement Issues

Assessment is essential to the evaluation of humour interventions. Nevertheless, the assessment of 'humour' or sense of humour possesses some challenges: due to the yet not fully explored multifaceted nature of humour, no comprehensive instrument exists. As a minimal criterion, studies should at least assess the components of humour targeted by the intervention, although it is also instructive to determine if other facets do not change due to the intervention or training. Next, we briefly discuss some important assessment tools that either stem from positive psychology or have often been used in prior intervention studies (see Ruch 2007, 2008 for a more thorough review of measures).

The *Values in Action—Inventory of Strengths* (VIA-IS; Peterson and Seligman 2004) assesses humour as a character strength with 10 items on a 5-point Likert-style scale (from 1 = 'very much like me' to 5 = 'very much unlike me'). A high scorer is someone '…who is skilled at laughing and teasing, at bringing smiles to the faces of others, at seeing the light side, and at making (not necessarily telling) jokes' (Peterson and Seligman 2004, p. 530). This scale is particularly useful when training the benevolent forms of humour (on both the intra- and inter-individual level).

The *Benevolent and Corrective Humor* (BENCOR; Ruch 2012) is another newcomer guided by positive psychology. However, two forms of humour aiming at the 'good' are distinguished and tested by six items each that are answered in a 7-point Likert-style scale ranging from 1 = 'strongly disagree' to 7 = 'strongly agree'. Benevolent humour describes a humorous outlook on life that entails the realistic observations and understanding of human weaknesses (and the imperfection of the world), but also their benevolent humorous treatment. By contrast, corrective humour involves moral-based ridicule; that is, the use of mockery to fight badness and mediocrity (Ruch and Heintz 2016).

The *Sense of Humor Scale* (SHS; McGhee 1996) was designed to assess the different facets of sense of humour that can be trained through McGhee's *7 Humor Habits Program*. The SHS is also suitable to determine one's progress following the completion of a humour training. It consists of 40 items in a 7-point Likert-style scale (1 = 'strongly disagree' to 7 = 'strongly agree'), with eight items each measuring 'playful/serious attitude' and 'positive/negative mood' and 24 items measuring *sense of humour* (i.e., enjoyment of humour, laughter, verbal humour, finding humour in everyday life, laughing at yourself, and humour under stress). Similar to the VIA-IS humour scale, it is unipolar and unidimensional, and the two are highly positively correlated (e.g., Müller and Ruch 2011).

Several measures tap into multidimensional conceptualisations of humour, but at least two specifically assess styles of humour. The *Humorous Behavior Q-Sort-Deck* (HBQD; Craik et al. 1996) and the *Humor Styles Questionnaire* (HSQ; Martin et al. 2003), with the latter being often used in research and practice. The HSQ is designed to distinguish between adaptive (i.e., affiliative, self-enhancing) and maladaptive (aggressive, self-defeating) styles of humour. The HSQ is a self-report questionnaire composed of 32 items with a 7-point Likert-style scale (1 = 'totally disagree' to 7 = 'totally agree') measuring those four dimensions.

The *State-Trait-Cheerfulness Inventory* (STCI; see Ruch et al. 1996 or Ruch and Hofmann 2012 for an overview) assesses the temperamental basis of the sense of humour: *cheerfulness*, *seriousness*, and *bad mood.* The temperamental foundations of humour are assumed to be universal, even if the expression of humour varies across culture and time. Respondents answer questions on a 4-point Likert-style scale (1 = 'strongly disagree' to 4 = 'strongly agree'). The STCI has both trait (60 item) and state (30 item) versions. The state form is suited to evaluate the effects of humour trainings both before and after a single training session or a longer intervention period (see Ruch and Hofmann 2012 for an overview).

These measures assess self-reported changes in mood or humour as a trait. Furthermore, interventions that aim at increasing *humour ability* (i.e., humour production) or *appreciation* (i.e., the liking of certain kinds of humorous stimuli) may want to use: (a) humour production 'tests', where the quality of the produced humour is rated by experts or judges; or (b) humour appreciation measures, where typically different kinds of humorous stimuli are rated for the degree of funniness and aversiveness (see Ruch 2008 for an overview). Such tests can provide behavioural measures for whether the humour training enhanced wittiness and enjoyment of humour.

Types of Humour Interventions

Humour interventions have emerged from the tradition of humour research (i.e., founded on humour theory or practice), as well as from a positive psychology tradition (i.e., adopting established interventions to humour). The interventions and trainings generally differ on three dimensions: (1) they may be designed for *individuals* (and individual use) or focusing on *groups*, (2) they may be administered *offline* (i.e., face-to-face or through manuals) or *online* (i.e., through websites or software), and (3) they may be *standardised* (i.e., following guidelines or a strict plan) or *ad hoc* (i.e., tools and strategies are defined but the procedure of the session is open; e.g., clinic clowns working in groups and responding to the situation without an a priori schedule). In the following, we describe the most prominent humour training and intervention programmes that emerged in the recent past (see Ruch 2008; Ruch et al. 2011; Ruch and McGhee 2014 for an overview on early humour intervention studies).

Self-Administered Individual Humour Interventions from a Positive Psychology Tradition

Starting with Seligman et al. (2005) the effectiveness of online presented positive interventions were tested using a double blind, placebo controlled design. Interventions lasted for 1 week and happiness and depression served as dependent variables. Interventions like using one's signature strengths in a new way proved to be effective and so was 'three good things'; that is, writing down three good things that happened during the day, remembering the situations, and the feelings associated with them. For some individuals humour is a signature strength (i.e., a very central strength), but no such analysis (using humour among those with humour as one of the top five strengths) has been conducted so far. Humour was not involved in the Seligman et al. (2005) study, but effective interventions were varied to incorporate humour. Gander et al. (2013) introduced an online, self-administered variant of the three good things intervention by instructing participants to think of 'three *funny* things' each day (for 1 week). When comparing the levels from pre to postintervention, a decrease in depressive symptoms, but no effect on self-rated happiness, was found. However, increases in self-reported happiness were found for the follow up measures after 1 and 3 months.

Wellenzohn et al. (2016a, b, c) conducted several placebo-controlled individual online humour interventions basing on the three funny things intervention. They replicated the findings of Gander et al. (2013), but also extended the repertoire of humour-based online interventions by creating five variants of humour interventions (all of them lasting for 1 week). The five variants built on existing interventions (such as counting kindness or the gratitude visit) and consisted of: (1) collecting funny events and sharing them with the people involved, (2) counting funny things, (3) applying humour (like using ones signature strength), (4) solving stressful situations in a humorous way, and (5) the three funny things exercise. All interventions enhanced happiness, three of them for up to 6 months (i.e., three funny things, applying humour, and counting funny things), whereas only short-term effects on depression were found.

In a next set of studies, Wellenzohn et al. (2016a, b) investigated potential working mechanisms and moderators of the online humour-based interventions. In a first study, they manipulated the time focus in the instruction of the three funny things intervention, focusing on the past, present, or future in order to investigate two potential working mechanisms (the attentional shift to the positive and savouring positive emotions). In line with the hypotheses, the 'present' variant was associated with both mechanisms (attentional shift and savouring positive emotions), while the 'past' variant only related to savouring and the future only related to the mechanism of attentional shift. Yet, all three variants enhanced self-reported happiness and lowered depressive symptoms from pre to postintervention (compared to the control group).

In a second study, they tested the three funny things intervention and tested for moderation effects of basic personality traits (i.e., psychoticism, extraversion, and neuroticism) and the sense of humour (as conceptualised by McGhee 1996). The results showed that only extraversion moderated the effects on self-reported happiness and depressive symptoms, but not sense of humour. However, if the participants experienced an increase in their sense of humour from pretest to the 1-month follow-up, this change did predict changes in happiness and depressive symptoms. Thus, increases in self-reported sense of humour were associated with the interventions' effectiveness at the follow-up measure.

Self- or Group-Administered Interventions from a Humour Research Tradition

For Individuals or Groups: McGhee's 7 Humor Habits Program

McGhee (1996, 2010a) developed a humour intervention programme that emphasises strengthening key humour habits and skills in a hierarchical order (establish a playful attitude, laugh more often and heartily, create verbal humour, look for humour in everyday life, laugh at yourself, find humour in the midst of stress). The *7 Humor Habits Program* (7HHP) is a standardised training, which can be completed individually through a manual, or guided by an instructor in a group. Both forms are accompanied by individual 'home play' exercises (behavioural component) and 'humor log exercises' (cognitive/reflective component), which help consolidating the new knowledge and assist the transfer into every day life. The key goals of the programme are to: (1) demonstrate the malleability of humour, (2) boost humour, (3) increase the frequency of positive emotions, (4) decrease the frequency of negative emotions, and (5) to increase emotional resilience and the ability to cope with stress. The programme aims to first build or strengthen the core habits and skills on 'good days' and then gradually apply the same habits in the midst of stress (when angry, anxious, depressed, etc.). Because sense of humour is often lost in the midst of stress, a minimum of 1 week of repetition of the habits on good days is considered crucial to the ability to later sustain the habits on bad (stressful) days.

Several studies have evaluated the 7HHP Program. The exact procedures vary across studies (number of trainers, setting in which the training took place, contents of the meeting, time points of follow-up measures, and number of follow ups), but all approaches trained the 7 Humor Habits in group settings (i.e., adults in a rehabilitation clinic Sassenrath 2001), healthy adults (Crawford and Caltabiano 2011; Rusch and Stolz 2009), clinically depressed adults (Falkenberg et al. 2011). The results show that the 7HHP increases positive emotions and subjective well-being. In detail, it increases playfulness (Andress et al. 2010; Crawford 2009; Sassenrath 2001), positive mood or positive affect (Andress et al. 2010; Crawford 2009; Sassenrath 2001), trait cheerfulness (over 2 months, Rusch and Stolz 2009; also for clinically depressed, Falkenberg et al. 2011), life satisfaction (Rusch and Stolz 2009), optimism, perceived sense of self-efficacy, and sense of control over one's internal states (over 3 months, Crawford and Caltabiano 2011). Moreover, it decreases seriousness and negative mood (Sassenrath 2001), depression (in healthy adults, Beh-Pajooh et al. 2010; Crawford and Caltabiano 2011; but not in clinically depressed individuals, Falkenberg et al. 2011), anxiety, and perceived stress (Crawford and Caltabiano 2011). Due to the encouraging findings from the clinical context, an adaptation of the manual for the use in therapy was developed (Falkenberg et al. 2012).

For Individuals or Groups: Training Cheerfulness as a State and Trait

Papousek and Schulter (2008) discussed that enhancing cheerfulness as a state and trait (as conceptualised in the state-trait model of cheerfulness; see Ruch et al. 1996 and Ruch and Hofmann 2012) may improve coping with future adversities, which in turn may promote psychological well-being. They developed a cheerfulness training that follows a behavioural therapy approach. The core of the training programme is to learn and practice techniques to efficiently self-induce cheerful moods (by imagination and voluntary production of nonverbal expressions of cheerfulness). By repeating the newly learned behaviours, imaginations of subjective weaknesses and unpleasant situations are coupled with the positive moods through conditioning mechanisms. A fundamental postulate of the training is that participants actively practice to self-induce cheerful moods, instead of just passively appreciating an instructor's jokes or humorous material. It is expected that imaginations of adversities and later real situations, automatically trigger a cheerful mood after having undergone the training. Results indicated enhanced cheerfulness levels increased due to the training programme. Mood changes were not only present during or shortly after the training sessions, but also 2 days after the training period, without further emotional stimulation. There was also a more general improvement in psychological well-being (more good-humoured, calm, fresh, and less anxious mood) as well as a reduction of feelings of stress and tenseness.

For Groups: Training the Sense of Humour in Clinical Groups

Hirsch et al. (2010) investigated the effect of a 'humour group' in elderly individuals with a depression. Each humour group consisted out of 7–12 participants who met twice a week for 4 weeks. Each session targeted a different humour related topic, coupled with exercises and games, as well as home assignments that should improve the transfer of the humour skills into daily life. The intervention increased the resilience and life satisfaction of the participants from pre to post. Especially patients with severe symptoms of depression profited from the intervention, as they further experienced an increase in state cheerfulness and a decrease in state seriousness (see Konradt et al. 2013 for a replication).

Clinic Clown Interventions

Within health care institutions, clinic clowns are the most commonly found 'humour practitioners' pursuing humour interventions repeatedly to varying groups of patients. These clown groups or clown visits follow certain rules, hospital regulations, and rituals and are usually conducted by trained clinic clowns. The clinic clowns may work alone or in pairs and follow their clown 'routine' or come with a set of skills and tricks (i.e., magic, puppetry, slapstick) that they use to amuse individuals or groups. Although the repertoire is somewhat fixed, the interventions are not fully standardised, as the clowns respond to the situation and the people (patients, relatives, hospital staff). Whereas most early empirical research based on qualitative data and reports, the recent years have brought about an increase in quantitative empirical research assessing the positive effects such clinic clown interventions have.

Research on clowning in health care settings focused mainly on the impact of clinic clowns on the patients, looking at the reduction of negative outcome variables in clown intervention groups compared to control groups (see Auerbach et al. 2014 for an overview; Vagnoli et al. 2010). Some studies show increases in trait and state ratings of cheerfulness (Hirsch et al. 2010) and short-term increases in self- and parent-reported psychological well-being (Pinquart et al. 2011). Moreover, clown interventions were found to be effective in reducing disruptive behaviour (Higueras et al. 2006) and symptoms of depression in geriatric patients (Hirsch et al. 2010), as well as self-reported pain (e.g., Bertini et al. 2011).

Other studies looked at the influence of clinic clowns on physiological changes: these studies showed positive effects reducing hyperinflation in severe obstructive lung disease patients (Brutsche et al. 2008) and one yet unreplicated study even reported increased pregnancy rates in women who were entertained by a clown after in vitro fertilisation compared to women with no entertainment by a clown (Friedler et al. 2011). Furthermore, a few studies focused on the interaction between clowns, patients, families, and staff. These studies found positive attitudes towards and acceptance of the clowns on the part of patients and staff (see Auerbach 2016 for an overview).

Auerbach et al. (2014) studied the differential effect on emotional states induced by clinic clown interventions compared to interventions of empathic nurses and clinic clowns. They developed a broad research instrument the *29 Clown Emotion List* (CLEM-29) allowing for the assessment of emotional states induced by clinic clown interventions (amusement, transcendence, arousal, unease). They could show that clinic clowns elicited mostly amusement and feelings of transcendence (e.g., feeling appreciated by the clown, elevation and awe when observing the clown). While the circus clown also elicited amusement (or hilarity), this type of clown failed to elicit the 'moral goodness'. Furthermore, while the clinic clown and the nurses elicited feelings of transcendence, the nurses did not elicit amusement. Thus, the clinic clowns unite the elicitation of feelings of amusement and hilarity, as well as transcendence. Moreover, the CLEM-29 predicted global positive and negative outcomes after the interventions better than traditional instruments for the assessment of mood and emotional states. Auerbach et al. (2016) partially replicated their findings in an experimental setting studying clinic clown and nurse interventions in a physical rehabilitation centre for adults. They found that clinic clown interventions elicited amusement and arousal from pre to postintervention, but no change in unease was found. Interestingly, the effects did not change for individuals observing the interventions or individuals being directly involved in the intervention, thus showing that the positive effect of clinic clowns is present for patients as well as bystanders.

Although the CLEM-29 proved to be useful for assessing self-reported emotional states by clinic clowns, it has one major limitation: It relies on the patients and observers to being able to report about their feelings, while notably the two groups of individuals most often encountering clinic clown interventions are not able to fill in questionnaires (albeit for different reasons). For example, young children (which cannot speak yet) and elderly adults with dementia (which cannot speak anymore). Clinic clowns utilise a variety of interaction strategies, which not only involve verbal, but also sensory interventions (e.g., balloons, bubbles, music, touching soft fabrics, human touch, etc.). Those strategies are aimed to elicit positive emotions in patients and seem to be particularly well suited for individuals who have problems with processing verbal information. With respect to patients with dementia, a decrease in cognitive functions can be observed within the course of the illness. Still, the sensory techniques might still elicit positive affect in dementia patients. Furthermore, long-term memory remains stable much longer than the short-term memory and individuals with dementia will still profit from clowning techniques that involve music, riddles, and stories linked to their past.

Hofmann et al. (2017) investigated the effects of a clinic clown group intervention on spontaneous facial emotion expression in two samples of elderly adults with mild to severe Alzheimer's type dementia. Moreover, they assessed peer-rated short- and mid-term changes in the residents' behaviour and mood. By applying the *Facial Action Coding System* (FACS; Ekman et al. 2002), the spontaneous expression of seven basic emotions and different types of smiles and laughs in the participants' face while interacting with the clinic clown alone or in the group was assessed. The results showed that the clown did elicit positive emotions, such as amusement, sensory pleasure, and *schadenfreude*, which went along with the expression of smiles and laughs. Moreover, the care staff completed peer-ratings on the patients' thoughts, feeling, behaviours on mornings, lunchtimes, and evenings on the days of the clown visits, as compared to control days with no clown. The ratings showed that on days with a clown visit, the increase of negative affect over the course of the day was less steep than on control days and the elderly individuals showed several changes in behaviours, such as reporting less pain and increased communication to caretakers.

Recommendations for Future Research and Practice

Research on Concept and Instruments

It seems futile to plan and conduct interventions studies when the components of a sense of humour are not defined and measured in a satisfactory way. It is not yet clear how to best represent the different actions, feelings, and cognitions in relation to humour in a structural model. While we moved away from unidimensional models to multidimensional ones, no model exists that incorporates all the identified components of humour. In personality research hierarchical models have proven successful. Many, narrower correlated concepts are combined at a higher level to form a few general concepts, which, in turn, might even result in a general factor (in this case a *general humour ability*). The bottom of such a model involves humour skills that may be trained. They define a component of, for example, 'making fun' which, together with other components form a stronger 'playful-cheerful' cluster. Such a model is currently being tested. It contains three further components (tentatively called mockery, play with ideas, and mastery) and prototypical components of humour (e.g., laughing at yourself, satire, sarcasm, nonsense, fun) are located in it. New initiatives should also relate to measure the same humour traits by different means (e.g., self-report, peer-report, structured interview, behavioural observation) to see how much substance and how much noise is in each of the measures.

Interventions

Future Technologies

New emerging technologies may be changing the face of individualised online humour interventions and training programmes. In the recent past, virtual agents (and their corresponding avatars) have been developed to not only detect a human users' laughter and expression of amusement, but also to adequately respond to it with laughter. Such interfaces have now been started to being implemented into simple humour induction settings (e.g., Hofmann et al. 2015). First evidence shows that the presence of a laughing virtual model enhances the overt expression of amusement, particularly for individuals with heightened thresholds for the experience of cheerfulness and amusement. Thus, the laughing virtual agents may assist the fostering and induction of amusement online. Laughing and amusement expressing virtual companions might increase the participant's motivation to complete the intervention and lead to more amusement. This is not trivial, as Goeritz (2007) showed that not all established induction methods of positive affect work in online settings, and a laughing virtual companion could help in overcoming such problems. Also, it might be interesting to assist the elicitation and up-regulation of amusement in online interventions for outcomes like enhanced pain thresholds and stress reduction (e.g., Cohn et al. 2009; Giuliani et al. 2008; Papa and Bonanno 2008;

Zweyer et al. 2004). In such interventions, a virtual companion could serve as an accompanying online tutor, social partner, or instructor next to amusement fostering exercises, or being part of the exercise itself.

Different Interventions for Different People?

The results of several studies have shown that trait cheerfulness predicts how much individuals profit from humour interventions (e.g., Hofmann et al. 2015; Papousek and Schulter 2008), thus, one might want to consider that trait cheerful individuals respond differently compared to non-trait cheerful individuals when being confronted with a humour intervention. Interventions may need to be adapted in terms of intensity, duration, and content to allow for a 'person-intervention fit'. For example, it might be indicative to start with less intense stimuli in low-trait cheerful individuals, but prolonging the training, as low-trait cheerful individuals might need longer to get their cheerfulness heightened and may profit from a less intense, gradual approach (see Ruch and Hofmann 2012). Furthermore, the preintervention score in cheerfulness or sense of humour may be indicative of who will have the strongest (or weakest) gains in humour or various well-being assessments as a result of the training.

How Long Is Long Enough?

Research systematically exploring the length and intensity of humour interventions is warranted. Brief interventions lasting for only a few minutes over 7 days, as reported in Gander et al. (2013) or Wellenzohn et al. (2016a, b), may be effective. Their participants reported reduced self-reported depressive symptoms at the end of the 7 days, as well as at a 1- and 3-month follow-up (but not at a 6-month follow-up). Self-reported happiness scores did not increase (relative to pretest scores) at day 7, but did increase at the 1- and 3-month follow-up (but not at the 6-month follow-up). Also group interventions, such as humour groups or clinic clown interventions, usually just last for about an hour in weekly cycles and are repeated for usually 2 months. Thus, although the actual time spent on the interventions is relatively short within the course of a week, these interventions have been shown to be effective in increasing self-reported positive outcomes, such as cheerfulness, resilience, and well-being, and/or decreasing negative outcomes such as stress and depressive symptoms.

Can Morally Good Forms of Humour Be Promoted?

As mentioned before, humour may also contain critical views of others and may be more related to vice than virtue. Indulging in negative forms of humour correlated inversely with both meaningfulness of life and satisfaction with life (see Ruch 2012) and hence a training module is needed that helps participants to identify virtue (and vice) in humour and then enables them to generate humour that is in the service of these virtues, for example, expressing humanity or justice, rather than exposing shortcomings and follies skilled but mercilessly. Needless to say that only after completing a full structural model of humour we will know what components (neutral, or relating to vice or virtue) can be trained.

Conclusion

Humour is not centre place in positive psychology and did not get a lot of attention. Nevertheless, the research conducted so far confirms that humour can be trained and that doing so in turn leads to desirable outcomes (e.g., increased positive affect and decreased negative affect, life satisfaction). Changes induced by training prevail at least for a few months. Long-term changes are not documented so far. Intervention studies should also go beyond examining effects on well-being and examine increases in variables that are associated with the use of humour (e.g., smoother interactions, popularity as a friend, partnership quality). While correlations exist such variables have yet to be examined in humour intervention studies. Future research on humour trainings should also test their boundaries. Are humour trainings useful for everyone, or moderated by certain factors? For example, is the same programme fitting independent of the level of humour? Maybe special modules will have to be developed for use with 'humour starters' and 'advanced humour users'. In any case, humour should be in the toolbox of applied positive psychologists.

Acknowledgements The preparation of this chapter was facilitated by the support of the Swiss National Centre of Competence in Research LIVES—*Overcoming Vulnerability: Life Course Perspectives*, which is financed by the Swiss National Science Foundation.

References

Andress, W. C., Hoshino, M., & Rorke, S. C. (2010, July). *Empirical evidence for therapeutic laughter courses on a university campus*. Paper presented at the 35th Annual National Wellness Conference, Stevens Point, WI, USA.

Auerbach, S. (2016). *Send in the clowns? Emotional reactions to hospital clown interventions*. Unpublished dissertation, University of Zurich, Switzerland.

Auerbach, S., Hofmann, J., Platt, T., & Ruch, W. (2014). An investigation of the emotions elicited by hospital clowns in comparison to circus clowns and nursing staff. *European Journal of Humor Research, 3*(1), 26–45.

Auerbach, S., Ruch, W., & Fehling, A. (2016). Positive emotions elicited by clowns and nurses: An experimental study in a hospital setting. *Translational Issues in Psychological Science, Special Issue on "The Psychology of Humor", 2*(1), 14–24.

Beh-Pajooh, A., Jahangiri, M., & Zahrakar, K. (2010). Humor skills training and reducing depression in patients with spinal chord injury. *Journal of Iranian Psychologists, 6*(1), 227–236.

Bertini, M., Isola, E., Paolone, G., & Curcio, G. (2011). Clowns benefit children hospitalized for respiratory pathologies. *Evidence-Based Complementary and Alternative Medicine, 2011*, 1–9.

Brutsche, M. H., Gossmann, P., Mueller, R. E., Wiegand, J., Pello, Baty, F., & Ruch, W. (2008). Impact of laughter on air trapping in severe chronic obstructive lung disease. *International Journal of COPD, 3*, 185–192.

Cohn, M. A., Fredrickson, B. L., Brown, S. L., Mikels, J. A., & Conway, A. M. (2009). Happiness unpacked: Positive emotions increase life satisfaction by building resilience. *Emotion, 9*, 361–368. doi:10.1037/a0015952.

Craik, K. H., Lampert, M. D., & Nelson, A. J. (1996). Sense of humor and styles of everyday humorous conduct. *Humor: International Journal of Humor Research, 9*, 273–302. doi:10.1515/humr.1996.9.3-4.273.

Crawford, S. (2009). *Humor skills enhancement: A positive approach to emotional well-being*. Unpublished doctoral dissertation, James Cook University, North Queensland, Australia.

Crawford, S., & Caltabiano, N. J. (2011). Promoting emotional well-being through the use of humour. *The Journal of Positive Psychology, 6*, 237–252. doi:10.1080/17439760.2011.577087

Deaner, S. L., & McConatha, J. T. (1993). The relation of humor to depression and personality. *Psychological Reports, 72*, 755–763. doi:10.2466/pr0.1993.72.3.755.

Ekman, P., Friesen, W. V., & Hager, J. C. (2002). *Facial action coding system: A technique for the measurement of facial movement*. Paolo Alto, USA: Consulting Psychologists Press.

Falkenberg, I., Buchkremer, G., Bartels, M., & Wild, B. (2011). Implementation of a manual-based training of humor abilities in patients with depression: A pilot study. *Psychiatry Research, 186*, 454–457. doi:10.1016/j.psychres.2010.10.009.

Falkenberg, I., McGhee, P. E., & Wild, B. (2012). *Humorfähigkeiten trainieren: Ein Manual für die psychiatrisch-psychotherapeutische Praxis* [Humor skill training: A manual for psychiatric and psychotherapeutic practice]. Stuttgart, Germany: Schattauer.

Friedler, S., Glasser, S., Azani, L., Freedman, L. S., Raziel, A., Strassburger, D., Ron-El, R., & Lerner-Geva, L. (2011). The effect of medical clowning on pregnancy rates after in vitro fertilization and embryo transfer. *Fertility and Sterility, 95*, 2127–2130. doi:10.1016/j.fertnstert.2010.12.016.

Gander, F., Proyer, R. T., Ruch, W., & Wyss, T. (2013). Strength-based positive interventions: Further evidence on their potential for enhancing well-being and alleviating depression. *Journal of Happiness Studies, 14*(4), 1241–1259.

Giuliani, N. R., McRae, K., & Gross, J. J. (2008). The up-and down-regulation of amusement: Experiential, behavioral, and autonomic consequences. *Emotion, 8*(5), 714–719. doi:10.1037/a0013236.

Goeritz, A. (2007). Mood induction in the www. *Motivation and Emotion, 31*, 35–47. doi:10.1007/s11031-006-9047-4.

Higueras, A., Carretero-Dios, H., Muñoz, J. P., Idini, E., Ortiz, A., Rincon, F., et al. (2006). Effects of a humor-centered activity on disruptive behavior in psychiatric patients in a general hospital psychiatric ward. *International Journal of Clinical and Health Psychology, 6*, 53–64.

Hirsch, R. D., Junglas, K., Konradt, B., & Jonitz, M. F. (2010). Humortherapie bei alten Menschen mit einer Depression. Ergebnisse einer empirischen Untersuchung [Humor therapy in the depressed elderly. Results of an empirical study]. *Zeitschrift für Gerontologie und Geriatrie, 43*(1), 42–52.

Hofmann, J., Platt, T., Ruch, W., Niewiadomski, R., & Urbain, J. (2015). The influence of a virtual companion on amusement when watching funny films. *Motivation and Emotion, 39*, 434–447. doi:10.1007/s11031-014-9461-y.

Hofmann, J., Ruch, W., & Platt, T. (2017). *Clinic clown intervention for elderly with dementia*. Manuscript in preparation. University of Zurich, Switzerland.

Konradt, B., Hirsch, R. D., Jonitz, M. F., & Junglas, K. (2013). Evaluation of a standardized humor group in a clinical setting: A feasibility study for older patients with depression. *International Journal of Geriatric Psychiatry, 28*(8), 850–857.

Kuiper, N. A., & Martin, R. A. (1998). Laughter and stress in daily life: Relation to positive and negative affect. *Motivation and Emotion, 22*, 133–153.

Lefcourt, H. M., & Martin, R. A. (1986). *Humor and life stress: Antidote to adversity*. New York, NY: Springer.

Martin, R. A. (2001). Humor, laughter, and physical health: Methodological issues and research findings. *Psychological Bulletin, 127*, 504–519. doi:10.1037/0033-2909.127.4.504.

Martin, R. A., & Lefcourt, H. M. (1983). Sense of humor as a moderator of the relation between stressors and moods. *Journal of Personality and Social Psychology, 45*, 1313–1324. doi:10.1037/e330252004-002.

Martin, R. A., Puhlik-Doris, P., Larsen, G., Gray, J., & Weir, K. (2003). Individual differences in uses of humor and their relationship to psychological well-being: Development of the humor styles questionnaire. *Journal of Research in Personality, 37*, 48–75. doi:10.1016/s0092-6566(02)00534-2.

Marziali, E., McDonald, L., & Donahue, P. (2008). The role of coping humor in the physical and mental health of older adults. *Journal of Mental Health and Aging, 12*, 713–718. doi:10.1080/13607860802154374.

McGhee, P. E. (1996). *Health, healing and the amuse system: Humor as survival training*. Dubuque, IA: Kendall/Hunt.

McGhee, P. E. (2010a). *Humor as survival training for a stressed-out world: The 7 Humor Habits Program*. Bloomington, IN: Author House.

McGhee, P. E. (2010b). *Humor: The lighter path to resilience and health*. Bloomington, IN: Author House.

Moran, C. C., & Massam, M. M. (1999). Differential influences of coping humor and humor bias on mood. *Behavioral Medicine, 25*, 36–42. doi:10.1080/08964289909596737.

Müller, L., & Ruch, W. (2011). Humor and strengths of character. *The Journal of Positive Psychology, 6*, 368–376. doi:10.1080/17439760.2011.592508.

Nezu, A. M., Nezu, C. M., & Blissett, S. E. (1988). Sense of humor as a moderator of the relation between stressful events and psychological distress: A prospective analysis. *Journal of Personality and Social Psychology, 54*, 520–525. doi:10.1037/0022-3514.54.3.520.

Papa, A., & Bonanno, G. A. (2008). Smiling in the face of adversity: The interpersonal and intrapersonal functions of smiles. *Emotion, 8*, 1–12. doi:10.1037/1528-3542.8.1.1.

Papousek, I., & Schulter, G. (2008). Effects of a mood enhancing intervention on subjective well-being and cardiovascular parameters. *International Journal of Behavioral Medicine, 15*, 293–302. doi:10.1080/10705500802365508.

Park, N., Peterson, C., & Seligman, M. E. P. (2004). Strengths of character and well-being. *Journal of Social and Clinical Psychology, 23*, 603–619.

Peterson, C., & Seligman, M. E. P. (2004). *Character strengths and virtues: A handbook and classification*. Washington, DC: American Psychological Association.

Peterson, C., Park, N., & Seligman, M. E. P. (2006). Greater strengths of character and recovery from illness. *The Journal of Positive Psychology, 1*, 7–26. doi:10.1080/17439760500372739.

Pinquart, M., Skolaude, D., Zaplinski, K., & Maier, R. F. (2011). Do clown visits improve psychological and sense of physical well-being of hospitalized pediatric patients? *Klinische Pädiatrie, 223*, 74–78. doi:10.1055/s-0030-1267932.

Proyer, R. T., Gander, W., Wyss, T., & Ruch, W. (2011). The relation of character strengths to past, present and future life satisfaction among German-speaking women. *Applied Psychology: Health and Well-Being, 3*, 370–384. doi:10.1111/j.1758-0854.2011.01060.x.

Ruch, W., Köhler, G., & van Thriel, C. (1996). Assessing the "humorous temperament": Construction of the facet and standard trait forms of the State-Trait-Cheerfulness- Inventory–STCI. *Humor: International Journal of Humor Research, 9*, 303–339. doi:10.1515/humr.1996.9.3-4.303.

Ruch, W. (2004). Humor. In C. P. Peterson & M. E. P. Seligman (Eds.), *Character strengths and virtues: A handbook and classification* (pp. 583–598). Washington, DC, USA: American Psychological Association.

Ruch, W. (Ed.). (2007). *Sense of humor: Explorations of humor as a personality characteristic*. Berlin, Germany: Mouton de Gruyter.

Ruch, W. (2008). The psychology of humor. In V. Raskin (Ed.), *A primer of humor* (pp. 17–100). Berlin, Germany: Mouton de Gruyter.

Ruch, W. (2010, June). *The seriousness and fun about humor*. Paper presented at the 5th European Conference on Positive Psychology, Copenhagen, Denmark.

Ruch, W. (2012, April). *Humor and positive psychology: A matching couple?* Paper session presented at the 25th Annual Conference of the Association for Applied and Therapeutic Humor, Chicago, USA.

Ruch, W., & Heintz, S. (2016). The virtue gap in humor: Exploring benevolent and corrective humor. *Translational Issues in Psychological Science: Special Issue on "The Psychology of Humor", 2*(1), 35–45.

Ruch, W., & Hofmann, J. (2012). A temperament approach to humor. In P. Gremigni (Ed.), *Humor and health promotion* (pp. 79–113). Hauppauge, NY: Nova Science.

Ruch, W., & McGhee, P. E. (2014). Humor intervention programs. In A. C. Parks & S. M. Schueller (Eds.), *Handbook of positive psychological interventions* (pp. 179–193). Oxford, UK: Wiley-Blackwell.

Ruch, W., & Proyer, R. T. (2015). Mapping strengths into virtues: The relation of the 24 VIA strengths to six ubiquitous virtues. *Frontiers in Psychology, 6*, 460. doi:10.3389/fpsyg.2015.00460.

Ruch, W., Proyer, R. T., Harzer, C., Park, N., Peterson, C., & Seligman, M. E. P. (2010a). Adaptation and validation of the German version of the Values in Action Inventory of Strengths (VIA-IS) and the development of a peer-rating form. *Journal of Individual Differences, 31*, 138–149. doi:10.1027/1614-0001/a000022.

Ruch, W., Proyer, R. T., & Weber, M. (2010b). Humor as character strength among the elderly: Theoretical considerations. *Zeitschrift für Gerontologie und Geriatrie, 43*, 8–12. doi:10.1007/s00391-009-0080-2.

Ruch, W., Proyer, R. T., & Weber, M. (2010c). Humor as a character strength among the elderly: Empirical findings on age-related changes and its contribution to satisfaction with life. *Zeitschrift fur Gerontologie und Geriatrie, 43*, 13–18. doi:10.1007/s00391-009-0090-0.

Ruch, W., Rodden, F. A., & Proyer, R. T. (2011). Humor and other positive interventions in medical and therapeutic settings. In B. Kirkcaldy (Ed.), *The art and science of health care: Psychology and human factors for practitioners* (pp. 277–294). Göttingen, Germany: Hogrefe.

Rusch, S., & Stolz, H. (2009). *Ist Sinn für Humor lernbar? Eine Anwendung und Evaluation des 8 Stufen Programs (McGhee, 1999)* [Can a sense of humor be learned? An application and evaluation of the 8-Step Program (McGhee, 1999)]. Unpublished master's thesis, University of Zurich, Switzerland.

Sassenrath, S. (2001). *Humor und Lachen als* Stressbewältigungsstrategie [Humor and laughter as coping mechanism]. Unpublished master's thesis, University of Vienna, Austria.

Seligman, M. E. P., Steen, T. A., Park, N., & Peterson, C. (2005). Positive psychology progress: Empirical validation of interventions. *The American Psychologist, 60*, 410–421. doi:10.1037/0003-066x.60.5.410.

Vagnoli, L., Caprilli, S., & Messeri, A. (2010). Parental presence, clowns or sedative premedication to treat preoperative anxiety in children: What could be the most promising option? *Pediatric Anesthesia, 20*, 937–943. doi:10.1111/j.1460-9592.2010.03403.x.

Wellenzohn, S., Proyer, R. T., & Ruch, W. (2016a). Humor-based online positive psychology interventions: A randomized placebo-controlled long-term trial. *The Journal of Positive Psychology, 11*(6), 584–594. doi:10.1080/17439760.2015.1137624.

Wellenzohn, S., Proyer, R. T., & Ruch, W. (2016b). *Who profits from humor-based positive psychology interventions? The moderating effects of personality traits and sense of humor.* Manuscript submitted for publication.

Wellenzohn, S., Proyer, R. T., & Ruch, W. (2016c). How do positive psychology interventions work? A short-term placebo-controlled humor-based study on the role of the time focus. *Personality and Individual Differences, 96*, 1–6. doi:10.1016/j.paid.2016.02.056

Yovetich, N. A., Dale, J. A., & Hudak, M. A. (1990). Benefits of humor in reduction of threat-induced anxiety. *Psychological Reports, 66*, 51–58. doi:10.2466/pr0.66.1.51-58.

Zweyer, K., Velker, B., & Ruch, W. (2004). Do cheerfulness, exhilaration, and humor production moderate pain tolerance? A FACS study. *Humor: International Journal of Humor Research, 17*, 85–119. doi:10.1515/humr.2004.009.

Part II
Education and Development

Chapter 6
Well-Being and Well-Doing: Bringing Mindfulness and Character Strengths to the Early Childhood Classroom and Home

Thomas J. Lottman, Sarah Zawaly, and Ryan Niemiec

Abstract The science of character strengths and mindfulness has increased voluminously in the last couple decades but the application of each in the classroom, especially character strengths, has been limited and shallow. We outline four distinct areas of learning around mindfulness and character strengths to enable teachers to bring forth an optimal impact on the strengths of children. Special attention is given to parents in this model as well. We argue that the zeitgeist of social-emotional learning in the classroom offers particular value around well-doing as children learn prescribed skill-sets and the building of positive relationships. What is missing from social emotional learning (SEL), however, is a focus on well-being that speaks to the positive identity of each unique child. Research and practices from the new science of character serves as a pathway for supporting and boosting child well-doing and well-being which leads to child flourishing. To this end, we adapt Niemiec's (2014) integration programme (Mindfulness-Based Strengths Practice; MBSP) to an individualised coaching model. We share some of these adaptations and offer numerous concepts for teachers to use personally and with students (e.g., strength-sight, the autopilot mind), exercises to support teachers (e.g., 'catch AP-ASAP', 'the 10 second pause', the use of signature strengths), and offer new research (partial replication study) on the most common 'emergent' character strengths in young children. We discuss a framework devised to boost strengths-based thinking and positive beliefs in children that flows from moment-making to meaning-making to memory-making, and on to mindset-making.

T.J. Lottman (✉) • S. Zawaly
Children, Inc., 333 Madison Avenue, Covington, KY 41011, USA
e-mail: tom@childreninc.org; szawaly@childreninc.org

R. Niemiec
VIA Institute on Character, 312 Walnut Street, Cincinnati, OH 45202, USA
e-mail: ryan@viacharacter.org

C. Proctor (ed.), *Positive Psychology Interventions in Practice*,
DOI 10.1007/978-3-319-51787-2_6

Abbreviations

Catch AP-ASAP	Autopilot minds-as soon as possible
MBSP	Mindfulness-Based Strengths Practice
MTT	Mental time travel
SEL	Social emotional learning

Introduction

This chapter focuses on what's best in young children and examines the attitudes and actions of teachers and parents that nurture the development of positive characteristics. The best in children are their inner strengths, happiness, and goodness and the outer expression of corresponding traits and values. Parents' wishes for their children are grounded in these strengths, and those wishes are both universal and timeless. And while these parental hopes are timeless, the scientific study of the nature of character strengths, especially in young children, is relatively recent. The purpose of this chapter is to capture the crucial insights from this field and bring them to the classroom and the home.

In just 15 years, positive psychology, the science of well-being, has developed a large and growing body of empirical evidence. Its backbone, the science of character strengths, has built an impressive array of findings linking character strengths to life satisfaction, health, achievement, and numerous other positive outcomes (Niemiec 2013). While the application of character strengths in the field of education has been a popular topic (e.g., Linkins et al. 2014; Proctor et al. 2011; Proyer et al. 2012; Quinlan et al. 2014; Seider et al. 2013; White and Waters 2014), there remains a great deal yet to learn about the implications of this research for the optimal development of children.

The application of character science in education (and early childhood education in particular) means identifying and promoting the unique constellation of emergent character strengths in each child. What character strengths are young children most likely to express? How can these strengths be identified by important adults in the child's life? How will these character strengths be optimally nurtured and reinforced by teachers and parents? Helping children to be aware of their emergent strengths and to apply these strengths in the classroom not only reinforces the likely repetition of strength-driven prosocial 'well-doing' but also the acquisition of positive 'well-being' convictions about themselves and their place in the world.

So what are these character strengths so essential to our happiness and goodness? In what is arguably the largest and most wide reaching project in positive psychology to date, Chris Peterson, a researcher at the University of Michigan, and Martin Seligman, the father of positive psychology, led a group of 55 renowned scholars to review essential literature, catalogues, and texts over more than two millennia dealing with human virtues. This daunting 3-year project yielded consensus on six

Table 6.1 VIA Classification of character strengths and virtues

Wisdom	Courage	Humanity
Creativity	Bravery	Love
Curiosity	Perseverance	Kindness
Judgment	Honesty	Social intelligence
Love of learning	Zest	
Perspective		
Justice	Temperance	Transcendence
Teamwork	Forgiveness	Appreciation of beauty
Fairness	Humility	Gratitude
Leadership	Prudence	Hope
	Self-regulation	Humour
		Spirituality

major categories of core virtues that were consistent across many disparate traditions. These six virtue categories are: wisdom, courage, humanity, justice, temperance, and transcendence. These virtue classes were then organised around 24 subsidiary character strengths that met various scientific criteria and were comprehensively described in the pivotal book, *Character Strengths and Virtues: A Handbook and Classification* (Peterson and Seligman 2004). Cross-cultural validation of this classification was also performed to confirm this as a universal classification of human strengths and not confined to any one culture or group (see Biswas-Diener 2006; McGrath 2014; Park et al. 2006). See Table 6.1 to review the VIA Classification (Peterson and Seligman 2004), which includes the 24 character strengths and 6 virtues.

As part of this project to assemble a 'common language' of character strengths, the scientists also developed and tested assessment instruments to measure these character strengths in adults (VIA Survey; Peterson and Seligman 2004), and in youth (VIA Youth Survey; Park and Peterson 2006a). Access to the free VIA Survey and VIA Youth Survey, and their many translations, as well as a review of over 200 research studies on character strengths, and application resources are available at the website of the VIA Institute on Character: http://www.viacharacter.org.

One primary contribution of this classification system is that it provides researchers, teachers, and parents a common 'lens and language' to examine and discuss character strengths in the lab, in the school, and in the home. For *researchers*, it's a framework for operationally defining, measuring, and testing character strengths and interventions designed to promote them. For *teachers* it's a way to focus efforts to spot and encourage emerging strengths. And similarly for *parents* it's a way to identify and understand the unique constellation of strengths that represent the best that is within their child. Having this classification system enables new research, new educational concepts in social and emotional learning, and new insights for parents invested in nurturing the development of their child's character.

Many character strengths emerge in early childhood (Hoffman 1975). However, they often emerge without the awareness of the significant adults in the lives of children. Parents and teachers recognise and support concrete prosocial behaviours, but they often are blind to their underlying character strengths and the child's core beliefs about themselves, other people, and the world in general. And even until recently, research in general, and positive psychology in particular, have been largely silent on character strengths in young children (Park and Peterson 2006b). If we are intentional about applying insights from the science of character strengths to a developmental frame in early childhood, we must create tools that help teachers and parents understand and facilitate this process in young children. Some of what good teachers and parents already do is consistent with the insights of character science so an important task is to first, make the invisible 'visible' and second, make the visible 'intentional'.

In recent years, the link between social and emotional learning (SEL) and academic success has been well established. SEL has become an accepted and celebrated component of educating the whole child. However, we suggest that 'what' is being learned in SEL is artificially narrow. The SEL field is heavily concerned with the acquisition of prescribed prosocial skill sets at the expense of acquiring individual positive mindsets. Said another way, SEL focuses on behavioural well-doing and not sufficiently on experiential well-being. Indeed, both are important for children and character strengths are equally crucial for positive identity development/who the child is (well-being) and acting-with-strength/healthy connecting (well-doing).

In preschool, kindergarten, and early primary grades, it is clear that the skills of turn-taking, cooperation, and perspective-taking are crucial to academic and life success. However, far less focus is given to the core beliefs the child is learning as strengths develop, and how these beliefs can be identified and nurtured by the adults in the child's life. Herein, important questions remain: How are core character strengths experienced and 'owned' by the child? How do character strengths become a positive and enduring component of who the child is? How do character strengths define the narrative self for the child?

A child's belief systems are the 'subjective' filters through which the 'objective' world is perceived and understood. Yet SEL pays little attention to how these belief systems develop. The field has not explained how *events* in the life of a child are sufficiently attended to so that they become meaningful *experiences* that are connected to other events to become part of narrative *memories* that in turn *are* rehearsed through self-talk so that they become *beliefs* by which he or she understands his or her world. The fields of neuroscience and positive psychology describe the brain's negativity bias through which a child is more likely to attend to, process, and remember negative events than positive events (Hanson 2013; Rozin and Royzman 2001). Educators would benefit from understanding how to help children attend to and process positive events into impactful experiences that are encoded in memory and nurtured to beliefs. Strategies of 'moment-making', 'meaning-making', 'memory-making', and 'mindset-making' should be acquired and applied by all SEL practitioners.

Nurturing Well-Being and Well-Doing in Early Childhood

Daniel Siegel (1999, 2010), a Harvard-trained neuroscientist, coined the term 'mindsight' to describe an attentional focus that allows us to observe our own mental activity. He described mindsight as our 'seventh sense' that allows us to see and reflect on our internal world. This concept, well-grounded in neuroscience, is confirmed in the growing literature on mindfulness. Siegel refers to several kinds of 'mindsight maps' (me-maps and you-maps) that provide insight into ourselves and others. Mindsight, whether emerging from skilled parenting, attained through clinical interventions, or nurtured through contemplative practices, is essential to our sense of well-being.

We sought to amplify the benefits of mindsight derived from neuroscience with the development of 'strengthsight', which emerges from the relatively new field of character science. Strengthsight refers to the attentional focus on our own character strengths and the character strengths of others. In the book *Mindfulness and Character Strengths* (2014), Niemiec brings together mindfulness practice and strengths practice, or mindsight + strengthsight to connect the yin and yang of well-being and well-doing. Niemiec uses the metaphor of two large entwined trees to represent the traditional separation of mindfulness and character strengths, in which each tree has its own deeply grounded historical and substantive root system and each with their own extensive, yet entwined branching to describe the integration of mindfulness and character strengths. As Niemiec states:

> Mindfulness opens a door of awareness to who we are and character strengths are what is behind the door since character strengths are who we are at our core. Mindfulness opens the door to potential self-improvement and growth while character strengths use is the growth itself. (p. 344)

One of the results of this integration is mindfulness-based strengths practice (MBSP), which integrates the best practices of character strengths, mindful living, and mindfulness meditation. As described by a leading mindfulness scientist, Ruth Baer (2015), MBSP is the only intervention programme specifically designed to cultivate both; in other words, MBSP takes a unique approach differentiating itself from other mindfulness-based programmes as it uses mindfulness to target what is strong (e.g., character, well-being) rather than what is wrong (e.g., stress, chronic depression). It helps participants become stronger in their mindfulness practices, engage more deeply in mindful living, and boost their consciousness around strengths use (Niemiec 2012; Niemiec et al. 2012). Early research on MBSP is promising, revealing substantial benefits to flourishing, happiness, engagement, and strengths use (Briscoe 2014; Niemiec 2014) and unique benefits for positive relationships and problem management (Niemiec and Lissing 2015).

Recognising the needs of parents and teachers and the power of mindfulness and character strengths therein, we adapted the MBSP programme as an individualised coaching model for early childhood educators and parents. Our intent is for teachers to develop the skills to recognise their own strengths, spot strengths of co-workers and students, nurture these strengths, and help parents recognise and encourage the growth of strengths within their children. We discuss some of these adaptations on the following pages as well as weave in critical theoretical underpinnings that support the use of mindfulness and character strengths in the classroom.

We envision four distinct learning phases that are pivotal for bringing the science of mindfulness and character strengths to early childhood development:

1. Teachers learn mindfulness practice and strengthsight with their own character strengths.
2. Teachers use mindful awareness to 'strength-spot' in children.
3. Teachers skilfully nurture emerging character strengths in children.
4. Teachers teach parents to spot and nurture strengths in their children.

For teachers, children, and parents, this effort combines implications of research in both mindfulness and character development. The goal is to promote both awareness of internal experiences and insight about both the cause and effect of internal experience on external expressions and behaviour.

Phase 1: Teachers Learn Mindfulness Practice and Strengthsight with Their Own Character Strengths

In phase one of this model (typically six to eight sessions), teachers develop a mindfulness practice and become aware of their character strengths through exercises adapted from Niemiec's (2014) MBSP.

Catch AP-ASAP

Cultivating mindfulness is a prerequisite for teachers' greater awareness of their own strengths and their ability to spot emerging strengths in the classroom. The general concepts of mindfulness are taught through explanations and exercises. The operational definition of mindfulness from leading scientists in the field describes the essence of mindfulness as being captured in two-parts: (1) the self-regulation of attention, with (2) an attitude of curiosity, openness, and acceptance (Bishop et al. 2004). Teachers are challenged to take greater control of their attention, and enhance awareness across three levels—their own autopilot tendencies, the here and now experience for their young learners, and the moment-to-moment interactions between them.

One way to further the teacher's ability to internalise the concept of mindfulness is building an awareness of autopilot. Autopilot is described as the human mind wandering off to thoughts and feelings (Segal et al. 2002). The autopilot mind is adaptive, the brain's way of simplifying daily living. Deliberate mind wandering has been associated with some positive outcomes, such as creative problem-solving (Mooneyham and Schooler 2013). However, this efficiency comes at a price. And that price, in addition to diminished well-being for many, is missed opportunities in life—opportunities to savour the small moments, such as the beauty of a sunrise or the large moments of truly feeling ourselves or our loved ones in the flow of being the best version of ourselves. Therefore, in MBSP participants are encouraged to 'catch AP-ASAP', to catch their autopilot minds as soon as possible so they can then determine the best course of action—creative mindlessness, a return to the here and now, or another course of action.

Mindfulness should not be a tool for teaching, but rather a tenet of teaching. Jennings (2015) suggests that mindfulness is 'the heart of teaching' (p. 214). There is no more powerful pedagogy than the compassionate presence of a teacher attentive and attuned to a child's curiosity and a child's desire to learn. When teachers catch autopilot and become aware of the present moment, they are giving themselves a greater chance to explore opportunities and have deeper connections with children, parents, and themselves. In Phase 1 of this MBSP coaching model, teachers explore activities in their day in which autopilot takes over. Cultivating mindfulness is illustrated through stories that are relatable to everyday life. Participants gain a better understanding of how autopilot affects their interactions with their students and in their personal life. Simple strategies such as choosing one activity a day to focus your attention on, taking a break from multi-tasking, and catch AP-ASAP are a few ways teachers learn to incorporate mindfulness practices into their daily routine.

When one teacher was asked to choose an area in her life where mindlessness has a negative impact, she chose the paper route her and her daughter do every Sunday. This was a time she described as an autopilot mode. Their paper route was filled with Amanda creating her to-do list in her head and making her schedule for the week. As she described, it was very difficult to be present to her daughter. Often times she would get caught in 'reactive mode' because of the long list of to-dos on Sundays and would rush her daughter through the route causing stress and often ending in arguments. Amanda chose to be mindful during this time with her daughter and reduce her mind wandering. She rooted her attention in her breath and listened carefully to her daughter's words, observed body language, and monitored her own thoughts and feelings; when her mind wandered, she returned her focus to her breath and the interaction with her daughter. She was elated about the connection she was able to make with her daughter. Amanda began to see the love her daughter had for nature and noticed how she stopped to smell the flowers (i.e., the character strength called 'appreciation of beauty'). They talked about planting bulbs in the autumn to create their own garden filled with all the flowers they loved. This became a regular practice for Amanda and she described a deeper connection and understanding that was made between her and her daughter. This story demonstrates how when we are in autopilot we often don't connect with others in our life on a level that can be achieved when we are able to get out of our head and into our heart. Awareness of autopilot had served as a catalyst for Amanda's character strengths use.

The 10-Second Pause

Autopilot is often described as a shift from a reactive to a responsive mode of experiencing (Hanson 2013; Segal et al. 2002). In a responsive mode, we feel calm, at ease, are able to express ourselves creatively, and are caring towards others. In a reactive mode our brain 'overestimates threats and underestimates opportunities' (Hanson 2013, p. 136). In simple terms we 'overreact or avoid'. Our brains are built to perceive threats—this is how we are able to react in life-threatening situations. It is however the overreaction and habitual reaction to non-threatening situations that we seek to improve in the classroom. When we pause and take a breath we activate the parasympathetic nervous system allowing us to shift into responsive mode. This pause allows teachers to get out of reactive mode in the classroom and respond to situations in a calm way. This acquired skill helps teachers respond to the feelings behind the actions of the children in their classroom. Hanson describes a number of ways to increase responsive mode, for example, teachers are asked and reminded to develop this mode by having self-compassion, and reliving the best moment of their day.

Creating a 'pause' is a key concept for teachers throughout these sessions. In order for teachers to spot strengths in themselves, reflect on these strengths, and ultimately appreciate and recognise them in themselves and their students, it is imperative that teachers 'take in the moment'. We live in such a distracting and busy world that often times we can go throughout the day without stopping and 'being in the moment'. Without these moments, it is much more difficult to cultivate and practice your own strengths and nurture the strengths of young children.

Teachers are asked to create a cuing strategy that reminds them to pause throughout the day for as little as 10 seconds. One teacher described what she found most useful in MBSP was creating this pause in her life:

> I pause for at least 30 seconds several times a day now. It seems to clear away the traffic jam in my head and forces me to redirect my attention. I have found that pausing before speaking makes a difference in how I respond to my students and family.

Mindfulness practices help to balance out the brain's negativity bias. Such practices allow us to be more aware of and appreciative of positive events. And the positive emotions evoked by these events in turn help us to become more mindful. Fredrickson's (2001, 2004, 2013) research on her 'broaden-and-build theory' demonstrates that the experience of positive emotions actually enhances and broadens attention and awareness. This, in itself, can have significant effects on a teacher's effectiveness in spotting and nurturing character strengths in young children.

Building a Common Language: Aware, Explore, Apply

The majority of the MBSP coaching model involves participants understanding and developing their mindfulness and character strengths. Since character strengths are capacities for thinking, feeling, and behaving, they can be built up. The teachers learn to deepen their understanding of mindfulness and strengths in order to boost their overall strengths capacity. The aware-explore-apply model (Niemiec 2013, 2014) is a process for working with and developing character strengths and mindfulness supports for each of the three phases.

The first step to helping teachers become aware of their strengths is to take the VIA Survey. The survey results act as a guide to understanding each participant's signature strengths (i.e., those strengths highest in one's character strengths profile that are most core and essential to identity). It is important for the coach to utilise his or her own strengths throughout the sessions to provide compassion to the teachers and be mindful while listening to how the teachers react to discovering their strengths. Deploying one's signature strengths at work is linked to greater work satisfaction, greater well-being, and higher meaning in life. Moreover, expressing four or more signature strengths at work is linked with more positive work experiences and meaningful work (Harzer and Ruch 2012). To explore the use of signature strengths, teachers are asked to think of a time when they felt they were at their best professionally and personally. This exercise from MBSP is a way for the teachers to become more aware of when they are using their strengths and how they feel when their signature strengths are used. Talking positively about oneself can often feel foreign and at times uncomfortable. This consensual nomenclature or common language of strengths give teachers a new way to see themselves and become aware of when and how they use their strengths.

Exploring strengths is central to every session. Teachers spend time reflecting on times they have used their signature strengths and savouring these moments. This savouring fills teachers 'emotional bank accounts' counterbalancing the struggles they face with students, coworkers, and with themselves. This balance becomes an important reflection for teachers and how their relationship with themselves is connected to self-kindness and their relationship with others is connected to 'other-oriented strengths' (e.g., kindness, fairness, forgiveness) and connectedness with others. Loving kindness meditation and the character strengths breathing space (i.e., a 3 min meditation that targets the essence of mindfulness practice through the strengths of curiosity, self-regulation, and perspective) become part of the sessions and teachers are asked to cultivate these practices throughout the week. One teacher stated:

> I am surprised how much I got into loving kindness meditation. I am practicing it regularly before starting the day. When I start my day with this meditation I feel more positive and in tune with the children in my classroom. My connection to my students is deeper, and I am able to stay calmer. I bring to the forefront of my day two of my signature strengths, love and kindness.

Teachers take these meditations and strengths exploration exercises to the next level by making a conscious effort to appreciate the strengths of the people around them. This is particularly powerful because most people are unaware of their strengths. Only one-third of people have a meaningful awareness of their strengths (Linley 2008) and 100% of people have some types of strength blindness around their strengths (Niemiec 2014). Mindfulness has been shown to be a pathway to break through and improve upon blind spots in self-knowledge (Carlson 2013).

In order to build the teacher's capacity to become aware of their strengths, explore them, and apply them in and out of the classroom, MBSP uses several exercises: (1) strength interview; (2) character strengths 360; (3) using signature strengths in a new way; and (4) spotting strengths in movies, books, and other people. A strength interview is an exercise in which the teacher interviews someone in their life about their strengths. This helps the teacher gain perspective on how people utilise strengths and gives them an opportunity to practice mindful listening. Next, teachers ask several people in their life to fill out the 'character strengths 360' in which informants note the character strengths that they see as most core to who the teacher is and offer one example for each strength spotted. Having another's perspective shows teachers what strengths they may underutilise and what strengths they might not see in themselves that others value.

The exercise called 'using signature strength in a new way' is a rigorously studied intervention that has been shown in randomised, double-blind, placebo-controlled studies to boost happiness and decrease depression for as long as 6 months (Gander et al. 2012; Seligman et al. 2005). By intentionally using signature strengths in a new way teachers can deepen their awareness of signature strengths by discovering new ways to use them. One teacher surprised her coworkers by leaving short thank you notes on their desks expressing how grateful she is for each of their signature strengths.

Strengths-Spotting in All Activities

We teach teachers to use any interaction or life experience as an opportunity for not only mindfulness, but also for strengths-spotting. One exercise involves teachers practicing strengths-spotting in movies, books, and the people around them (Niemiec and Wedding 2014). Oftentimes it is easier to use a strengths 'lens' when watching movies or reading books. We find that this personal work quickly transfers over to the classroom and becomes part of the teachers' daily routine.

In addition to spotting children's strengths use, teachers will also spot an 'overuse' of strengths. For example, a perseverant child who is getting ready for outdoor playtime is holding up the line because they insist on zipping their own coat or tying their own shoe. Frustration may emerge for the child because he or she is determined to complete the task. Teachers can mentally connect the character strength of perseverance (even though it may be an overuse) with the task at hand. This exemplifies the importance of teachers recalibrating their 'radar screen' to see the perseverance and change the way they view a 'stubborn' child. These strengths are indeed

Table 6.2 Comparison of prevalent character strengths in two studies

Park and Peterson (2004)		Lottman and Zawaly (2014)	
Character strength	Prevalence rank	Character strength	Prevalence rank
Love	1	Love	1
Kindness	2	Kindness	2
Creativity	3	Curiosity	3
Humour	4	Humour	4
Curiosity	5	Perseverance	5
Love of learning	6	Creativity	6
Perseverance	7	Love of learning	7
Self-regulation	8	Social intelligence	8
Social intelligence	9	Bravery	9

visible and teachers can intentionally recognise and encourage these strength mindsets.

Phase 2: Teachers Learn to Spot Emerging Strengths in Young Children

Early Manifestations of Character Strengths

As children begin to develop cognitively and emotionally, character strengths begin to emerge. Park and Peterson (2006) collected parents' written descriptions of their children (ages 3–9) and then rated for character strengths. This is the first study that looks at the early manifestations of strengths and their association with happiness. The first two authors of this chapter partially replicated the Park and Peterson study coding free parent narratives for character strengths of children ages 3–6 using the same instructional set as the first study (Lottman and Zawaly 2014). The raters independently coded the narrative descriptions for each of the 24 character strengths using a binary code of 1 (mention of strength) or 0 (no mention of strength). Using a test sample of 20 narratives, the independent raters demonstrated 0.95 interrater agreement calculated using the Fleiss Kappa statistic.

The results mirrored those of Park and Peterson (2006) in several ways. First, there was great variation in the length of free descriptive narratives, however even the short narratives were useful because they often listed traits. Secondly, the prevalence of traits was very similar to those of Park and Peterson. Examples of sections from parent narratives scored for each of the strengths in the Lottman and Zawaly (2014) study is presented in Tables 6.2 and 6.3.

Strengths in young children emerge in a variety of settings. Through observations and teacher reporting one significant outlet for using strengths is play. Pretend

Table 6.3 Examples of narrative sections scored for each strength (Lottman and Zawaly 2014)

Character strength	Parent narrative section
Love	'Extremely loving, loves to be held'
	'Very loving and caring'
Kindness	'Likes to help others'
	'Wants to comfort you when you are upset or feeling down'
Curiosity	'Curious and love to explore nature'
	'Not afraid to try new things on her own'
Humour	'Loves to make her brother laugh'
	'Hilarious, silly, goofy'
Perseverance	'Knows what he wants and what's needed to get it'
	'Determined, very strong willed'
Creativity	'Always devising something remarkable to make out of found objects'
Love of learning	'Regularly pulls out advanced math and alphabet books on her own'
	'Loves to hear how things go together and how they work'
Social intelligence	'Good at reading others' feelings'
	'High levels of empathy for others'
Bravery	'Isn't afraid of anything'
	'Stands up for himself'

play is an important developmental skill that encourages thinking and problem-solving skills. Observers can readily see children's character strengths, such as teamwork, creativity, perseverance, and curiosity, when the child pretends to open up an ice cream shop or pizza parlour. When role-playing, children play 'house' or 'school' and become the mom, dad, teacher or sibling and an abundance of character strengths can be seen if the teacher is mindful and present using their strength-sight. Teachers observe kindness and love when they observe a student care for a baby. When a teacher can point out those positive experiences by relating the child's action to a feeling the child can internalise the positive beliefs about themselves (all through pretend play). For example, *'Jimmy, you are being so gentle with the baby. You are showing so much love to that baby just like your mommy loves you'*.

Teachers can see character strengths in almost all young learners, such as when sharing a ball at recess to more complex skills like understanding others' feelings. Many teachers observe that the 2- and 3-year-olds they are teaching demonstrate social intelligence. Even at these ages children can understand how another is feeling and are able to know when a child with special needs in the room needs an extra hand. The older children may nurture young ones in the class while others make it their 'job' to ensure that children with special needs are included. Teachers have also suggested that with social intelligence, humour often develops. Humour appears throughout the preschool day and the kids can make the teachers laugh through silly songs, telling a joke, and appreciating others' jokes. Creativity in art projects is easy to see, as are the acts of kindness and love when children send home love notes to their mom and dad. When teachers take the time to appreciate these moments it is much easier to redirect negative behaviours and understand the feelings behind them.

Some children have been described in the classroom as having an unrelenting need for understanding how something might work—from a marble run to keeping a tower from crashing. Their curiosity and love of learning urges them to get the teacher involved to further their knowledge and understanding. One parent described her 4-year-old son's curiosity as the 'fuel to his fire'. When teachers focus on strengths as opposed to deficits, they discover a fuel that can ignite a spark in young children. When that spark is lit a child can own their strengths, have pride in what they do, and become a confident child inside and outside the classroom. This ownership becomes part of the child's identity that not only enables well-doing, but also well-being. We have observed that classrooms of young learners who hear positivity are more likely to have positive self-talk and develop a positive mindset.

The lack of research on emerging character strengths makes it all the more important that teachers become aware of and make an intentional effort to identify even subtle behaviours that signal emerging strengths in young children. In this phase, teachers are given an observation protocol that identifies relevant behaviours associated with each strength. In the next phase, teachers are given the tools to nurture these emerging strengths that will be part of the belief system of the child.

Phase 3: Teachers Learn to Nurture Emerging Character Strengths

As discussed in Linkins et al. (2014), Neal Mayerson, Chairman of the VIA Institute on Character, provides valuable insight on how teachers, parents, and researchers might think about promoting the development of character strengths in young children. He suggests that teachers especially, too often see themselves as 'sculptors' attempting to 'mould' children's development of preferred strengths. Rather, teachers should see themselves as 'gardeners' nurturing and optimising the soil or environment in which the unique strengths of each child can grow and flourish.

Creating an early childhood environment for the flourishing of character strength development is an element of all good, developmentally appropriate practice. And one of the first tasks of a character strength coach is to help the teacher understand that much of which what good coaches are already doing is exactly what is needed to nurture character growth. The coach helps make the invisible visible. But beyond that, the coach seeks to help the teacher learn and apply new skills that will optimise the flourishing of these emerging strengths. The coach helps make the visible more intentional through the skill sets we call moment-making, meaning-making, memory-making, and mindset-making. In other words, becoming intentional about orchestrating the number of positive events in the early childhood environment; helping to make those events meaningful experiences for the child; helping those events get coded as enduring memories; and rehearsing those memories so that they become core beliefs the child has about herself, others, and the world in general.

Prerequisites for orienting a classroom to the use and growth of character strengths include: (1) introducing character strength language and examples, and (2) making character strengths a part of daily classroom routine. For example, during story time children can note character strengths they relate to in the story and a teacher might prompt for this by saying something like, *'The owl babies' mommy was very brave to go out for food in the night. Does anybody ever feel brave?'* or *'Wow, this little bunny is really working hard! That bunny is perseverant! I see you all working hard throughout the day. Are you perseverant like the little bunny?'* Just as MBSP uses characters from movies and books to facilitate strengthsight in adults, children can practice strengthsight from their own literature.

During the day, the teacher might say, *'Who feels proud of themselves when they use lots of zest and energy to finish their work?'* or *'If you made someone laugh with your strength of humour today then line up over here'*. Teachers might send home a note to parents saying, *'Give me a hug today because I was very kind when I helped a friend'* or *'Give me a high five I because I was brave today on the playground when I tried out a new game'*. Bridging the connection from school to home fosters further development of each child's unique character strengths.

Moment-Making

There is no doubt that orchestrating positive experiences for the child in the preschool classroom is the foundation for a number of positive outcomes. Fredrickson (2001, 2004, 2013) proposed a broaden-and-build theory to explain these positive effects. Positive emotions expand the child's thought-action pool of potential responses, such that momentary joy triggers an urge to play, interest leads to the desire to explore, and so on. Emotion begets experience and experience begets skills.

In positive moment-making, frequency and consistency trump intensity and complexity. Small, consistent events, such as simple eye contact, a smile, and an encouraging word, have greater impact than infrequent intense encounters. Creating positive events in the preschool classrooms often takes three forms. First, and most important, is the intentional personal engagement that the teacher orchestrates for each child. Being intentional about getting down to the level of the child, engaging in mutual gaze, and using a soft voice to recognise the child's accomplishments, are all essential to creating the critical mass of attention, attachment, and attunement necessary for the child to feel valued. The second form of positive moment-making is being intentional about creating opportunities for mutual, cooperative play and achievement. And finally, it involves being intentional about orchestrating situations in which the child is able to apply their own character strengths in the service of themselves and others. When a teacher is intentional about increasing the frequency of positive moments for each child, good things happen. However, this is easier said than done. Even for the best teacher, the preschool environment is not always harmonious. Teachers often find themselves intervening in negative events rather than creating positive events. It is often beneficial for the teachers to devise a cueing system to remind themselves to actively engage each child with positive moments. One way is the 'penny transfer' technique (Cairone et al. 2007). For example, the teacher begins with five pennies in her left hand pocket. The jingling of the coins provides a good reminder to positively engage five children. Each time she connects with a child, she transfers one of the coins to her right pocket. When she has transferred all of the coins, she begins again with five new children. Soon the positive engagement becomes automatic and the cueing is unnecessary.

Creating positive events for young children is necessary but not sufficient in helping them engage in and benefit from strengths practice. Dreikurs and Soltz (1964) reminded us that young children are wonderful observers but rotten interpreters. It's not enough to make the moment—the teacher must also help make the meaning.

Meaning-Making

One prerequisite for a child's meaning-making is to develop what Tulving (2002) called a subjective perspective, the ability to attend to and make sense of mental states across time. Teachers and parents can nourish that ability by engaging consistently in mental state talk or mind-talk with the child. Referencing your own thoughts and feelings or wondering about the inner thoughts or feelings of a character in a book help the child orient their own inner life, their own mindfulness (Adrian et al. 2005; Taumoepeau and Ruffman 2008). Mental state talk promotes theory of mind, the awareness that others have thoughts, feelings, and intentions that can be different from your own. And that can become a developmental skill chain (mind-talk promotes theory of mind which then leads to perspective taking which eventually enriches to empathy). A classroom or home enriched with mind-talk is an environment that helps a child make meaning of life events, both positive and negative.

One significant obstacle for a positive event to become a meaningful experience for the child is the brain's negativity bias. The fields of neuroscience and positive psychology describe this negativity bias through which a child is more likely to attend to, process, and remember negative events than positive events (Hanson 2013; Rozin and Royzman 2001). Educators benefit from understanding how to help children attend to and process positive events and turn them into impactful experiences that are encoded in memory and nurtured to beliefs.

First, the teacher or parent can create the *pensive pause* for the child. A touch, a gaze, a thoughtful comment that gives positive valence to the child's behaviour is often all that it takes to help the child make meaning from the positive event. The teacher has helped the child to make an event an experience: *'Jamal, I just wanted to tell you how happy I was to watch you help Chris put the blocks away. That's using your kindness'*.

Another meaning-making strategy by the teacher or parent is to connect the event in the child's external environment to consequent emotions in the internal world: *'I'll bet you felt proud that you worked so long and hard in finishing that puzzle. Persevering with a hard job really makes you feel good'*. Young children do not automatically link external events to internal experiences and they benefit from the teacher's or parent's assistance to connect those dots.

And finally, the teacher can help the child link the current positive event and experience to other similar events or experiences in the past: *'When you shared your grapes with Julia and she smiled, it reminded me of when you let Michael have the first turn on the computer yesterday. You're really good at kindness and fairness'*. This strategy involves three elements: (1) labelling the strength(s), (2) identifying the resulting positive impact on others, and (3) reinforcing the strength(s) by linking it (them) to a past example(s) of strength use.

Memory-Making

As early as 18 months of age children begin to talk about the past and by age 3 they can talk about the past in a relatively coherent style (Hudson 1990). The work of Nelson and Gruendel (1986) marked a fundamental shift in the understanding of children's memory that has been continued with the work of the Family Narrative Lab at Emory University (Quas and Fivush 2009). They collectively emphasise a functional perspective in which children as young as preschoolers use memory to guide motivated behaviour to attain cognitive and social goals. Further, the way adults, especially mothers, reminisce with children impacts autobiographical memory and identity (McLean and Syed 2014; Perfect and Lindsay 2013). Our approach attempts to use the insights from a substantial body of research on reminiscing (Wareham and Salmon 2006) to help young children begin to weave emerging character strengths as thematic elements of their personal narrative.

In her pivotal treatise on the development of autobiographical memory, Fivush (2011) details the layers of representation that move beyond simple episodic memory of 'what happened' to the more personalised memory of 'what happened *to me*'. First the child must have a sense of the subjective self that experienced the event that includes personal thoughts and feelings about the event. And it is not simply that 'in that moment in the past I had thoughts and feelings', but also that 'they are *mine*. They are *owned by me*'. And finally, 'I can connect those past thoughts and feeling that were mine to the thoughts and feelings I have now' in remembering the events and even to the future in the self that will plan for them and experience them. This conceptualisation of autobiographical memory has generated a great deal of child development research in behavioural and neurological correlates of mental time travel (MTT) involved in recalling the past and predicting the future (Schacter et al. 2007; Busby and Suddendorf 2009).

Important recent research (Cleveland and Morris 2014; Cleveland and Reese 2005; Cleveland et al. 2007) has shed light on not only the importance of parent-child interactions about reminiscing in the formation of autobiographical memory, but also how parents can be trained in strategies for enriching the reminiscing experience. Children want to feel both confident and competent, and that means feeling that they have both opportunities for choice as well as the skills to make good choices. While young children can make sense of the past, they tend to struggle with reminiscing. Cleveland and Morris (2014) demonstrated that parents' language in support of reminiscence can serve both functions of encouraging autonomy and scaffolding structure in the formation of autobiographical memory. We adapted the parent training in autonomy-support and elaborative structure techniques developed by Cleveland and Reese to help teachers connect character strength use memories as thematic threads in the formation of the narrative self. Examples of such techniques include:

Autonomy Support

- In talking about strength use, follow the child's lead in the conversation.
- Expand on the child's specific strength use topic.
- Listen carefully to the child's talk about strength use and encourage her to elaborate. This might mean using back-channel responses such as 'I see' or 'Uh-huh' to confirm interest.
- Do not change the topic of conversation as long as the child is talking about strength use.

Elaborative Structure

- Ask many *Wh-* questions (what, when, where, who, why) to scaffold the child's recall of a strength use memory.
- Include statements that provide the child with new information about the event. For example, *'When you shared your blocks with Steven, he seemed very happy, and I bet you felt good'* (connects memory of behaviour to positive feeling consequences for another child and to positive feeling consequences for herself).
- Affirm the child's contributions to the reminiscence to help them own it as part of their narrative self.

We believe that teachers and parents can learn to scaffold narratives about past experiences of emerging character strength use for children such that they become organising principles for the life narrative that shapes the child's retrospective understanding of their past and their prospective understanding of their future. Teachers and parents are encouraged to: (1) identify emerging strengths, (2) call the child's attention to moments of strength use, and (3) scaffold the child's understanding of the connection between strength use and positive inner experiences as well as external outcomes. These will increase the likelihood that character strengths will help to generate the child's mindsets and beliefs about themselves, others, and the world in general.

Mindset-Making

Dweck's (2006) pioneering work on growth versus fixed mindsets provides potential insights into how adult-child interactions can shape enduring beliefs about a child's essential character strengths. For example, the way parents talk to their children shapes their associations to effort and perseverance. When a parent consistently praises intelligence rather than effort (*'Look how fast you did that puzzle... you're so smart!'*) the more likely the child is to avoid tasks that don't come fast and easy and to associate effort with failure. Using the scaffolding strategies mentioned in the previous section, teachers and parents can reinforce children's emerging character strengths.

One area of developmental research specific to preschoolers is their use of private speech or 'self-talk'. Vygotsky (1986) first pointed out the benefits of private speech. Private speech helps the child connect words, thoughts, and feelings in the service of critical thinking and self-regulation (Winsler et al. 2007). It is the forerunner of more complex executive functions and metacognition. We sought to develop unique ways of reinforcing a child's private speech about character strengths, namely through songs. While music may seem to be a peculiar pedagogical strategy, think about how you learned the alphabet. We have discovered that music is a powerful teaching tool particularly around character strengths. Eight years ago, Children Inc. launched a venture, Growing Sound (http://www.growing-sound.com), that develops and disseminates research-based children's music designed to promote social and emotional development from preschool through elementary grades. Over the last several years, Growing Sound published seven albums of songs informed by the field of positive psychology: (1) *Feeling positive: Songs of positive psychology for young children* (Kisor and Lottman 2010)—songs of curiosity, kindness, and gratitude; (2) *New day: Songs of hope and optimism for young children* (Hulefeld et al. 2010); (3) *Here, now, know-how: Songs of mindfulness for young children* (Kisor and Lottman 2012); (4) *Imagination generation: Songs of creativity for young children* (Kisor and Lottman 2011); (5) *Songs of resilience* (Kisor and Lottman 2006)—songs of perseverance, bravery, and zest; (6) *Take care,* songs of kindness, social intelligence, and love (Lottman 2012); and (7) *Everyone is someone*, songs of teamwork, fairness, and compassion (Lottman 2012).

While much of the content is described earlier, we also differentiate songs by their type and intent. For example, self-talk songs help a child learn and internalise private speech about character strengths. '*I can do it*' (Kisor 2006, track 1) and '*I'm gonna find a way*' (Kisor 2006, track 5; see Fig. 6.1) foster perseverance. Experiential songs such as '*Smell the flower, blow the candle out*' (Kisor 2010, track 9) allow the child to experience the strength of self-regulation and mindfulness practice. Story songs such as '*Miriam*' (Kisor 2010, track 13) and '*What if everyone did it too?*' (Kisor 2012, track 4) promote perspective taking and empathy. Concept songs such as '*Everyone is someone*' and '*Living in my own skin*' (Kisor 2012, track 6 and 10) encourage children to connect to their own unique strengths.

With moment-making, meaning-making, memory-making, and mindset-making we provide a menu of strategies for teachers and parents to nurture the well-doing

Fig. 6.1 Lyrics to a song about building perseverance (Kisor 2006)

I'M GONNA FIND A WAY
I keep on working till I figure it out
Figure it out, figure it out
I keep on working till I figure it out
I'm gonna find a way
I might have to do it again and again
5 6 7 8 9 10
I might have to do it again and again
But I'm gonna find a way
I keep on working till I figure it out
Figure it out, figure it out
I keep on working till I figure it out
I'm gonna find a way
I might have to turn things inside out
Inside out, inside out
I might have to turn things inside out
But I'm gonna find a way
I keep on working till I figure it out
Figure it out, figure it out
I keep on working till I figure it out
I'm gonna find a way

and well-being that is the constellation of character strengths that define the unique positive core of each child.

Phase 4: Teachers Support Parents' Strength-Spotting and Nurturing

The last phase involves training teachers and directors to have the competence and confidence in strength-spotting and strength appreciation so they can transfer these skills to parents. One of the most effective strategies for transferring parenting information and skills is through peer-to-peer learning. We utilise the Parent-Café model which has been used extensively across the United States in the Strengthening Families Program. Parent-Cafes are conducted by teachers and directors and use videos to introduce concepts, build skills to grow strengths, and to help their children acquire a positive mindset. The process is designed to generate meaningful conversations about examples of emerging character strengths in their children as well as their awareness of their own strengths and how they use them in their parenting practices.

The videos energise and motivate parents to take the first step in strengthsight which is completing the VIA Survey to gain insight into their own strengths. For parents, as well as teachers, this is often the first time they have thought about their child's character strengths and the first time anyone has helped them discover and use their own strengths. Niemiec (2014) discusses the phenomenon of 'strength blindness' where individuals are unaware of the strengths that others see in them. This is particularly true of many parents who are experiencing significant stressors and are questioning their own capacity to cope. Additionally many parents experience schools as problem-focused when communicating about their children. The opportunity to gain and apply strengthsight in reflecting more about themselves and their child, is not only informational for parents, but also motivational. It gives them a new lens and language to engage each other about their children and parenting. Initially reluctant parents quickly warm up to and embrace the chance to talk about their child's unique set of strengths, and their newly acquired awareness of their own strengths.

Conclusion

True social and emotional learning for children, parents, and teachers is not a process of bringing something from the outside in, but rather bringing something from the inside out. It is not just learning prescribed social skill sets, but more importantly tapping into strengths-based mindsets. And the new insights of character science and mindfulness provide tools for facilitating that process. The early childhood years are the incubator for character strengths, and until recently the important adults in the child's life lacked the effective monitors to detect and promote those strengths. In this application of character science to early childhood, this deficit is remedied and the pathways open up for tuning into, exploring, and expressing the best qualities of oneself and others.

References

Adrian, J. E., Clemente, R. A., Villanueva, L., & Rieffe, C. (2005). Parent-child picture-book reading, mother's mental state language and children's theory of mind. *Journal of Child Language, 32*, 673–686.

Baer, R. (2015). Ethics, values, virtues, and character strengths in mindfulness-based interventions: A psychological science perspective. *Mindfulness, 6*, 956–969. doi:10.1007/s12671-015-0419-2.

Bishop, S. R., Lau, M., Shapiro, S. L., Carlson, L., Anderson, N. D., Carmody, J., Segal, Z. V., Abbey, S., Speca, M., Velting, D., & Devins, G. (2004). Mindfulness: A proposed operational definition. *Clinical Psychology: Science and Practice, 11*, 230–241.

Biswas-Diener, R. (2006). From the equator to the North Pole: A study of character strengths. *Journal of Happiness Studies, 7*(3), 293–310. doi:10.1007/s10902-005-3646-8.

Briscoe, C. (2014). *A study investigating the effectiveness of mindfulness-based strengths practice (MBSP).* Thesis submitted to University of East London.

Busby, G. J., & Suddendorf, T. (2009). Preschoolers begin to differentiate the times of events from throughout the lifespan. *European Journal of Developmental Psychology, 6*(6), 746–762.

Cairone, K., Huber, D., & Likins, L. (2007). *Facing the challenge disc 2 (DVD).* Wilmington, DE: Video Active Productions.

Carlson, E. N. (2013). Overcoming the barriers to self-knowledge: Mindfulness as a path to seeing yourself as you really are. *Perspectives on Psychological Science, 8*(2), 173–186.

Cleveland, E. S., & Morris, A. (2014). Autonomy support and structure enhance children's memory and motivation to reminisce: A parental training study. *Journal of Cognition and Development, 15*(3), 414–436.

Cleveland, E. S., & Reese, E. (2005). Maternal structure and autonomy support in conversations about the past: Contributions to children's autobiographical memory. *Developmental Psychology, 41*, 376–388.

Cleveland, E. S., Reese, E., & Grolnick, W. S. (2007). Children's engagement and competence in personal recollection: Effects of parents' reminiscing goals. *Journal of Experimental Child Psychology, 96*, 131–149.

Dreikurs, R., & Soltz, V. (1964). *Children: The challenge*. New York: Hawthorne Books.

Dweck, C. (2006). *Mindset: The new psychology of success*. New York: Random House.

Fivush, R. (2011). The development of autobiographical memory. *Annual Review of Psychology, 62*, 559–582.

Fredrickson, B. L. (2001). The role of positive emotions in positive psychology: The broaden-and-build theory of positive emotions. *American Psychologist, 56*(3), 218–226.

Fredrickson, B. L. (2004). The broaden-and-build theory of positive emotions. *Philosophical Transaction of the Royal Society B, 359*, 1367–1377.

Fredrickson, B. L. (2013). Positive emotions broaden and build. In P. Devine & A. Plant (Eds.), *Advances in experimental social psychology* (Vol. 47, pp. 1–53). Burlington, VT: Academic Press.

Gander, F., Proyer, R. T., Ruch, W., & Wyss, T. (2012). Strength-based positive interventions: Further evidence for their potential in enhancing well-being. *Journal of Happiness Studies, 14*, 1241–1259. doi:10.1007/s10902-012-9380-0.

Hanson, R. (2013). *Hardwired for happiness: The new brain science of contentment, calm, and confidence*. New York: Harmony.

Harzer, C., & Ruch, W. (2012). When the job is a calling: The role of applying one's signature strengths at work. *The Journal of Positive Psychology, 7*(5), 362–371. doi:10.1080/17439760.2012.702784.

Hoffman, M. L. (1975). Developmental synthesis of affect and cognition and its implications for altruistic motivation. *Developmental Psychology, 11*(5), 607–622.

Hudson, J. A. (1990). The emergence of autobiographical memory in mother-child conversation. Knowing and remembering in young children. In R. Fivush & J. A. Hudson (Eds.), *Emory symposia in cognition* (Vol. 3, pp. 166–196). New York: Cambridge University Press.

Hulefeld, M., Kisor, D., & Lottman, T. (2010). *New day: Songs of hope and optimism for young children*. Covington, KY: Growing Sound.

Jennings, P. A. (2015). *Mindfulness for teachers: Simple skills for peace and productivity in the classroom*. New York, NY: W.W. Norton.

Kisor, D. (2006). *Songs of resilience*. Covington, KY: Growing Sound.

Kisor, D. (2010). *Feeling positive: Songs of positive psychology for young children*. Covington, KY: Growing Sound.

Kisor, D. (2012). *Here, now, know-how: Songs of mindfulness for young children*. Covington, KY: Growing Sound.

Kisor, D., & Lottman, T. (2006). *Songs of resilience*. Covington, KY: Growing Sound.

Kisor, D., & Lottman, T. (2010). *Feeling positive: Songs of positive psychology for young children*. Covington, KY: Growing Sound.

Kisor, D., & Lottman, T. (2011). *Imagination generation: Songs of creativity for young children*. Covington, KY: Growing Sound.

Kisor, D., & Lottman, T. (2012). *Here, now, know-how: Songs of mindfulness for young children*. Covington, KY: Growing Sound.

Linkins, M., Niemiec, R. M., Gillham, J., & Mayerson, D. (2014). Through the lens of strength: A framework for educating the heart. *The Journal of Positive Psychology, 10*(1), 64–68. doi:10.1080/17439760.2014.888581.

Linley, A. (2008). *Average to A+: Realising strengths in yourself and others*. Coventry, UK: CAPP Press.

Lottman, T. (2012). *The A.F.T.E.R. school program: Songs and activities promoting acceptance, friendship, teamwork, empathy and responsibility*. Covington, KY: Growing Sound.

Lottman, T., & Zawaly, S. (2014). *The character strengths of young children: A partial replication of Park & Peterson (2006)*. Unpublished data from Children, Inc.

McGrath, R. E. (2014). Character strengths in 75 nations: An update. *The Journal of Positive Psychology, 10*(1), 41–52. doi:10.1080/17439760.2014.888580.

McLean, K. C., & Syed, M. (Eds.). (2014). *The Oxford handbook of identity development*. New York: Oxford University Press.

Mooneyham, B. W., & Schooler, J. W. (2013). The costs and benefits of mind-wandering: A review. *Canadian Journal of Experimental Psychology, 67*(1), 11–18. doi:10.1037/a0031569.

Nelson, K., & Gruendel, J. (1986). *Event knowledge: Structure and function in development*. Hillsdale: Erlbaum.

Niemiec, R. M. (2012). Mindful living: Character strengths interventions as pathways for the five mindfulness trainings. *International Journal of Wellbeing, 2*(1), 22–33.

Niemiec, R. M. (2013). VIA character strengths: Research and practice (The first 10 years). In H. Knoop & A. Delle Fave (Eds.), *Well-being and cultures: Perspectives on positive psychology* (pp. 11–29). New York, NY: Springer.

Niemiec, R. M. (2014). *Mindfulness and character strengths: A practical guide to flourishing*. Cambridge, MA: Hogrefe.

Niemiec, R. M., & Lissing, J. (2015). Mindfulness-based strengths practice (MBSP) for enhancing well-being, life purpose, and positive relationships. In I. Ivtzan & T. Lomas (Eds.), *Mindfulness in positive psychology: The science of meditation and wellbeing*. London: Routledge.

Niemiec, R. M., & Wedding, D. (2014). *Positive psychology at the movies 2: Using films to build character strengths and well-being*. Boston, MA: Hogrefe.

Niemiec, R. M., Rashid, T., & Spinella, M. (2012). Strong mindfulness: Integrating mindfulness and character strengths. *Journal of Mental Health Counseling, 34*(3), 240–253.

Park, N., & Peterson, C. (2006a). Moral competence and character strengths among adolescents: The development and validation of the values in action inventory of strengths for youth. *Journal of Adolescence, 29*, 891–905.

Park, N., & Peterson, C. (2006b). Character strengths and happiness among young children: Content analysis of parental descriptions. *Journal of Happiness Studies, 7*(3), 323–341.

Park, N., Peterson, C., & Seligman, M. E. P. (2006). Character strengths in fifty-four nations and the fifty US states. *The Journal of Positive Psychology, 1*(3), 118–129.

Perfect, T. J., & Lindsay, D. S. (Eds.). (2013). *The SAGE handbook of applied memory*. London: Sage.

Peterson, C., & Seligman, M. E. P. (2004). *Character strengths and virtues: A handbook and classification*. New York, Washington, DC: Oxford University Press, American Psychological Association.

Proctor, C., Tsukayama, E., Wood, A. M., Maltby, J., Fox Eades, J., & Linley, P. A. (2011). Strengths Gym: The impact of a character strengths-based intervention on the life satisfaction and well-being of adolescents. *The Journal of Positive Psychology, 6*(5), 377–388.

Proyer, R. T., Sidler, N., Weber, M., & Ruch, W. (2012). A multi-method approach to studying the relationship between character strengths and vocational interests in adolescents. *International Journal for Educational and Vocational Guidance, 12*(2), 141–157.

Quas, J., & Fivush, R. (Eds.). (2009). *Emotion in memory and development: Biological, cognitive, and social considerations*. New York: Oxford University Press.

Quinlan, D. M., Swain, N., Cameron, C., & Vella-Brodrick, D. A. (2014). How 'other people matter' in a classroom-based strengths intervention: Exploring interpersonal strategies and classroom outcomes. *The Journal of Positive Psychology, 10*(1), 77–89. doi:10.1080/17439760.2014.920407.

Rozin, P., & Royzman, E. B. (2001). Negativity bias, negativity dominance, and contagion. *Personality and Social Psychology Review, 5*(4), 296–320.

Schacter, D. L., Addis, D. R., & Buckner, R. L. (2007). Remembering the past to imagine the future: the prospective brain. *Nature Reviews Neuroscience, 8*(9), 657–661.

Segal, Z. V., Williams, J. M. G., & Teasdale, J. D. (2002). *Mindfulness-based cognitive therapy for depression: A new approach to preventing relapse*. New York, NY: Guilford.

Seider, S., Novick, S., & Gomez, J. (2013). The effects of privileging moral or performance character development in urban adolescents. *Journal of Early Adolescence, 33*(6), 786–820.

Seligman, M. E. P., Steen, T. A., Park, N., & Peterson, C. (2005). Positive psychology progress: Empirical validation of interventions. *American Psychologist, 60*, 410–421.

Siegel, D. (1999). *The developing mind: Toward a neurobiology of interpersonal experience*. New York: Guilford Press.

Siegel, D. (2010). *Mindsight: The new science of personal transformation*. New York: Bantam Books.

Taumoepeau, M., & Ruffman, T. (2008). Stepping stones to others' minds: Maternal talk relates to child mental state language and emotion understanding at 15, 24, and 33 months. *Child Development, 79*(2), 284–302.

Tulving, E. (2002). Episodic Memory: From mind to brain. *Annual Review of Psychology, 53*, 1–25.

Vygotsky, L. (1986). *Thought and language* (A. Kozulin, Trans.). Cambridge, MA: MIT Press.

Wareham, P., & Salmon, K. (2006). Mother-child reminiscing about everyday experiences: Implications for psychological interventions in the preschool years. *Clinical Psychology Review, 26*(5), 535–554.

White, M. A., & Waters, L. E. (2014). A case study of 'The good school:' Examples of use of Peterson's strengths-based approach with students. *The Journal of Positive Psychology, 10*(1), 69–76. doi:10.1080/17439760.2014.920408.

Winsler, A., Manfra, L., & Diaz, R. M. (2007). "Should I let them talk?" Private speech and task performance among preschool children with and without behavior problems. *Early Childhood Research Quarterly, 22*(2), 215–231.

Chapter 7
Applying Positive Psychology in the Primary School: Celebrating Strengths, a UK Well-Being Project

Jenny Fox Eades and Judith Gray

Abstract This chapter describes the evolution and impact of a well-being project which was co-created by an educational adviser with experience of positive psychology and psychodynamic theory and a cluster of schools in areas of urban deprivation in the north of England. It argues that such projects need to be underpinned by a philosophy of education and suggests that there are three important levels of thinking and action for education—theory, framework, and practice. Finally, it argues for a specifically educational theory of well-being and what that might contain.

Abbreviation

WWW What went well

The Evolution of Celebrating Strengths

Celebrating Strengths (2008) evolved from a mental health project running in four schools in an area of urban deprivation in the North East of England. The original project focused on the importance of teachers telling traditional stories to children and also on how the daily and yearly rhythms of school life might contain anxiety and nurture relationships. After completing a distance learning course with Martin Seligman and discussing it with the schools, I (JFE) incorporated elements of positive psychology into the project.

J. Fox Eades (✉)
Edge Hill University, St Helens Road, Ormskirk, Lancashire L39 4QP, UK
e-mail: jennyfoxeades@gmail.com

J. Gray
Frodingham Infant School, Rowland Road, Scunthorpe, North Lincolnshire DN16 1ST, UK
e-mail: head.frodingham@northlincs.gov.uk

C. Proctor (ed.), *Positive Psychology Interventions in Practice*,
DOI 10.1007/978-3-319-51787-2_7

Celebrating Strengths has now been practiced by a number of schools in the UK for over 10 years and by schools in Australia and New Zealand for 6 years. Therefore, unlike many school initiatives, it is proving to be durable. The elements that might contribute to this durability—and whether these might be transferred to other approaches to well-being—will be discussed below.

Applying Positive Psychology in Schools

Character Strengths

The most obvious idea from positive psychology that is applied within Celebrating Strengths is a focus on the 24 VIA character strengths (Peterson and Seligman 2004). We took the 24 character strengths and linked them to the traditional stories we were telling and to the annual cycle of festivals we were creating. We wanted to focus explicitly on the strengths—by playing games or doing exercises we called 'strengths builders' which draw attention to and create opportunities to use the strengths.

We also wanted the strengths to implicitly influence the life of the school—by filling the auditory environment and the physical environment of the school with the language of strengths. So teachers learned about their *own* strengths, they used the words with children and with parents and with each other and classroom and corridor displays often referred to the character strengths.

In addition to the character strengths, an underlying theme of creating *positive habits of thought, speech, and behaviour* was woven into the strengths builders, the stories and traditions we created. This underlying theme incorporated other positive psychology concepts, such as flow (Csikszentmihalyi 1999), the importance of autonomy (Deci and Ryan 2008; Deci and Flaste 1995), Frederickson's (2001) 'broaden-and-build' theory on the importance of positive emotions, Dweck's (1999) work on mind-set, and Gable et al.'s (2004) work on active constructive responding.

We didn't teach children *about* these theories. We built the theories into the strengths builders, into the stories we told and into the traditions we created. For example, one of our earliest and simplest ideas, 'what went well' (WWW; Fox Eades 2006), was an adaptation of Seligman's (2011) three blessings exercise, with a deliberate focus on telling the story of what had gone well at the end of the day. The *Mood Booster*, a simple box of games/stories/exercises that boost the mood of the group or the individual (Fox Eades and Catt 2012b), was a way of building positive emotions (Frederickson 2001). A classroom exercise called *Speakers and Listeners* drew on the idea of responding constructively or enthusiastically to good news from the speaker (Gable et al. 2004) and involved telling and retelling that good news to enjoy it all the more (Fox Eades and Catt 2012a).

Positive Psychology Plus

Psychology and psychological methods of research are a dominant voice in education (Smeyers and Depaepe 2012), though this dominance is perhaps now being challenged by that of neuroscience (Kraft 2012). Historically however, education theory and practice have been influenced by a number of different disciplines besides psychology, including psychoanalysis, the history of education, theology, and philosophy. Celebrating Strengths follows in this tradition by drawing on theories and practices from a number of disciplines and combining them with positive psychology, to create what we feel is an educational philosophy and practice for schools.

Psychodynamic Theory

Psychodynamic theory derives originally from the work of Sigmund Freud (1930). It places emphasis on the unconscious dynamics and influences present in human interactions. Freud's ideas are still influential. For example, attachment theory is widely known about in education and is psychodynamic, deriving from the work of psychoanalyst John Bowlby (1969). Attachment theory proposes that children suffer in later life if they have failed to develop a secure attachment to a primary caregiver during early infancy and it is one of the theories behind Celebrating Strengths.

Another key psychodynamic influence on Celebrating Strengths was Bruno Bettelheim (1975). Bettelheim argued that the metaphors and symbols in fairy tales were important in helping children to make sense of their lives and to find hope in difficult situations.

Theology

In the past, theology or religion was an important influence on education—it is where questions of 'right' and 'wrong' have traditionally been addressed and is a source of sacred myths and hopeful stories (Rohr 2012). The schools that helped to develop Celebrating Strengths were secular schools in the UK. Precisely *because* they were secular schools and because few, if any, of their pupils were practising members of a faith community, they wanted the children to hear the rich, powerful, life giving stories of different faith traditions and to teach them to experience silence, beauty, and ritual. So we told faith stories as well as traditional tales and adopted practices, like silence and an annual rhythm of celebrations, into Celebrating Strengths.

The Impact of Working with Character Strengths on Staff and Children

Judith is the head teacher of an infant school in an area of high social deprivation in the north of England. She has worked with Celebrating Strengths for 7 years. Judith has described Celebrating Strengths as the *'platform from which we function'* (personal communication December 10, 2014). In my opinion, Judith is the UK head teacher who has embraced Celebrating Strengths the most and has embedded it into every facet of school life. It is not really a *'psychological intervention'*—it is, as Judith says, *'a basic philosophy to live by'* (personal communication December 10, 2014).

On a practical level, Celebrating Strengths is present in every classroom, in the corridors and in weekly assemblies. In the classroom there might be a WWW display on the wall, or a display asking how the children have used their strengths. The corridors are full of displays that show strengths in action in traditional stories and fairy tales. Every week starts with a whole school assembly where Judith retells a traditional or faith story that shows one of the character strengths in action (Fig. 7.1).

In addition, Judith constantly revisits the character strengths with staff and, at least once a term, staff do a 'strengths spotting' exercise at a staff training evening, where they encourage their colleagues by saying what strengths they have seen in each other in the past weeks.

The result of this consistent focus is that staff are able to draw quite naturally on a language of strengths in their everyday interactions with one another and with the children, even when working, as they frequently do, under extreme stress. Teachers are supported in looking for the best in children at all times. For example, Judith told me a story about a child who, because they had not really been taught any differently, kept looking in a teacher's handbag. Rather than see this as a purely negative action, the teacher reframed it in terms of the child's quite natural *curiosity* and allowed the child to observe some of the contents of the bag before gently explaining that, in the future, the bag was private to the teacher. The teacher had affirmed the child's curiosity, while redirecting their behaviour in a more appropriate way.

Celebrating Strengths has given adults and children in this school a language to speak about and reflect on positive, good, and beautiful things—and the opportunities to do so. It has changed what they talk about and what they focus on.

One of the class teachers, Kayley, told me a story about a little girl whose behaviour was unusual. When listening to classical music she would see vivid pictures in her mind and talk about them. The other children initially laughed at her unusual behaviour but Kayley quietly commented on the girl's intense imagination and *creativity* and, as Kayley said, *'the children didn't laugh anymore'* (personal communication December 10, 2014).

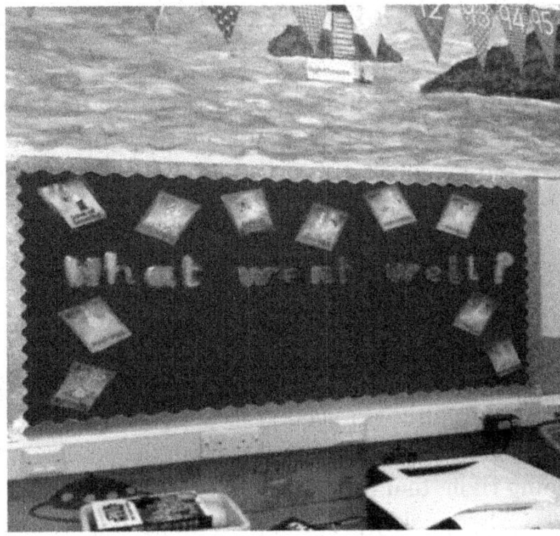

Fig. 7.1 A classroom display of 'what went well?' (WWW), using post cards of selected character strengths

Research into Celebrating Strengths

An Evaluation Report

Celebrating Strengths was evaluated by Reena Govindji and Professor Alex Linley of the Centre for Applied Positive Psychology (now the Centre of Applied Positive Psychology, http://www.cappeu.com) in 2008. They spoke to head teachers, teachers, pupils, and parents at five participating schools in the north of England. One theme that emerged from the evaluation was an increase in the children's self-confidence and motivation to achieve. This was seen as resulting from greater awareness of, and ability to use, their strengths. The report also highlighted significantly improved behaviour both in the school and home environment. Staff involved in using the approach highlighted how it had significantly impacted children's cognitive, emotional, and behavioural development.

Celebrating Strengths was linked to specific improvements in literacy skills because of the focus on story-telling, and to the creation of a calmer school environment that helped students at examination times. One school noted how exclusions from school had been reduced by half following its introduction. The report also noted improvements in the relationships between children, and said that Celebrating Strengths had helped children to understand that everybody has strengths. It had also improved the quality of staff relationships and interactions and increased their resilience in dealing with difficult students.

Telling the Story of Celebrating Strengths

In my own research I have asked teachers and pupils to *tell the story* of what Celebrating Strengths has meant to them and to their pupils. One of Judith's teachers told me the story of a little boy I shall call Colin.

Colin's Story

When I spoke with his teacher, Colin had only been with the school about 6 weeks. He was a boy with a traumatic family history, very high levels of anxiety and a deep fear of failure. He needed to get everything right in order to feel safe and he also needed constant reassurance from the adults around him that he *was* getting everything right, that he was ok.

Colin quickly picked up on the strengths language he heard all around him at the school. At first he learned to spot strengths in other children and did so, very generously and spontaneously. Gradually, he learned to recognise and believe that he had strengths of his own. Colin's teacher described the language of strengths as *'a tool he uses to get through the day'* (personal communication December 10, 2014). He was learning to tolerate failure because even when not getting things 'right' he knew he was using his strengths and those around him recognised and affirmed him for doing so. He now needed less reassurance because he was coming to believe that he had strengths which he could draw on. He was learning to see the good in himself.

Bethany's Story

Bethany was a little girl who had never really been anywhere outside the town where she lived. She had never seen the sea. She had never visited the countryside. She had never seen a forest. So when her school took her to a 'forest school' (http://www.forestschoolassociation.org) she was filled with awe. She walked around, listening to the sound of the rain on the leaves repeating to herself: *'Beautiful. It is so beautiful'* (personal communication December 10, 2014). She did not want to join in with the activities or the other children. She just wanted to walk and look and wonder.

It would have been easy for Bethany's teacher to react with concern—Bethany was being 'anti-social' after all, she was apparently not 'engaging in learning'. But Bethany's teacher has worked at celebrating children's strengths for over 7 years now and so instead of seeing Bethany or her behaviour as a problem, she saw that Bethany was using some important strengths and respected her desire for solitude. Later, she said to Bethany: *'Your love of beauty, your spirituality, are just amazing'*.

I don't know, of course, but I suspect that Bethany will always remember that day. She will remember it as her first real encounter with beauty and she will remember being allowed to enjoy that beauty in her own way. She will also remember having a teacher who valued her, who recognised the importance of what was happening, and who saw and commented on her strengths.

John and George's Story

John and George are a little older than Colin and Bethany. They are in Year 6 at another school I have worked with and they have helped to lead *Celebrating Strengths* at their school since they were in Year 3. I interviewed them as part of my research.

John and George decide on the strength of the week for the whole school. They take a lead in looking for examples of that strength in their peers, or *strengths spotting*, and award certificates or stickers at the end of the week in assembly. They keep the language and idea of strengths alive for their hard-working teachers. Since they were both in Year 6 when we spoke, they were preparing to help the younger ones take a lead when they left the following year. Not only were they exercising leadership within the school through Celebrating Strengths they were encouraging other pupils to become leaders too.

Their thoughts and reflections are worth sharing in detail. *'It has helped us so much…like out in the playground if people are getting left out…people see how strengths help… it's made people think more about what they do…they reflect more on their actions and stuff…it makes kids...like…want to do kind things more...they know about the strengths and how to do them so it makes them do them more… we've learned how to use strengths more…it's taught them what the strength is and how to use it…'* (personal communication July 18, 2015).

Speaking of what they, personally, had learned from Celebrating Strengths the boys said: *'We've learned patience…we've sort of grown…we've learned to work with people better…'* (personal communication July 18, 2015).

And in the following comment, one of them sums up Aristotle's belief that we learn how to use the character strengths and virtues by using them: *'I think it's actually helped people's teamwork...like they do teamwork to get a sticker…but then they really know how to do teamwork'* (personal communication July 18, 2015).

The Teachers' Story

Their teacher, like other teachers interviewed, focused on the importance of the character strengths as a language: *'It gives you a language to talk about what you're good at'* (personal communication July 18, 2015). Other teachers have said it gives children *'a way of thinking about themselves'* or *'something to fall back on in times of difficulty'* (personal communication May 19, 2014). They also comment that it helps children *'learn to value each other'* (personal communication December 10, 2014).

Two teachers whose school had gone through a very turbulent period said that *'this got us through'* that it was *'a commonality holding things together'* (personal communication December 9, 2014).

A head teacher from Australia noted that, *'this is all about relationship'* (personal communication May 19, 2015). This comment suggests an important question to ask of any school project on positive psychology whatever its focus—does it support and enhance relationships? Relationships are at the core of well-being and at the heart of learning, so enhancing relationships must be a priority for any project that seeks to improve well-being in an educational context. Then the questions become: Does this positive psychology project help children and young people form better relationships with one another and with themselves? Does it improve teachers' relationships with one another and with their students? Is there an impact on the school's relationship with parents?

Creating Durable Well-Being Projects or Interventions

Celebrating Strengths has proved to be a durable project. One colleague called it a 'sticky' project (personal communication June 1, 2015). It has persisted in schools that have experienced changes of head teacher, change of building, and even changes of name and identity—and it is still around when other projects have faded and been forgotten. There may be many reasons for this durability. I suggest that one is the focus on stories and storytelling and another is the link that is made between concepts and *practices*.

Stories to Live by

The Franciscan writer, Richard Rohr (2012), notes that the Western world has replaced the inspiring stories of myth and legend with the stories of economics and materialism and consumerism. One might add the story of celebrity to that list. Such stories do not inspire—they hold no wisdom and little hope. Humans need stories to make sense of their lives and each generation passes on its values to the next through story. Psychological frameworks and techniques, concepts like resilience, flow, and positive emotion are important—but not, I would argue, enough to inspire us to lead a fulfilling life or to enjoy well-being. For that, we need a sense of purpose and a sense of meaning.

Bettelheim (1975) said that stories help children—and adults—in 'the struggle for meaning' (p. 3). By linking the character strengths to particular traditional folk and faith stories and by embedding concepts, such as flow and positive emotions in the *practice* of storytelling, we helped to embody positive psychology into school in a way that teachers found supportive on a daily basis—and which was clearly educational—and therefore they kept on doing it. The characters in the stories served to

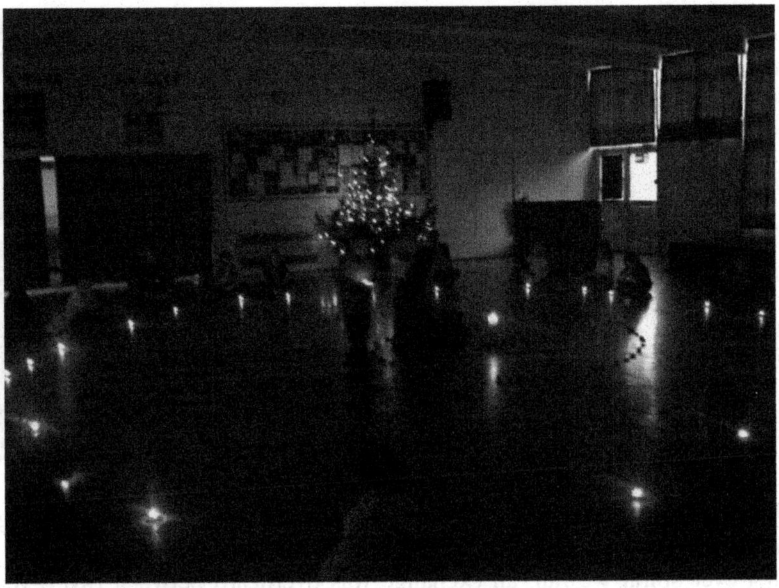

Fig. 7.2 The spiral of lights

bring the strengths 'to life' for children. They can remember Anansi, the spider, when they think of wisdom, or the shy monk Caedmon when they need some courage. Stories and storytelling turn concepts from positive psychology—and from psychodynamic theory—into practices teachers can use every day.

Traditions and Institution Wide 'Habits'

Another way that we embodied positive psychology in Celebrating Strengths was by making links between concepts and regular celebrations or 'traditions'. Human institutions are, by nature, quite conservative. Once something has happened several times we feel as if we have always done it this way. We took deliberate advantage of this trait and built or created traditions or customs that became, essentially, institution wide *habits*, practices that happened each day or each week, each term or each year. We then made a link between that custom and particular character strengths or ideas from positive psychology so that, each time the custom was repeated, the character strength or idea was also revisited in an explicit way.

For example, one of the most powerful and beautiful traditions we developed was a walking meditation called *The Spiral of Lights*. Once a year, in the run up to Christmas, each class takes it in turns to spend 30 min in the hall, walking a spiral made of pebbles and creating a circle of candlelight—in silence—with Allegri's Miserere playing in the background (Figs. 7.2 and 7.3).

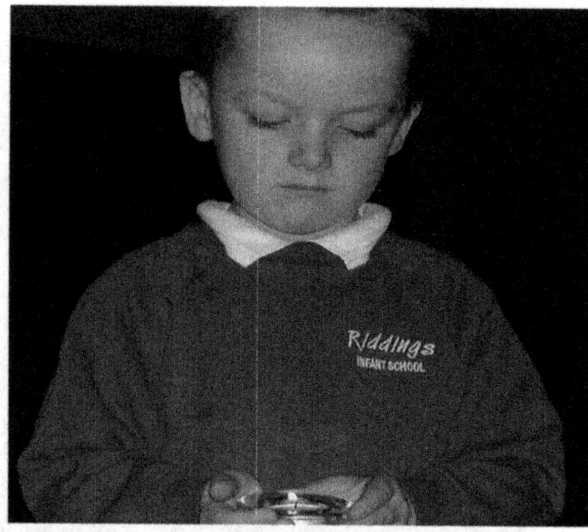

Fig. 7.3 A pupil showing complete absorption in The Spiral of Lights walking meditation

We linked the spiral walk to the strengths of hope and spirituality, though we might also have made a link to love of beauty since it is a beautiful practice. After the first ever spiral we ran, an exchange was overheard between two 6-year-old boys. One said: *'That was nice'*. The other replied: *'No, that was beautiful'* (personal communication December 6, 2004).

Other assemblies and activities in the same term pick up on the themes of hope and spirituality. Ten years later, the schools that helped develop the spiral walk are still practicing it and therefore still thinking, explicitly, about hope and about spirituality. They have essentially forgotten that there was ever a time when their school did *not* do the spiral of lights in the run up to Christmas. We have firmly embedded the concepts of hope and spirituality—and the importance of silence to well-being—because they are linked to a durable practice or tradition.

Three Levels of Educational Thinking and Practice

In addition to the presence of stories, storytelling, and the deliberate use of tradition, I suggest that there is a third reason why Celebrating Strengths has proved to be a durable method for applying concepts from positive psychology in schools. And that is because it works at three different levels or in three different ways:

- It is rooted in a theory and philosophy of *education*.
- It provides a framework of practical ideas and suggestions for teachers.
- It allows teachers to be creative—to turn the ideas and suggestions into personal and classroom practices, adapted to their own environment.

All of these ways of working, or levels of thinking and practice are, I think, essential if positive psychology is to make a lasting contribution in schools.

The Importance of a Theory and Philosophy of Education

Positive psychology has its own theory and philosophy behind it, but it is the theory and philosophy of psychology. The philosophy of education and the goals of schools are not necessarily identical with either the philosophy or the goals of psychology. If positive psychology is applied in schools, it needs to begin to address the question of the purposes of education and how a particular 'intervention' might support or detract from one or more of these purposes. Often the purposes of education are assumed rather than made explicit and 'being happy' is assumed to be one such purpose. But is it? Should it be?

Discussion of the purposes of education—and how positive psychology supports one or more of those purposes—would help ensure that positive psychology does not prove to be a passing fad but makes a mature contribution to the education of the next generation. You need to have thought about *why* you are doing something—what values you are trying to implement—in order to assess whether a particular practice helps to embody those values or achieve that goal.

Celebrating Strengths was rooted in certain fundamental educational ideas. These included:

- Teachers are the most important part of the child's environment.
- All learning happens in relationships and our emotions affect our learning.
- Children need to be securely attached to their teachers to learn well.
- The body, the mind, and the emotions are all linked.
- All behaviour is a kind of communication and some of it is unconscious.

I do not claim that when we started out we had a coherent, comprehensive, philosophy of education. However, part of what evolved in the development of Celebrating Strengths was what Judith has called *'a philosophy to live by'* (Personal communication December 10, 2014). We were asking questions about what education was for, what school might be like—philosophical questions and educational questions. We have continued—and continue—to ask these questions and the questions inform what we do within Celebrating Strengths and how we do it.

A Framework of Practical Ideas

In addition to thinking about *why* we engage in education and why we might use positive psychology within education, it is also important to think about *how* we might do that. In the case of Celebrating Strengths, we developed a corpus of stories, a series of traditions, and a language of strengths that gave teachers and pupils a framework to work within and suggestions for how they might implement ideas from positive psychology.

Importantly, the framework was there to provide structure and guidance, not to prevent innovation or stifle creativity. What teachers do in their classroom, how they tell stories, follow traditions, and make use of the language of strengths is left to their personal judgement and individual enthusiasms and has to be adapted to the needs of the particular situation, group, or child they are working with.

It is important to provide a framework so that teachers feel supported in attempting to implement abstract concepts like flow, strengths, or positive emotions in real situations. At the same time, it is also important to refrain from over prescription, from attempting to legislate exactly what teachers should say and do in the classroom. A handbook can be useful but simply following a handbook is not teaching—teaching is the moment by moment creative response to the changing situation and needs of the people you are with.

A Creative Personal Response

The third and arguably the most important part of any initiative, is how it is put into action by each teacher—what actually happens on a daily basis, what do teachers *do* with these ideas, this framework, today, this morning, with this child or group of children? And these daily practices need to be crafted by individual teachers because only they can know the needs of their class and what their own particular strengths and enthusiasms are.

I would also argue that these practices need to be implemented by the teacher in their own life first and only then used with pupils. As Judith puts it, *'it depends on how the teacher and the teaching assistant in the classroom keep it alive'* and she adds that staff *'embody'* it (Personal communication December 10, 2014). For example, Judith's staff spot strengths in one another and in themselves before they try to practice strengths spotting with pupils.

If we don't practice these ideas in our own lives, then we may teach *about* positive psychology but we cannot model it for our pupils and modelling has always been seen as one of the most powerful of teaching techniques. Do we talk about gratitude or do we feel and show it? Do we expect children to show a growth mindset or do we cultivate one for ourselves? In other words, do the adults in the school practice positive psychology for themselves, first, or is it something they try to *do* to the children while ignoring its implications for their own lives?

At the schools I work with there is no question that, at their best, positive psychology has become a daily practice, a school wide positive habit.

Conclusion: An Educational Concept of Well-Being

From my own research and from 11 years of working in well-being in schools, I suggest that it is not enough to assume that we know what 'well-being' means in the context of education. It is a term that has many meanings, from the purely physical, to the emotional and spiritual. If we are going to promote well-being in schools, what kind of well-being is it that we are going to promote? Do we want pupils to feel cheerful all the time and experience no sadness, or struggle, or failure? Do we want them to do whatever they can to achieve success, even at the expense of their health or the happiness of those around them?

If the answer to these questions is 'no', and I suspect that for most educators it will be, then the well-being we actually seek to promote must contain some notion of virtue or morality, must encompass the ability to cope with challenges, and must involve the physical body as well as the disembodied mind.

Virtue: Beauty and Pleasure

For the ancient Greek philosophers, whose influence is acknowledged by positive psychologists (Peterson and Seligman 2004), it simply made no sense to consider happiness apart from virtue or goodness. The happy or fulfilled life just *was* the virtuous life. If education is about preparing children to lead a fulfilling life then how to live well, how to be moral, is a necessary part of that preparation.

I am not suggesting that we impose a particular morality or view of morality onto children. I am suggesting that we give them a language in which to think about virtue and about right and wrong—that is, a language of character strengths and virtues. I also suggest that we tell them stories that explore these ideas and that we give children tools like philosophical enquiry (http://www.philosophy4children.co.uk/) that will allow them to engage in discussion and to reach their own conclusions. An educational well-being cannot avoid engaging with ideas about virtue if it is serious about preparing the next generation to lead a fulfilling life.

I also want to argue that our educational concept of well-being should be about beauty as much as it is about health. There is a great deal of emphasis on health in our culture—and in education. One writer talks about our 'obsession with health' which 'tends to medicalize every moment' (Bruckner 2000, p. 52). Alongside the ancients' view that morality was an intrinsic part of well-being, they also saw beauty as an intrinsic part of it. If we focus on promoting well-being as a way to stem the perceived rising tide of youth depression, we paradoxically make ill-health and depression the centre of our attention. Since it is often said that we get more of what we focus on, I suggest that we need to focus instead on putting more beauty and more simple pleasures into the classroom—and on teaching pupils to stop and appreciate them. A simple story well-told is a work of art—and we can stop, enjoy it, and benefit from it together. We are not, then, involved in a 'health intervention' at all but in doing education—beautifully—and in a way that will help us to thrive.

Challenging

Learning is not, nor should it be, always easy, always comfortable. Neither is life. One of our reasons for including traditional tales in Celebrating Strengths is precisely their inclusion of the struggles and challenges of life. These are always set in a hopeful context—the stories we tell have happy endings—but death, misfortune, and failure are all present.

Dewey (1922) argues that learning only happens when we are out of step with our environment—if all is well, we coast and we do not grow or learn. So discomfort is an inherent part of the learning process and pupils need to learn to fail and how to come back from failure. As Colin's story above illustrates, understanding that we have, like all other human beings, character strengths and virtues, means that we can afford to fail and know that we have resources to fall back on in times of trouble.

Resilience, according to Judith, is not a particular strength but is a result of our ability to draw on all the strengths at the right time. An educational concept of well-being has to involve the ability to fail and to take risks in learning. Without that, there is no education.

Embodied

Western ideas of psychological well-being largely ignore the body and its intimate connection with mind and emotion (Christopher 1999; Sugarman 2007). I suggest that a concept of well-being or flourishing that is educational must attempt to avoid Cartesian assumptions of a disembodied mind and acknowledge the embodied nature of flourishing and of education itself.

Richard Shusterman (2008), a philosopher who specialises in thinking about the body, argues that it is because we fail to notice simple, physical pleasures and increasingly seek stimulation through the consumption of mass media that we are suffering from over stimulation. This leads, he says, to an inability to engage in 'tranquil, steady and sustained attention'(Shusterman 2008, p. 7).

In Celebrating Strengths, we have adopted deliberately low tech practices, which use the body, the mind, and emotions together, like the use of silence, walking meditations, and oral storytelling. In this way we try to counter-balance children's increasing use of technology and to ensure that they and we can engage in 'tranquil, steady and sustained attention' (Shusterman 2008, p. 7).

At Judith's school they embody the character strengths and virtues by making the British Sign Language sign for each strength whenever they say it and the children pick this up quite naturally. When I interviewed Judith for my research she signed all the way through the conversation without noticing because she simply cannot say *'love'*, or *'courage'*, or *'self-control'*, without making the corresponding signs. You can, quite literally, see character strengths and virtues being celebrated all day, every day in the classroom and in the playground, by teachers, support staff, and by the children themselves.

References

Bettelheim, B. (1975). *The uses of enchantment: The meanings and importance of fairy tales*. London: Penguin.

Bowlby, J. (1969). *Attachment and loss: Vol.1. attachment*. New York: Basic Books.

Bruckner, P. (2000). *Perpetual euphoria: The duty to be happy*. Princeton: Princeton University Press.

Christopher, J. C. (1999). Situating psychological well-being: Exploring the cultural roots of its theory and research. *Journal of Counseling & Development, 77*, 141–152.

Csikszentmihalyi, M. (1999). *Flow: The psychology of optimal experience*. New York: Harper & Row.

Deci, E., & Flaste, R. (1995). *Why we do what we do: Understanding self-motivation*. London: Penguin.

Deci, E. L., & Ryan, R. M. (2008). Hedonia, eudaimonia, and well-being: An introduction. *Journal of Happiness Studies, 9*, 1–11.

Dewey, J. (1922). Human nature and conduct. 2012 ed. Digireads.com Publishing.

Dweck, C. (1999). *Self-theories: Their role in motivation, personality and development*. New York: Psychology Press.

Fox Eades, J. M. (2006). *Classroom tales: Using storytelling to build emotional, social and academic skills across the primary curriculum*. London: Jessica Kingsley Publishers.

Fox Eades, J. M. (2008). *Celebrating strengths: Building strengths-based schools*. Coventry: CAPP Press.

Fox Eades, J., & Catt, B. (2012a). *Our Community festival*. Kirkby-in-Ashfield: TTS.

Fox Eades, J., & Catt, B. (2012b). *Performing arts festival*. Kirkby-in-Ashfield: TTS.

Frederickson, B. L. (2001). The role of positive emotions in positive psychology: The broaden-and-build theory of positive emotions. *American Psychologist, 56*, 218–226.

Freud, S. (1930). Civilisation and its discontents. In I. Smith (Ed.), *Freud—Complete works* (pp. 4462–4532). http://www.valas.fr/IMG/pdf/Freud_Complete_Works.pdf.

Gable, S., Reis, H., Impett, E., & Asher, E. (2004). What do you do when things go right? The intrapersonal and interpersonal benefits of sharing good events. *Journal of Personality & Social Psychology, 87*, 228–245.

Kraft, V. (2012). Neuroscience and education: Blind spots in a strange relationship. *Journal of Philosophy of Education, 46*(3), 386–396.

Peterson, C., & Seligman, M. E. P. (2004). *Character strengths and virtues: A classification and handbook*. Washington, DC: American Psychological Association.

Rohr, R. (2012). *Falling upward*. London: SPCK.

Seligman, M. E. P. (2011). *Flourish: A new understanding of happiness and well-being and how to achieve them*. London: Nicholas Brealey.

Shusterman, R. (2008). *Body consciousness: A philosophy of mindfulness and somaesthetics*. Cambridge: Cambridge University Press.

Smeyers, P., & Depaepe, M. (2012). The lure of psychology for education and educational research. *Journal of Philosophy of Education, 46*(3), 315–331.

Sugarman, J. (2007). Practical rationality and the questionable promise of positive psychology. *Journal of Humanistic Psychology, 472*, 175–197.

Chapter 8
Transforming Our Schools Together: A Multi-School Collaboration to Implement Positive Education

Denise M. Quinlan

Abstract This chapter outlines the story of the decade-long collaboration by a cluster of low- to mid-SES state schools that implemented positive education and transformed their school cultures. In the process they developed more cohesive staff teams and supported leadership development at principal and teacher level, as well as enhancing student and teacher well-being. The Cluster schools embedded gratitude, strength spotting, and appreciative inquiry as core practices in their schools and introduced and developed programmes and activities aligned with positive education. Factors contributing to the success of this collaboration included the shared values of a leadership group committed to improving student flourishing, an inclusive and flexible approach to planning and implementation, and recognition of each school's particular context and priorities. This group of schools overcame numerous challenges providing evidence that low- to mid-SES schools can successfully collaborate to implement positive education with significant benefits for students and staff.

Abbreviations

AI	Appreciative inquiry
RTLB	Resource, teacher: learning and behaviour
SES	Socioeconomic status
SWPB4L	School Wide Positive Behaviour for Learning
VIA-IS	Values in action—inventory of strengths

D.M. Quinlan (✉)
4 Sim Street, Māori Hill, Dunedin 9010, New Zealand
e-mail: denise@drdenisequinlan.com

C. Proctor (ed.), *Positive Psychology Interventions in Practice*,
DOI 10.1007/978-3-319-51787-2_8

Introduction

He oranga ngākau he pikinga waiora.
[Positive feelings in your heart will enhance your sense of self-worth].

It is almost a decade since the label *positive education* was coined to describe the adoption of positive psychology in schools with the explicit goal of supporting student well-being (Norrish 2015). Since the mid-2000s the scientific literature on positive education has grown as programmes and practices for schools have been developed and researched (e.g., Green et al. 2007; Norrish et al. 2013; Oades et al. 2011; Seligman et al. 2009; Waters 2011). Schools however, are not laboratories and the myriad of factors on which they can differ means conducting randomised controlled trials is problematic. Programmes that are not effective in a brief controlled trial may work well over a longer time period, as a component of a broader well-being effort, in a different teacher's classroom, or in a different school environment. Fortunately, there is much we can learn from the experiences of schools that have implemented positive education.

The positive education journeys of schools provide important information and inspiration for other schools. Geelong Grammar School, an elite Australian school that pioneered implementation of positive education, has shared valuable case studies, rich details of activities, and insights from staff and students in the story of its decade-long journey (Norrish 2015). However, less is known about how lower-SES schools have managed to support well-being on limited budgets or how schools have collaborated to achieve their well-being goals. This chapter[1] outlines the story of the decade-long collaboration of a cluster of low- to mid-SES (socioeconomic status) state schools that successfully implemented positive education to transform their school cultures. To our knowledge, this is the first collaborative cluster to implement positive psychology across their schools. This collaboration has helped build cohesive staff teams, supported leadership development, and enhanced student and teacher well-being. We hope that some of the lessons learned and benefits obtained may be of use to others in education that serve similar communities.

Background to the Well-Being Cluster

The South Dunedin Schools Well-Being Cluster was formed in late 2006 to support student well-being through social and emotional learning. The Cluster comprised nine primary and intermediate schools ranging in size from approximately 100–300 students. All schools were coeducational and one school was affiliated to a church. The schools served low- to mid-SES populations in a city of 130,000 people in New

[1]This chapter is dedicated with heartfelt gratitude to the principals of Te Wai Pounamu Well-Being Cluster: W. Cormick, M. Hillerby, R. McQuillan-Mains, J. Sinclair, D. Smith, G. Tenbeth, and S. Turnbull.

Zealand where the school year comprises four 10-week terms that run from February to December.

Almost one in five New Zealand children live in medium to risk households (exposure to 3–4 risk factors) and a further 6% live in households exposed to five or more risk factors (high risk) such as living in an area of high deprivation, being victims of crime or discrimination, having poor mental health, feeling isolated, or having multiple housing problems (Statistics New Zealand 2012). Cluster principals were concerned for the welfare of their students, a number of whose families experienced intergenerational unemployment, drug and alcohol addiction, domestic abuse, or poverty. Principals observed the growing number of students with socio-emotional behavioural and learning difficulties, without a corresponding increase in school behavioural support resources.

The Cluster successfully applied for a government education funding stream to address learning difficulties (including emotional and behavioural difficulties) and used this funding to implement a circle time (Mosley 2005; Roffey 2006) programme across the Cluster. Teachers learned how to lead classroom circle or group discussions about feelings, challenges, or conflict. This process created opportunities for children to practice respectful communication, and empowered students to find peaceful ways to resolve conflict. As an extension of the programme, the schools also introduced playground games and activities that encouraged cooperative play and reduced playground conflict.

Within 2 years, Cluster schools' principals could see positive changes in students and staff. Students were learning to take turns, listen, and express their feelings in a safe environment. Teachers were leading classroom discussions about feelings and values, and becoming more understanding of the factors underlying challenging student behaviour. A number of schools had implemented values-based programmes and were working to embed them through circle time discussions. The Cluster schools were united in their desire to continue in this direction. The commitment, through circle time, to a safe environment and development of socioemotional competency of teachers and students prepared the ground for positive education to take root successfully in the Cluster schools.

The Implementation of Positive Education Across the Cluster

This section outlines how positive education was implemented in Cluster schools from 2009 to 2014. It describes the main professional development undertaken by the schools and some of the activities introduced for staff and students. A presentation on positive psychology in March 2009 by the author sparked teacher interest and enthusiasm. The author's focus on gratitude (Emmons and McCullough 2004), strengths (Peterson and Seligman 2004), and appreciative inquiry (AI; Cooperrider et al. 2003) as tools for growth and change resonated with Cluster principals (illustrated in Fig. 8.1). Discovering a shared vision of compassion, connection, and mindfulness in schools and a commitment to 'looking for the best in each other

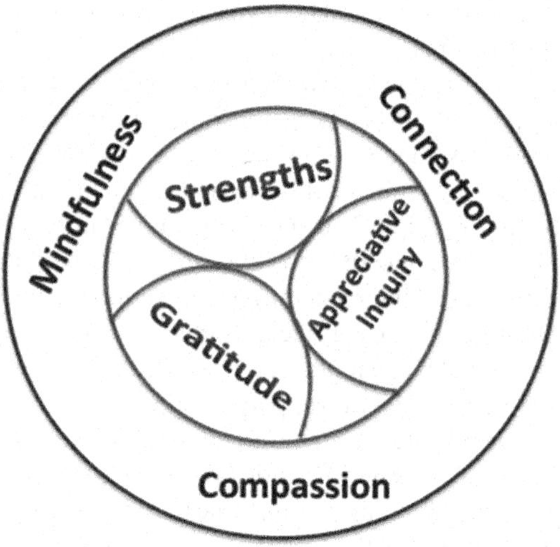

Fig. 8.1 Building a positive environment: Tools for growth and change (D. Quinlan ©)

rather than fixing the worst', the Cluster began what became a long-term partnership with the author to explore and embed positive education in their schools.

In October of 2009 principals and a senior behavioural support teacher from six Cluster schools visited schools implementing positive psychology in education in Melbourne, Australia. This week-long visit created a shared experience that brought this leadership group closer together and has been often referred to by the principals as pivotal in developing the trust and open communication that allowed the group to work effectively together.

The group were impressed with how Geelong Grammar School and other nearby private schools were implementing whole school programmes to support student and staff well-being. They were perhaps most inspired however by their visit to a low-SES Melbourne school whose charter of positive 'trademark behaviours' for the staffroom, supportive and warm staff interactions, classroom tools such as the 'catastrophe gauge' to help students find perspective, and confident, articulate students impressed them deeply. This school had a similar demographic with similar challenges and the Cluster was optimistic that if positive education could take root here, it could work as well in New Zealand.

Introducing Positive Education to All Staff

If positive education was to become embedded in their schools, then the principals believed it needed to be shared with all staff. In 2010, the renamed Te Wai Pounamu Well-being Cluster began its implementation of positive education at a professional development day for all staff including teacher aides, support staff, and caretakers. Staff were given an overview of positive psychology that outlined the contribution of well-being to beneficial life outcomes including academic achievement (Seligman et al. 2009), models of well-being (Ryff and Keyes 1995; Seligman 2002), and the role and influence of positive emotions (Fredrickson 1998; Fredrickson and Joiner 2002; Fredrickson et al. 2008). Staff had completed the Values in Action—Inventory of Strengths (VIA-IS; Peterson and Seligman 2004) prior to the training day and explored how well-being can be enhanced by identifying and developing character strengths (Govindji and Linley 2007; Linley et al. 2010; Seligman et al. 2005; Quinlan et al. 2015a). They also learned why practices such as gratitude (Sheldon and Lyubomirsky 2006; Froh et al. 2009) and kindness (Lyubomirsky et al. 2004; Otake et al. 2006) influence well-being (Lyubormirsky et al. 2005).

Soon afterwards each school conducted staff meetings to discuss how they would begin to implement this information in their school. Plans emerged through responding to five questions:

- What have we learned?
- What are we most excited about?
- What's the best focus for our school? (Where in our school might we most easily and successfully implement this information?)
- What are our concerns?
- What's the next smallest step we can take?

These questions enabled staff to share their enthusiasm and concerns and to focus implementation on each school's particular context and the staff capacity to make immediate small-scale change. Priorities were to foster gratitude in children, to increase awareness and experience of positive emotions, and to focus attention on staff well-being. Across all schools there was enthusiasm for learning more about strengths and sharing this with students and staff.

The Cluster principals had agreed that teachers should be given time to learn about positive psychology and use it personally and as a staff group before introducing it to the classroom. The focus for the first year was staffroom behaviours, starting staff meetings by sharing 'what went well' for each participant, and using an AI approach (Cooperrider et al. 2003) for strategic planning and reviews. In practice, teachers were soon asking to take positive education to their students. Most teachers wanted to share gratitude practices and strengths information with the students, and supported noticing 'three good things' to start or end the day and the introduction of 'strengths assemblies'. A number of teachers introduced discussion of strengths into their classrooms. This was based on their own initiative and not part of a required programme.

Small-Scale, Teacher-Led Initiatives

Rather than focusing on the 24 character strengths of the VIA classification (which principals thought would be overwhelming for teachers as well as students), Cluster schools focused on developing five strengths shown in some research to support relationships and well-being (gratitude, love, hope, curiosity, and enthusiasm) (Park et al. 2004). Lead teachers from each school facilitated staff meetings to identify what staff could do to support these strengths in their interactions with each other and with students. Each school identified a range of activities that teachers and support staff implemented over that year. These included emphasising gratitude through the school day by looking for 'what's good' during challenges as well as good times and having more celebrations of successes. Among other suggestions were allowing time for students' 'burning questions' and tangents in the classroom; staff modelling positive behaviours to each other and to students; unpacking what each of the strengths meant with students; using inspirational figures/videos to inspire hope in students; encouraging students to take an active role within school decisions (e.g., school council and policies regarding toys and activities at school); having one of the strengths as a collective school 6-weekly goal; and having more games where teachers relinquished their leadership role to play directly with students. Implementing ideas proposed by teachers' enabled many small initiatives to be implemented in a short period of time. Teachers were supportive of the initiatives and engaged by the inclusive nature of the process used.

Over the next year schools gradually introduced the 24 VIA character strengths to students through school assemblies and class discussion. At some school assemblies, teachers told stories about times they had used a strength (or had failed to—self-deprecatory stories were popular with students!). In other schools, senior students led assemblies where they explained strengths to their peers and teachers through music, stories, or graphics.

Each school found language and examples appropriate for its context to explain the character strengths. For example, prudence was variously explained as 'making good choices' and 'saving for a rainy day' and by the daredevil skateboarders at one school, 'look before you leap'. Most Cluster schools acknowledged strengths in action at their weekly assemblies. Rewards were as simple as applause, time with the principal, or having their photograph added to the principal's 'wall of wonder'. At one school students could nominate another student and specify the strength they had observed.

Strengths and Stories

To help embed strengths language and understanding in the classroom, Cluster principals and lead teachers attended workshops on strengths spotting and on storytelling. Teachers learned to recognise strengths in themselves and in their students, using games and activities. They noted that sharing strengths stories with their colleagues brought them closer as a staff group. They found it helpful to see the strengths in their students' favourite activities and saw how being able to comment on these strengths could benefit their students and build connections with them. Teachers resonated with the author's description of the VIA strengths as '24 ways to like a difficult child'. They found the practice of identifying strengths in a challenging student was often instrumental in building connection and finding a way through previous impasses.

Lead teachers learned to tell stories and to teach students to do the same. Identifying and discussing the strengths of characters in stories usually led to discussion of issues in students' learning and home lives. For some of these teachers storytelling soon became an integral element of their teaching, while for others it was a new skill acquired slowly with practice and support. As with other aspects of positive education, each school encouraged teachers to try new approaches and see if they worked for them. No teacher was required to implement a practice or activity they were not comfortable with.

Positive Relationships: Strength Spotting, Kindness, and Respect

What quickly emerged as a priority for the Cluster, however, was the requirement for teachers to display kindness and respect in their interactions with students. To support this, teachers were encouraged and supported to notice strengths in their students. The Cluster emphasised this direction in 2011 when positive relationships were the focus for the year, beginning with a staff-training day on skills and strengths that support relationships. Staff shared their interpretations of love, fairness, friendship (the VIA nomenclature for the strength of social intelligence was adapted for school use), forgiveness, gratitude, and kindness. They discussed times they had been the recipient of these strengths and the effect of this on their relationships. Teachers discussed how they practised, noticed, and acknowledged these strengths in the classroom, identifying the strengths they found easiest or most challenging to express. The author shared with the group a model of different pathways through which strengths could influence behaviour and well-being in a classroom. Set out in Fig. 8.2, this model proposed that strength spotting by teachers (and students) could influence class morale, relationships, well-being, and learning (for simplicity the model does not show the influence of engagement and class climate on well-being). Subsequently, research has shown that almost all beneficial student outcomes from a strengths programme were mediated by teacher attitude, motivation towards, and frequency of strength spotting (Quinlan et al. 2015b).

The Cluster implemented the Awesome Us strengths programme in Terms 1 and 2 for Years 5 and 6 (9–12 year olds). Introduced to the classroom over a 6-week period, the programme used games and activities to help students work with their peers to identify their strengths, to recognise strengths in others, and to use strengths to pursue personal goals. Teachers enjoyed participating in the programme, observed positive changes in their classrooms, and were keen to continue using programme tools and activities, such as ending each day with *'what strengths have you spotted in this class today?'*, strength spotting in funny or inspiring video clips, and discussing current events from a strengths perspective. For example, students discussed what strengths would be helpful if you were trapped in a mine or above ground waiting for a family member and debated which strengths were most useful when

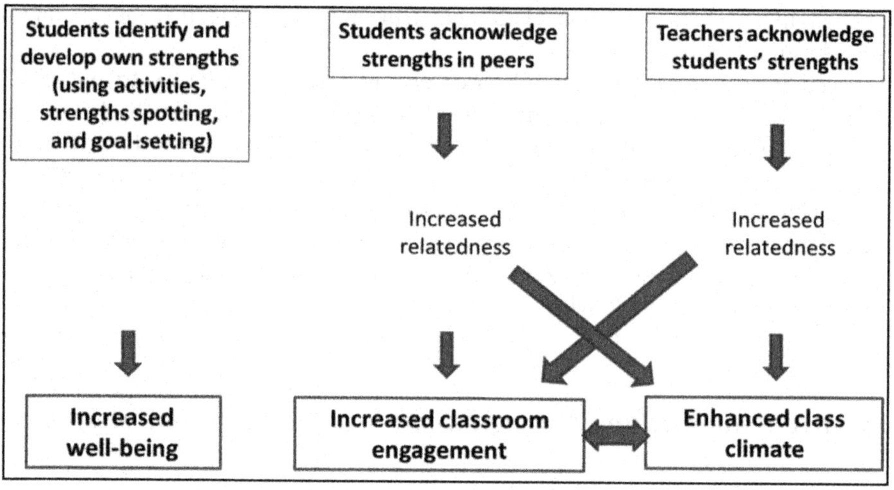

Fig. 8.2 Proposed model: Effects of strengths identification and strength spotting in the classroom

going shopping for family gifts at Christmas. The Awesome Us programme was demonstrated to enhance well-being, classroom engagement, class climate (reducing class friction and increasing class cohesion), and relatedness and autonomy need satisfaction (Quinlan et al. 2015a).

Relationship Management Rather than Discipline

As the Cluster developed its focus on relationships, characterised by kindness and respect, the leadership of the Cluster began evaluating school practices. They believed a punitive approach to discipline was inconsistent with the ethos of positive education and the principles they had adopted. They resolved to introduce a restorative approach to discipline issues (Blood and Thorsborne 2005) that were framed as relationship management. Cluster principals agreed that in managing any incident or challenge with a student the goal was for it to be resolved with the relationship intact or improved. Teachers were encouraged to presume positive intentions on the part of those involved in discipline and conflict management issues, and asked to consider the resources of the student and teachers involved to resolve the issue. Cluster training explained how relationship skills were at the heart of this approach to discipline. Lead teachers from a number of schools attended training in restorative practice during the year and Cluster workshops included training in strategies to enhance relationships (e.g., active constructive responding (Gable et al. 2004)), encourage perspective and forgiveness, and using strengths to build relationships and resolve challenges.

Implementing positive psychology in the classroom required self-awareness and reflection on the part of teachers. For a small number, it was challenging to adopt a way of thinking that emphasised the positive in a situation or a person. To support teachers to demonstrate greater flexibility in their thinking, staff participated in workshops that explored thinking styles and some common thinking traps (Reivich and Shatte 2002). Teachers recognised that being able to separate an event from their thoughts or beliefs about it was a skill that could help prevent angry outbursts or fighting for some of their students, and would support self-regulation, relationships, and resilience for all. Learning to be flexible in their thinking and identify more than one possible explanation for a problem situation was useful for teachers, both personally and to share with students. *'Have you fallen into a thinking trap?'* became a popular question in some schools.

Inquiry, Reflection, and New Development

In 2012, the theme of building connection and community was used to encourage reflection and sharing on past Cluster experiences. The Cluster used its annual staff training day to conduct an AI of Circle Time practices and share the results of the Awesome Us programme with all staff. Staff reported feeling inspired by this reflection that gave them new insights and ideas for classroom practice. Reflection and sharing continued through the year and helped staff groups maintain connection, engagement and enthusiasm for future plans.

By 2012, the strengths-focus, circle time, and storytelling, along with other practices, such as gratitude and kindness, were being used on an ongoing basis in each classroom as well as in assemblies, staff meetings, newsletters, and parent evenings. A new programme aligned with positive psychology was introduced in March when a lead teacher-training day was held on '*The Art of Possibility*' (Zander and Zander 2000). This programme provided teachers with alternative ways to think about finding the 'positive core' or strengths of each student. It encouraged teachers to examine the structures and routines of their classrooms to ensure they were consistent with the positive, enabling environment teachers wanted to create for their students. Storytelling in the classroom was boosted by a visit from a UK expert in storytelling and strengths (Fox Eades 2008). A storytelling workshop held for Year 5 potential young leaders was very effective. These students subsequently led storytelling in their classrooms the following year.

Relationships and Community

Relationships and community have been enduring priorities for the Cluster. From 2010, schools had shared information on positive education with families through school newsletters, assemblies, awards, and homework assignments.

Although schools focused primarily on students and staff they were looking for ways to share positive education with their parent community. The staff-training day in 2013 provided an opening to do so. An education psychologist specialising in the neuroscience of development and learning presented the scientific evidence for the importance of strengths-based practices, kindness, and love at home and in the classroom. The importance of loving parental relationships proved to be a topic of great interest to the community who engaged with a number of meetings on this topic through the year.

Community engagement increased in 2014 when the Cluster theme was 'inclusion and well-being'. Staff meetings explored how the schools could better support well-being and achievement for Māori students (New Zealand's indigenous people). Community and staff attended Māori-led workshops that shared what well-being means for Māori students and their families. There is a high degree of congruence between positive education and the holistic relationship-focused approach to education that Māori wish for their children. This is an area ripe for further exploration and development in New Zealand.

Professional Development Aligned with Positive Education

The Cluster responded to teachers' concerns over student anxiety stemming from learning or home challenges by introducing a new programme in 2013 that brought relaxation and mindfulness to the classroom. The programme used stretching, massage, breathing techniques, visualisations, and mindfulness to help students be relaxed and calm in the classroom. Introducing mindfulness to classrooms was consistent with the goals and vision of positive education and with the Cluster priorities for enhancing students' ability to learn. This programme provided new information and practices that were adopted by teachers who were comfortable with this approach and found it easy to integrate into their classroom routine. Further mindfulness programmes have subsequently been implemented in other Cluster schools.

By 2014, long-serving staff needed stimulation and development in positive education, and accordingly, programmes such as *Pause, Breathe, Smile* (a mindfulness in schools programme), *Relax Kids* (relaxation and mindfulness), and *Play is the Way* (social and emotional competency through play) were adopted to meet this need. However, staff turnover meant that there was also a need to introduce new staff to the basic tenets of positive education and up skill them in practices and approaches now standard across the schools (such as Circle Time, strengths, storytelling and Appreciative Inquiry). To meet this need experienced teachers were encouraged to take leadership roles on particular topics, developing their expertise and sharing it with staff. Lead teachers' meetings also began to dedicate time for sharing programmes and resources.

The Te Wai Pounamu Well-Being Cluster: Fertile Ground for Positive Psychology

Collaboration offers a way for schools to overcome funding difficulties and share scarce resources, such as staff expertise in specific areas. By combining their professional development budgets, the Cluster was able to attract overseas and national experts to train staff and to fund staff travel to training and development opportunities at home and internationally. Expert teachers regularly inspired their colleagues from different schools in staffroom presentations and training. However, pragmatic drivers may not be sufficient to ensure successful collaboration. A number of factors stand out as having enabled the Cluster's successful implementation of positive education, development of a network of supportive colleagues, and extended community of caring. These included shared values, shared leadership, an inclusive and flexible approach to planning and implementation, and recognition of each school's particular context and priorities.

Shared Values

The principals of the Cluster shared a passion for their children to become resilient children and flourishing adults. Each group member was committed to developing children's well-being and resilience. The state-funded school-based support services for children with emotional and behavioural challenges (i.e., Resource Teacher: Learning and Behaviour; RTLB) was doing good work for the most severely affected students but lacked sufficient resources for all students' needs. The group was in agreement that 'until these children are psychologically well, we can't teach them successfully'. They wanted to encourage more empathy from staff for children with challenging home situations and appreciation for the strengths some students were required to draw on just to get to school each day. The Cluster's guiding principles (set out below) reflected core beliefs and formed the standard against which proposals were evaluated.

Principles of the cluster

- The school deals with the whole child—a holistic approach.
- We all, children and adults, deserve respect.
- Children are not problems to be solved but mysteries to be understood.
- Everybody has strengths; we can use these to help with challenges and solutions.
- We believe that we deal best with problems when we identify and acknowledge strengths and look for solutions.
- Mistakes are part of learning.
- It's OK for every child and adults to make and learn from our mistakes.
- We can choose how we think about and respond to others and events.
- We have the capacity to be flexible in our thinking.

The strengths of individual principals encouraged sharing and growth. Each principal demonstrated great empathy and kindness for others, willingness to be vulnerable and reflect on their own practice. They were characterised as 'low ego people that didn't blow their own trumpets', were open to experience, had strongly held opinions but were always willing to listen to others and take on new information, and a commitment to grow and change.

Although Cluster schools collaborated closely they respected each other's autonomy. After initial shared training, each school separately identified how positive psychology could be implemented in their school. For some schools creating peace and calm in the classroom and the playground was an essential first step, while for others being able to express feelings and resolve conflict were top priorities.

Inclusive Emergent Development

From the start, positive education was implemented in an inclusive way. All staff were trained in the approach and over the years, staff have been an integral part of progress review and planning. In the first year of learning about well-being, the focus of professional development was on staff using positive psychology for themselves. This had the dual benefit of allowing teachers test this potential 'fad' and focus on their own well-being. The attention paid to staff well-being is credited with bringing school management and staff closer and building more cohesive teams. Furthermore, as support for positive education grew, it was teachers who pressed for earlier implementation in the classroom.

Although the Cluster had a clear well-being mission, it remained open as to the methods used. From the outset the Cluster held a full staff-training day to set the theme for the year. Together, each staff group agreed how new skills or practices would be implemented in their school. Lead teachers received further training through the year and shared successful implementation practices from each school. They returned to their schools with what one teacher described as 'a treasure trove of teacher-tested ideas and tools'. This model for developing skills and sharing information through the Cluster evolved over time. Quarterly principals' 'summit meetings' were added to the calendar and by 2014 several whole-Cluster meetings (after school or evening) were added to inculcate new staff in the ethos of positive education and to strengthen staff ties between schools.

Each year staff reviewed progress and agreed priorities for action. Programmes or training aligned with the Cluster principles and current priorities could then be proposed. This approach has enabled the Clusters' development to evolve in response to staff and community priorities and needs, and to take advantage of available resources and opportunities.

Support and Leadership Development

Principals and staff from each Cluster school work closely with their peers, offering support and advice across school issues beyond positive education. These close relationships became an important source of support as principals' group members encountered personal and professional challenges over the years. When group members faced school closures, mergers, and family illness, principals held weekly breakfast meetings and maintained close contact to sustain and support each other. The group provided invaluable leadership development opportunities, in contrast to the isolation experienced by many of their colleagues. It provided a safe forum in which to share concerns and challenges. The honest and sometimes challenging feedback available to each principal from trusted peers has been described as a 'taonga', a treasure beyond measure.

Through their role as pivotal drivers of positive education at the classroom level, lead teachers have gained valuable professional and leadership development. They, and other interested teachers, have been encouraged to develop and share their expertise in topics of interest, with professional development now frequently provided by staff. Teachers have presented on teacher well-being, restorative justice, and relationship management to a variety of audiences. Cluster schools have been asked to share their experiences with schools taking part in a Ministry of Education-led School Wide Positive Behaviour for Learning (SWPB4L) programme. The Cluster has also hosted visitors from New Zealand and Australia keen to see how schools can collaborate to support well-being for children from low-SES backgrounds.

An Appreciative Approach

It is fundamentally difficult for a school to implement positive education whilst operating from a deficit mindset, using deficit-focused thinking and administrative structures and policies. The Cluster principals adopted an appreciative approach to planning implementation of positive education, and over time aligned school practices with an appreciative approach.

The use of AI began in 2009 on the principal group's visit to Melbourne—where it was used to reflect on the strengths of each school, to identify what most captured people's attention, and the steps they would need to take to apply specific practices in their schools. Following the introduction of positive education in 2010, staff each school conducted small-scale AI processes, identifying the positive core of their school, staffroom, and classrooms. They then envisaged their ideal vision for the school, and identified the next smallest steps that would take them closer to the vision. This enabled each school to choose the elements of positive education that would best supporting their school vision.

When the Cluster agreed to move from a behaviour management or discipline paradigm to one of relationship management, staff mapped their way forward using appreciative questions:

- What has been your most positive experience of discipline in a school, where you saw self-esteem, relationships, and well-being rise for those involved as a result?
- What has been your most positive experience of a problem or conflict being dealt with at school? How was it handled? What was the result?
- What models or practices that are consistent with positive education do you already use?
- What steps to manage conflict or harm would be consistent with positive education?

To acknowledge its foundations in Circle Time, Cluster schools conducted an appreciative inquiry to distil circle time learning and identify its role in embedding positive education. Each year staff used an appreciative approach to review classroom and whole-school positive education, sharing their peak moments. These discussions then formed the basis for establishing priorities for the following year and fed in to school planning.

Challenges for the Cluster

The Cluster's shared values and commitment to well-being faced numerous challenges. Although government funding provided initial support in 2007, this one-off funding stream ended several years later when government priorities shifted to literacy and numeracy. Funding has been an ongoing challenge. In 2013–2014 the Cluster generated income by hosting training and events for other schools.

Introducing positive psychology to schools has its challenges. Some teachers were irritated by the label *positive education*, saying it devalued existing teaching practices as *negative education*. In introducing positive psychology, the Cluster emphasised how this research provided evidence supporting what good teachers have always done. One school began its positive education journey by celebrating the 'good work we already do'.

Most staff became supportive after learning about the science of positive education or when they realised their well-being was now a priority for school management. A number of staff found the principles of positive psychology of enormous benefit in their own lives, and the implementation of positive education was accompanied by development of self-awareness and openness for many staff. For a very small number, acknowledging the influence of their emotions and relationships on teaching outcomes remained a challenge.

One teacher expressed concern at introducing new models into an already crowded curriculum. One Principal mapped how positive education related to core elements in the school's operation and links between them (see Fig. 8.3). These included values, character strengths, curriculum programmes, and key competencies

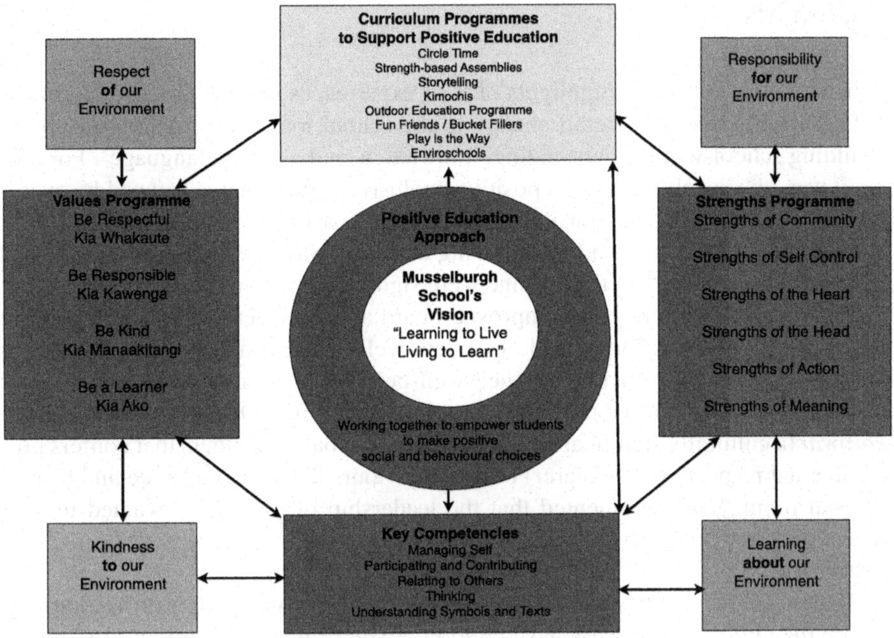

Fig. 8.3 Integration of positive education with School Vision (with permission from D. Smith, Principal, Musselburgh School, Dunedin, New Zealand)

(New Zealand's National Curriculum requires every school to demonstrate how it develop these competencies in students).

Principals acknowledged the ongoing importance of a supportive Board Chair to approve budgets for professional development and programmes required for successful implementation. One principal described winning Board of Trustees support after presenting research evidence and examples of leading schools using positive education. Very rarely, a challenge came from the community. A small number of families left one school concerned that positive education was 'too soft on kids' and didn't include sufficient punishment for inappropriate behaviour.

An ongoing challenge is the training of new staff not familiar with positive education. Some schools' staff job descriptions now requirement that staff are open to the positive education approach and knowledge of related programmes is an advantage. More significant than staff turnover however is the annual change in the school community. School values and practices need to be communicated to new families each year, without growing stale for the longer-standing community. The principal of one school commented, 'the strengths approach, kindness, and forgiveness are so embedded in our schools, that we sometimes forget how novel this approach is for some families'. Communicating with families and bringing them on board remains a significant challenge for some schools.

Highlights

When asked to reflect on highlights of their experiences in the Cluster, each principal commented on the overall change in the school tone. Some described this as 'building school-wide understanding, knowledge, and a shared language'. For others it was 'the development of a positive, inclusive culture that is "owned by everyone and is everybody's responsibility"'. One principal observed that 'staff, students, and parents learned new and more loving and kind ways to speak and listen', and that the flow on effects of this change were significant for the school.

Positive education research improved board and management understanding of the importance of teacher as well as student well-being. Teachers appreciated professional development focused on their well-being and increased awareness of their personal strengths and the role they can play in teaching. One school developed a *korowai* (a culturally significant traditional Māori cloak of feathers that confers protection and respect on the wearer) of the behaviours they wanted to see and hear in the staffroom. Staff commented that the leadership of the school wanted to hear their voice and 'they had a new language to express that voice and the feelings behind it'.

Benefits for students were identified from the beginning of the Cluster journey, where the circle time process gave children a voice and an opportunity to express their feelings and problem solve for themselves. As children's awareness of their strengths and those of their peers' strengths grew, how they viewed and interacted with each other also changed in many positive ways. Teachers reported that after the Awesome Us strengths programme not only had classroom teasing of one student stopped, but her classmates were standing up for her in the school playground.

The impact of teachers modelling strengths-focused language and positive relational behaviour was a powerful positive influence on students who in turn influenced each other. Younger students looked up to and learned from senior students who ran school assemblies. The strengths language gave students new ways to express themselves as well as viewing themselves more positively. Watching students show how their strengths 'look' at school assemblies, hearing teachers and students praising and encouraging each other, and seeing students confident enough to stand apart from their peers were all indicators for school principals of a more positive, supportive school culture. Senior students have had greater opportunities to develop leadership skills as students were encouraged to take on responsibilities within the school previously managed by teachers such as running assemblies, resolving peer conflict, and deciding on school policy regarding scooters and skateboards.

Future Directions for Cluster Schools

Since the Cluster began its well-being journey in 2007 two schools have been closed, a further three schools were merged, and one school dropped out of the programme after the original funding was exhausted. Each of the remaining schools has changed principals since that time. Against this backdrop of change it has been very challenging to maintain a cohesive group. New principals do not share the group history and understanding of the journey. They have their own priorities and naturally need to focus on getting to know their own staff.

A core group that included a current principal and two recently retired principals discussed the Cluster future earlier this year. They wondered if positive education would no longer be a priority for some Cluster schools. Attending Cluster meetings soon afterwards, they were surprised to hear how strongly lead teachers supported the positive education philosophy and continued to implement a strengths-based approach in their classrooms. In contrast to change at the principal level, lead teachers have remained the same. They offer continuity, commitment and connectedness for the Cluster.

There is an inevitable forward momentum in schools. Professional development budgets are allocated each year. Once the staff has been trained in an area over a number of years, there is a tendency to look for something new. The Cluster schools have focused on new areas aligned with their principles and the philosophy of positive education, and extend their ability to support student well-being and development. This has included training in the neuroscience of attachment and brain development (aligned with the Cluster focus on relationships), mindfulness, and relaxation (aligned with previous support for positive emotion, and resilience building through self-awareness and self-regulation), and guide physical play activities to support social and emotional learning (building self-awareness and self-regulation outside the classroom). The Cluster principals commented that it can be helpful to have a range of programmes aligned with positive education so that there is flexibility for both teachers and students in finding approaches that work well for them. However, staff and principals agree that kindness, gratitude, and a strengths-based approach with students are now an integral part of school functioning. These practices now underpin all new programmes.

One of the catch-cries for positive education has been 'live it, embed it, teach it' referring to the need for the philosophy to be lived by staff and embedded in school practice as well as being taught to students. Even if well-being were not to be taught explicitly in these schools in the future, it has been embedded in school practices and is lived in teacher behaviour towards students. It informs how students and staff are considered at the whole school level and how teachers interact with students in the classroom and playground. One cluster teacher appreciated the depth of the changes at their school when new students and staff were surprised by how tolerant and accepting students are of each other, while another realised it when a neighbouring home owner commented that the school playground was a happier place with fewer arguments and more positive language.

Conclusion

Ma whero ma pango ka oti ai te mahi.
[When everyone does their part the work will be complete].

In Te Wai Pounamu Well-Being Cluster everyone did their part and the outcome was more than the sum of the parts. The Cluster demonstrates that schools with limited budgets can successfully collaborate to implement positive education, bringing about significant positive change in school culture and practices. The shared vision and commitment of school principals was pivotal to initiate and provide momentum to the process of change. However, once change was underway, the commitment of lead teachers to drive the process at a classroom level was essential to keep it going. Now, after almost a decade, it may be these teachers that ensure the ongoing development of positive education in their schools.

Most importantly, teachers have seen how students can grasp concepts like strengths and gratitude and benefit from being encouraged to focus on what is right with them rather than what is wrong. Students have demonstrated repeatedly that they can engage with, understand and benefit from this appreciative approach to education. At times their understanding and insight has awed their teachers and increased their respect for students, such as when a 10-year old girl described going outside to see beauty in a cherry tree's blossom to calm her anger. Or when one 11-year old boy, previously bullied and from a challenging background, described feeling grateful 'because you know, we get to live this life'.

References

Blood, P., & Thorsborne, M. (2005, March). The challenge of culture change: Embedding restorative practice in schools. In *6th international conference on conferencing, circles and other restorative practices: Building a global alliance for restorative practices and family empowerment.*

Cooperrider, D. L., Whitney, D. K., & Stavros, J. M. (2003). *Appreciative inquiry handbook* (Vol. 1). San Francisco: Berrett-Koehler.

Emmons, R. A., & McCullough, M. E. (2004). *The psychology of gratitude.* New York: Oxford University Press.

Fox Eades, J. M. (2008). *Celebrating strengths: Building strengths-based schools.* Coventry: CAPP Press.

Fredrickson, B. (1998). What good are positive emotions? *Review of General Psychology, 2*(3), 300–319.

Fredrickson, B., & Joiner, T. (2002). Positive emotions trigger upward spirals toward emotional well-being. *Psychological Science, 13*(2), 172–175.

Fredrickson, B., Cohn, M., Coffey, K., Pek, J., & Finkel, S. (2008). Open hearts build lives: Positive emotions, induced through loving-kindness meditation, build consequential personal resources. *Journal of Personality & Social Psychology, 95*(5), 1045–1062.

Froh, J. J., Kashdan, T. B., Ozimkowski, K. M., & Miller, N. (2009). Who benefits the most from a gratitude intervention in children and adolescents? Examining positive affect as a moderator. *The Journal of Positive Psychology, 4*(5), 408–422.

Gable, S., Reis, H., Impett, E., & Asher, E. (2004). What do you do when things go right? The intrapersonal and interpersonal benefits of sharing positive events. *Journal of Personality & Social Psychology, 87*(2), 228–245.

Govindji, R., & Linley, P. A. (2007). Strengths use, self-concordance and well-being: Implications for strengths coaching and coaching psychologists. *International Coaching Psychology Review, 2*(2), 143–153.

Green, S., Grant, A. M., & Rynsaardt, J. (2007). Evidence-based life coaching for senior high school students: Building hardiness and hope. *International Coaching Psychology Review, 2*(1), 24–32.

Linley, P. A., Nielsen, K. M., Gillett, R., & Biswas-Diener, R. (2010). Using signature strengths in pursuit of goals: Effects on goal progress, need satisfaction, and well-being, and implications for coaching psychologists. *International Coaching Review, 5*(1), 6–15.

Lyubomirsky, S., Tkach, C., & Sheldon, K. M. (2004). *Pursuing sustained happiness through random acts of kindness and counting one's blessings: Tests of two six-week interventions*. Unpublished data, Department of Psychology, University of California, Riverside.

Lyubomirsky, S., King, L., & Diener, E. (2005). The benefits of frequent positive affect: Does happiness lead to success? *Psychological Bulletin, 131*(6), 803–855.

Mosley, J. (2005). *Circle time for young children*. London: Routledge.

Norrish, J. M. (2015). *Positive education: The Geelong Grammar School journey*. Oxford: Oxford University Press.

Norrish, J. M., Williams, P., O'Connor, M., & Robinson, J. (2013). An applied framework for positive education. *International Journal of Wellbeing, 3*(2), 147–161.

Oades, L. G., Robinson, P., & Green, S. (2011). Positive education: Creating flourishing students, staff and schools. *InPsych: The Bulletin of the Australian Psychological Society Ltd, 33*(2), 16–17.

Otake, K., Shimai, S., Tanaka-Matsumi, J., Otsui, K., & Fredrickson, B. L. (2006). Happy people become happier through kindness: A counting kindnesses intervention. *Journal of Happiness Studies, 7*(3), 361–375.

Park, N., Peterson, C., & Seligman, M. E. P. (2004). Strengths of character and well-being. *Journal of Social & Clinical Psychology, 23*(5), 603–619.

Peterson, C., & Seligman, M. E. P. (2004). *Character strengths and virtues: A handbook and classification*. New York: Oxford University Press.

Quinlan, D. M., Swain, N., Cameron, C., & Vella-Brodrick, D. A. (2015a). How 'other people matter' in a classroom-based strengths intervention: Exploring interpersonal strategies and classroom outcomes. *The Journal of Positive Psychology, 10*(1), 77–89.

Quinlan, D. M., Swain, N. S., Cameron, C., & Vella-Brodrick, D. A. (2015b). How 'other people matter' in a classroom-based strengths intervention: Exploring interpersonal strategies and classroom outcomes. *Journal of Positive Psychology, 10*(1), 77–89.

Reivich, K., & Shatte, A. (2002). *The resilience factor*. New York: Broadway Books.

Roffey, S. (2006). *Circle time for emotional literacy*. London: Sage.

Ryff, C. D., & Keyes, C. L. M. (1995). The structure of psychological well-being revisited. *Journal of Personality & Social Psychology, 69*(4), 719–727.

Seligiman, M. E. P. (2002). *Authentic happiness. Using the new positive psychology to realize your potential for lasting fulfillment*. New York: Free Press.

Seligman, M. E. P., Steen, T. A., Park, N., & Peterson, C. (2005). Positive psychology progress: Empirical validations of interventions. *American Psychologist, 60*(5), 410–421.

Seligman, M. E. P., Ernst, R. M., Gillham, J., Reivich, K., & Linkins, M. (2009). Positive education: Positive psychology and classroom interventions. *Oxford Review of Education, 35*(3), 293–311.

Sheldon, K. M., & Lyubomirsky, S. (2006). How to increase and sustain positive emotion: The effects of expressing gratitude and visualizing best possible selves. *The Journal of Positive Psychology, 1*(2), 73–82.

Statistics New Zealand. (2012). Vulnerable children and families: Some findings from the New Zealand General Social Survey. Retrieved from http://www.stats.govt.nz/browse_for_stats/people_and_communities/Children/vulnerable-children.aspx.

Waters, L. (2011). A review of school-based positive psychology interventions. *The Australian Educational & Developmental Psychologist, 28*(2), 75–90.

Zander, R. S., & Zander, B. (2000). *The art of possibility*. Boston: Harvard Business Press.

Chapter 9
Fostering Positive Changes in Health and Social Relationships in Children

Mariana Lozada, Natalia Carro, Marcela Kapelmayer, Viviana Kelmanowicz, Andrea Czar, and Paola D'Adamo

Abstract Several studies have demonstrated that altruism and gratitude may confer beneficial effects on psychophysical wellbeing. The present chapter describes how positive changes in health and social relationships can be fostered in 6- to 9-year-old children when participating in positive interventions. The findings show that the experience of working with others to attain shared goals and focusing on gratefulness positively modulated altruism and social interactions among peers, highlighting the great behavioural plasticity of children. Moreover, interventions involving cooperative playing not only increased positive relationships but also contributed to a decrease in chronic stress levels. The positive outcomes of participating in the described interventions were assessed by means of quantitative methods, such as physiological parameters, sociometric measures, and tests of altruism, the use of which, to our knowledge,

---

M. Lozada (✉) • N. Carro
INIBIOMA (CONICET-University of Comahue), Quintral 1250, 8400 Bariloche, Argentina
e-mail: mariana.lozada@gmail.com; lozadam@comahue-conicet.gob.ar; nadecar@yahoo.com.ar

M. Kapelmayer
Awe, Zapata 512 9c, CABA, Argentina
e-mail: marcela@grupoawe.com

V. Kelmanowicz
Awe, Zapata 512 9c, Buenos Aires, Argentina

University of Belgrano, Buenos Aires, Argentina

University of Palermo, Buenos Aires, Argentina
e-mail: viviana@grupoawe.com

A. Czar
Awe, Zapata 512 9c, Buenos Aires, Argentina

University of Palermo, Buenos Aires, Argentina
e-mail: andrea@grupoawe.com

P. D'Adamo
INIBIOMA (CONICET-University of Comahue), Quintral 1250, 8400 Bariloche, Argentina

Awe, Zapata 512 9c, Buenos Aires, Argentina
e-mail: paodadamo@gmail.com

C. Proctor (ed.), *Positive Psychology Interventions in Practice*,
DOI 10.1007/978-3-319-51787-2_9

has not been thoroughly explored in children. The present findings tie in well with the hypothesis that altruism is an embodied and situated human resource, which can convey intrinsic benefits. Furthermore, results from the studies mentioned indicate that positive transformations can be easily fostered through the performance of this type of intervention. Given that schools provide a stimulating environment that significantly influences children's development, our findings highlight the benefits of working in this way to promote positivity in formal educational contexts, which could certainly contribute to the enhancement of individual and social well-being.

Abbreviations

CEIC Clinical Research Ethics Committee
MAP Mindful awareness practice

Introduction

Altruism and social relationships are important aspects of human life, and as such have been studied extensively by positive psychology (e.g., Seligman et al. 2005). Social interaction begins at birth and plays a prominent role both in well-being and cognitive development (e.g., Eisenberg 2002; Seligman 2011; Vygotsky 1978). Several investigations have shown how empathic concern for others and social network diversity can promote health and well-being (Brown et al. 2005; Cohen and Janicki-Deverts 2009; Kok and Fredrickson 2010; Pace et al. 2009, 2010, 2012). Consistent with this beneficial effect, it has been found that altruism in human beings, which involves the acts of helping, sharing, comforting, informing, and so forth, tends to occur beyond reciprocity, kinship or reputation in a higher proportion than predicted by evolutionary theory (Fehr and Fischbacher 2003; Lozada et al. 2011). The fact that consideration towards others results in positive consequences not only for the receiver but also for the giver highlights the importance of our social nature, and questions the excessive emphasis often placed on cost rather than valuing the intrinsic benefits of these human attributes.

Numerous studies have shown that altruistic motivation emerges at an early age; for example, toddlers spontaneously help nonfamiliar individuals (Warneken and Tomasello 2006, 2008) and attempt to respond to the emotional needs of others, showing empathic concern for those in distress (Warneken and Tomasello 2009; Zahn-Waxler et al. 1992). Interestingly, it has been observed that children of less than 2 years of age exhibit greater happiness when sharing with others than when receiving treats themselves (Aknin et al. 2012), and that babies of 3–10 months prefer helping situations to neutral or hindering ones (Hamlin et al. 2007, 2010).

Embodied social experiences have a notable effect on children's prosociality. It has been found that assisting others favours prosocial attitudes (Eisenberg 1982; Eisenberg and Fabes 1998) and that playing cooperatively can decrease aggression and increase cooperation, whereas the opposite tends to occur after competitive games (Bay-Hinitz et al. 1994). Furthermore, cooperative activities have shown their usefulness in increasing self-confidence, creativity, and prosocial values (Garaigordobil 2004, 2005; Garaigordobil and Berrueco 2007). Along the same lines, it has been observed that after collaborating with a peer to attain a goal, 3-year-old children shared obtained resources equally (Warneken et al. 2011), although this egalitarian behaviour had previously been thought to occur later than 6 or 7 years old (Fehr et al. 2008). The studies above illustrate how these embodied experiences can foster prosocialness, emphasising the key role played by social contexts and highlighting the behavioural plasticity of young children.

There is much evidence to demonstrate the importance of experience in social cognitive processes (e.g., Di Paolo and De Jaegher 2012; Varela 2001). The embodied cognition and enactive theory (Varela et al. 1992) proposes that cognition is embodied, lived, and embedded in sociocultural contexts. It is inseparable from processes of perceiving and acting with others; i.e., cognitive agents are not passive data collectors who model the world, but active participants who enact a world in close coupling with others (e.g., Di Paolo and De Jaegher 2012; Held and Hein 1963; Varela 1999; Varela et al. 1992). Thus, cognition emerges from active participation with others (e.g., Di Paolo and De Jaegher 2012). This approach takes into account the search for meaning in participation ('participatory sense-making') in order to understand how mental states, intentions and actions are co-constructed while enacting with others (e.g., De Jaegher and Di Paolo 2007). Therefore, social cognition involves not only understanding others but also understanding with others (De Jaegher and Di Paolo 2007; Gallagher 2009).

Social interaction undergoes enormous changes throughout childhood (Winnicott 1979). During the first 8 years of life huge transformations occur, not only related to children's cognitive development but also to ways of interacting with others, and ways of playing and experiencing enjoyment. Games thus become a way of developing and enacting numerous virtues and attributes that enhance socialisation, involving the possibility of interaction with others, while incorporating and internalising external rules. Given the relevance of participatory sense-making (Di Paolo 2005; Di Paolo et al. 2010), group games can favour individual and social skills that become so important at this stage of development.

One way of evaluating social relationships in a group is through the sociogram, a sociometric parameter that describes and illustrates the dynamic nature of social processes (Garaigordobil 2005; Gutiérrez 1999; Lozada et al. 2014a; Moreno 1972). This reliable tool identifies the social network of each child in a group, assessed by means of a questionnaire asking each child to say which peers they want to play with, and which they do not. When this measure is applied at different moments within a certain group, dynamic social processes can be examined. In addition, as it analyses social exclusion, this indicator can also illustrate relational contexts in which antagonistic relationships might occur within a group. Thus, the analysis of all responses allows for a kind of X-ray of socioemotional ties within the group, facilitating understanding of subjects' relationships while they are immersed in complex and dynamic social contexts.

It has also been shown that experiences of gratitude, associated with empathic concern, can foster prosocial attitudes and the reduction of destructive interpersonal behaviour (Bono et al. 2004), and that grateful people tend to maintain more and better social relationships (Lyubomirsky 2008). Moreover, experimental studies have demonstrated that activities related to gratitude, such as writing a letter of appreciation, generate substantial positive changes in the writer (e.g., Seligman et al. 2005). Gratitude not only helps increase subjective well-being but also enhances altruistic motivation (Emmons and Shelton 2002). Thus, gratitude is considered a highly beneficial human strength, whose implementation might be of great significance. The development and promotion of these strengths, then, has been very much encouraged (e.g., Peterson 2006), given that they foster both subjective well-being and life satisfaction (Park et al. 2004; Proctor et al. 2011).

Positive interventions have proved to promote favourable change in educational settings and have therefore become more frequently applied worldwide (e.g., Flook et al. 2015; Quinlan et al. 2012; Schonert-Reichl et al. 2015; Seligman et al. 2009). Considering the importance of social interactions during childhood, and the intrinsic beneficial effects of prosocialness and gratitude, interventions that could promote the emergence of these positive qualities might be appropriate and desirable, given the complexity of social relationships nowadays. In this chapter we describe interesting findings related to positive interventions performed in primary classrooms, where empathic concern, cooperation, altruism, and gratitude were fostered in educational settings. Children participating in the studies showed positive changes, which were assessed using diverse methods including: physiological parameters, sociometric measures, and non-self-report altruism tests.

Our investigations aimed to evaluate whether the enactive experience of sharing and cooperating could facilitate the emergence of empathic concern and compassionate attitudes between peers. In line with this, we wanted to assess whether positive interventions that sought to enhance empathy and connectedness with others could promote physical and psychological well-being and also improve altruism and social interactions. We hypothesised that the enaction of mindful activities, cooperative playing or gratitude exercises would promote health, prosocialness, and better relationships between peers.

How Do We Work?

We work as an interdisciplinary team, composed of physicians, psychologists, teachers, and neurobiologists. In educational settings, we design experiential instances that allow 6- to 9-year-old children to learn about empathy and connectedness with peers. Before performing these activities, we generate instances that help children learn to listen to themselves, that is, learn to focus their attention on the present moment, so that this can help them listen to others.

We carried out two different types of intervention, that is, embodied experiences, both of which began with mindfulness practices to promote children's awareness of themselves and of others' feelings and needs. One kind of intervention implied a second instance involving cooperative playing, in which children worked towards collective goals and had an opportunity to experience the joy of sharing and helping each other, beyond self-centeredness; during a third, reflective, instance, children shared their impressions of the whole experience. The other kind of intervention involved activities that promoted gratitude among peers. Three case studies are explained below.

Case Study 1: Plasticity of Altruistic Behaviour

In the first study we evaluated the plasticity of altruistic behaviour in 6- to 7-year-old children (Lozada et al. 2014b). We carried out a short intervention in a school context, once a week, which included mindfulness practices and cooperative activities. Our aim was to assess whether this intervention positively modulated children's altruistic behaviour beyond reciprocation and reputation.

Methods

Participants

The research was performed in a public school in San Carlos de Bariloche, Argentina, where 41 six-year-old children participated. Given that the school had two first grade classes, we randomly chose one class as an experimental group and the other as a control. The experimental condition included 21 participants: 11 girls and 10 boys, and the control condition comprised 20 participants: 10 girls and 10 boys. All children were in good general health, and there were no significant differences in socioeconomic level. The research was performed according to the Declaration of Helsinki—the project had also previously been approved by the Clinical Research Ethics Committee (CEIC) and the Council of Education of Río Negro Province, Argentina. We explained the activities proposed for the intervention to the children's parents and all procedures were implemented only after parents and school authorities had provided their written consent. The participants' data were analysed anonymously and treated under confidential conditions. An individual interview was performed with each participant before and after the intervention.

Intervention

The intervention was carried out once a week during the timetabled art class and consisted of 10 sessions of 50 min. Three researchers and the art teacher performed the intervention in both groups. The activities in the experimental group involved three instances: An initial moment of mindful breathing, where children learnt to focus their attention on their inspirations and exhalations, counting them silently for approximately 2–3 min (and then the time was extended gradually), a second instance in which children played cooperatively in order to attain shared goals (Garaigordobil 2005), and a third instance in which artistic work was performed for 25–30 min. In the control group we performed environmental education classes including stories, movies, and pictures (extensively employed for primary school children), after which children carried out art class activities; that is, the instances involving mindful breathing and cooperative play were omitted.

Assessment

So as to evaluate the effects of the intervention we conducted a test of altruism between peers (Leighton 1992) similar to the Dictator Game[1], adapted for preschoolers (see Avinun et al. 2011). The test was carried out before and after the intervention in both groups by means of an interview conducted by one of the researchers. Each child was given 14 sweets for him/herself in an envelope and an empty envelope with the name of a peer, previously chosen at random. We said that the sweets were for him/herself, but if they liked, they could share some candies with the peer by putting them in the empty envelope; they were assured that the peer would not know about this. We left them alone for some minutes so that they could decide without pressure. The number of shared candies was compared before and after the intervention in both groups, evaluated by means of Wilcoxon matched pair test; we also compared the number of interruptions during the mindful practice of the first and last sessions in the experimental group through the Wilcoxon matched pair test.

[1] The Dictator Game involves two players. One player is the 'dictator' and the other is the 'recipient'. The dictator receives a certain amount of money and has to choose how to divide it between himself and the recipient, who has to accept the dictator's decision without an active role in the game. It is played under anonymous conditions, so that reputation and reciprocity do not affect decision-making.

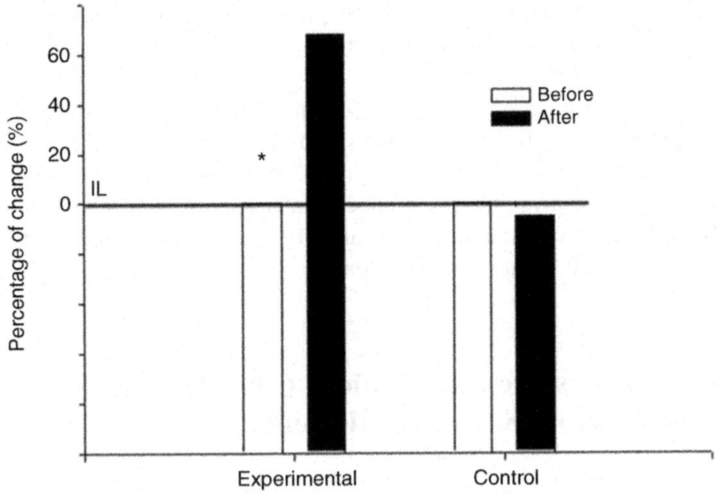

Fig. 9.1 Percentage of change in the altruism test before and after the intervention in the experimental and control groups; IL: initial level of response; * significant at $p < 0.05$

Results

The intervention program promoted significant changes in children's behaviour, which was reflected in several parameters such as: increased altruism, decreased aggressiveness, and an enhanced capacity to remain calm.

Altruism

We found significant differences in altruistic behaviour before and after the intervention in the experimental group, that is, at the end of the program children shared significantly more resources with their peer than prior to the intervention ($Z = 2.14$; $N = 19$, $p < 0.03$). In contrast, nonsignificant differences were found in the control group, that is, the intervention consisting of environmental education classes did not change altruism rates ($Z = 0.17$; $N = 20$, $p > 0.87$). No gender differences in altruism were observed in the control or experimental group prior to the intervention ($Z = -0.79$, $N_{1,2} = 21, 22$, $p > 0.45$), or after the intervention ($Z = -0.75$, $N_{1,2} = 11, 8$, $p > 0.49$) (see Fig. 9.1).

Mind-Body Integration Practices

The mindful breathing practice seemed to improve after the intervention in the experimental group, given that the number of interruptions were significantly reduced in the last session in comparison with the first one (0.83 vs. 0.17

respectively, $p < 0.0001$). Furthermore, the proportion of children who interrupted during the practice had decreased substantially by the last session (10%) in relation to the first practice (43%).

In conclusion, the experiences of playing cooperatively while developing empathic concern and achieving moments of mindful breathing enhanced altruistic attitudes in children of the experimental group, increasing awareness of themselves and of others and favouring the emergence of intrinsic altruism. These results are in line with our hypothesis that altruism is an embodied human resource, highly susceptible to experience within social contexts.

Case Study 2: Positive Interventions Can Decrease Stress Levels and Improve Social Relationships

The aim of this study was to evaluate the effects of a positive intervention, which included mind-body integration practices and cooperative activities, on salivary cortisol stress levels and social interaction in 7- to 9-year-old children (Lozada et al. 2014a).

Methods

The study was carried out over 8 months. We first interviewed each child individually, and then performed an intervention program once a week for 10 weeks, during which children carried out mind-body integration practices and cooperative play. At the conclusion of the intervention an individual interview was carried out and a final interview was also conducted 5 months later.

Participants

The study was carried out with children aged 7–9 in a private school in San Carlos de Bariloche, Argentina. As in Case Study 1, participants were all in good health, and there were no significant differences in body mass index or socioeconomic level. One class was selected at random as the experimental group, which included 26 participants (54% boys and 46% girls), and another class of 18 children (54% boys and 46% girls) formed the control group (which followed the regular school program). The intervention was performed in accordance with the Helsinki Declaration, as in Case Study 1.

Assessment

Salivary cortisol samples were collected on a normal school day between 8.00 and 8.30 a.m. in each group at three points in the study: previous to and immediately after the intervention, and again 5 months after the intervention had ended. Given that parents followed written instructions, children did not eat or drink for 30 min. previous to collection of salivary cortisol. Participants were asked to drool saliva into a collection tube. Cortisol samples were examined blind using spectrophotometric methods (Chemiluminescence, CLIA, Siemens). In order to compare relative differences in cortisol levels at the three points in the study for each group (i.e., experimental and control), we analysed the data by means of a 2 × 2 Factorial ANOVA test, evaluating interaction between variables (i.e., sample collection point and treatment group).

By means of a sociogram (Garaigordobil 2005; Moreno 1972) we evaluated social connectedness previous to and after the intervention. In an individual interview, children were requested to say which peers they would like to play with and which they would not like to play with. We used the social preference index (i.e., total number of positive choices minus the number of negative choices) to measure changes brought about by the intervention, and evaluated the results statistically by means of the Wilcoxon matched pair test.

Intervention

In the experimental group three researchers performed the intervention once a week, accompanied by the class teacher. We performed a total of 10 sessions of 60 min each. As in the first case study, the intervention entailed three consecutive instances, including: an initial stage of mind-body integration practices, a second stage of cooperative games, and a third stage of group reflection while sitting in a circle.

The first instance included breathing techniques and other mindfulness practices, and tai chi like exercises that involved slow, flowing and balancing movements, guided in a mindful way so that children could focus on these practices for several minutes. The breathing techniques were conducted as in Case Study 1. These practices helped children become more aware of moment-by-moment experiences (these resembled the mindful awareness practices (MAPs) which include forms of meditation, yoga, and tai chi) (Flook et al. 2010; Wall 2005). At the end of the intervention, by means of a questionnaire, each child was asked whether they continued practicing the learnt exercises in their homes, and under what circumstances.

Similar to the previous case study, the cooperative games entailed playing in a collaborative way in order to achieve group goals (Garaigordobil 2005). In the third instance, the children were invited to sit in a circle, and each child had the opportunity to express how they felt, say which parts of the game they enjoyed most and whether they preferred helping or being helped.

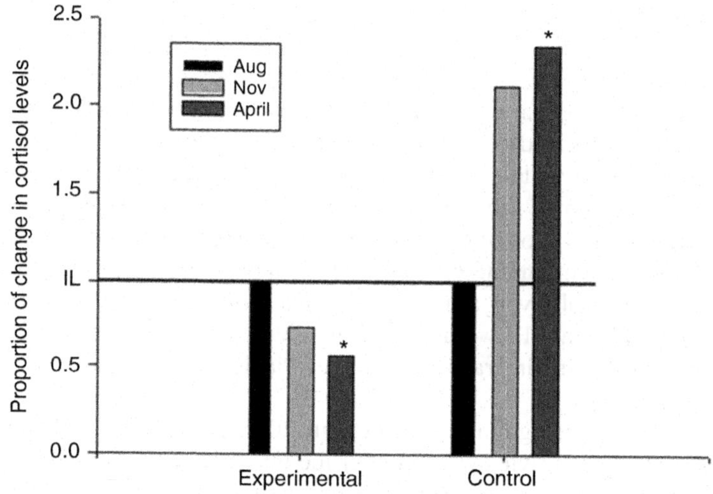

Fig. 9.2 Proportion of change in cortisol levels in the experimental and control groups, before the intervention (August), immediately after the intervention (November), and 5 months later (April). IL: initial level of response; * t test significant at $p < 0.05$ when comparing the experimental and control groups at each collection point

Results

Our findings showed that the intervention helped decrease salivary cortisol levels and helped improve social relationships between peers. Furthermore, most of the children reported that they continued practicing the learned exercises in their homes, in situations of emotional tension.

Salivary Cortisol

Relative cortisol levels measured before the intervention, at the end of the intervention, and 5 months after its conclusion, decreased significantly in the experimental group (Friedman ANOVA, $\chi^2 = 7.52$, $df = 2$, $p < 0.023$); the relative decrease in cortisol levels was 27.7% at the end of the intervention and 42.6% 5 months later. No significant differences were found, however, in the control group (Friedman ANOVA, $\chi^2 = 5.25$, $df = 2$, $p > 0.05$). A 2 × 2 ANOVA analysis demonstrated significant interaction ($df = 2$, $F = 3.1$, $p < 0.05$) between month (when cortisol was collected) and treatment (experimental or control), revealing a clear decrease in cortisol levels in the experimental but not in the control group (see Fig. 9.2).

Social Relationships

The intervention favoured positive changes in children's social interactions, given that in the experimental group children chose more peers to play with after the intervention than before it ($p < 0.019$), Wilcoxon pair test ($Z = 2.33$, $p < 0.002$). In contrast, changes were not found in the control group ($Z = 1.5$, $p > 0.13$).

Mind-Body Integration Practices

Immediately after the intervention, most of the children (93%) mentioned practicing the mind-body integration exercises in their homes when feeling fear, anguish, anger, pain, when trying to sleep, or when trying to regulate their aggression. Five months after the intervention, 85% of the children mentioned that they had continued practicing the exercises in their homes in difficult situations.

In sum, the intervention promoted positive changes in the children, given that chronic stress levels diminished in the experimental group but not in the control group; furthermore, after the intervention social relationships between peers were enhanced. Interestingly, children tended to incorporate the mind-body integration practices in their homes in order to cope with negative emotions. These findings highlight the great behavioural plasticity of children at this age and the positive impact that this kind of intervention can confer in a formal educational setting.

Case Study 3: Positive Interventions Based on Gratitude Can Improve Social Relationships

The aim of the present case study was to evaluate the effects of a positive intervention based on gratitude in social relationships in 8- to 9-year-old children.

Methods

Participants

The research was performed in a school context where 50 fourth graders (experimental group $n = 24$, control group $n = 26$) from a private school in Buenos Aires, Argentina, participated in the study. Of the total number of children, 62% were girls ($n = 31$) and 38% were boys ($n = 19$). Children's parents reported belonging to the middle class of Argentine society. Each of the two divisions was randomly assigned one condition: experimental or control. The experimental group consisted of 24 children ($n = 24$) of which 46% were boys ($n = 11$) and 54% were girls ($n = 13$). The control group had 26 children of which 8 were boys ($n = 8$, 31%) and 18 were girls ($n = 18$, 69%).

Assessment

As in the previous study, the sociogram was used to evaluate positive and negative social relationships through analysis of the following questions: a) Who would you choose as a playmate because you like to play with him/her? b) Who wouldn't you choose as a playmate because you do not like playing with him/her? Each item has 20 empty numbered spaces in which children write the names of the classmates chosen for each question. There is no minimum or maximum number stipulated for the completion of each item, so the number of partners chosen for each child is at their own discretion. The score obtained for each dimension is represented by the number of subjects chosen by each participant.

Intervention

The school in which the experiment was conducted assigned one class (50 min) once a week for the research. It was applied for six consecutive weeks with the two divisions of fourth grade, each of which was assigned a condition (experimental or control).

Children's parents signed their informed consent prior to the start of the research, the task, and work goals having been explained to them.

Initially, the gratitude questionnaire and sociogram were administered to both divisions before applying the research interventions. During all meetings, the experimental group used two instruments: storytelling and activities that children should prepare during the week. The stories were presented in PowerPoint format; the examiners read the stories aloud while the children followed the line by looking at the images on the screen. In the experimental group, each of the six meetings began with a story that encouraged children to relax and focus their attention on their breathing. This story aimed to provide a repetitive stimulus that would prepare children to initiate activities and get them ready for the next activity, which involved the mind-body integration practice and reading a story. Throughout the six meetings, three types of story were read, based on three different themes: solidarity, gratitude, and optimism. At each meeting, one story was read and the children were given a task designed to promote gratitude, which required them to think during the week about things or situations they appreciated in their lives. They had to record this at home and take it to the next meeting. In the second week, participants handed in the task they had done during the first week, which was read by the researchers. The task of the second meeting was to think of a positive feature of the first friend who had been chosen in the sociogram (first positive choice) and write it down for the next week. In the third week, the task was to think of a characteristic they felt grateful for, but this time belonging to the second friend they had chosen in the sociogram (second positive choice) and write it down. The focus of the fourth week was the negative choices that children had registered in the sociogram. The task was to think of a positive feature of the second classmate who was elected as a negative social relationship in the sociogram (second negative choice). The fifth week children

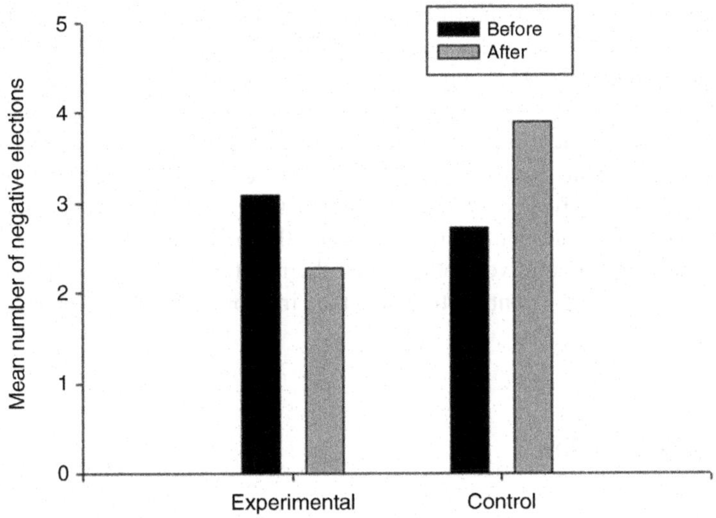

Fig. 9.3 Mean number of negative elections, before and after the intervention, for the experimental and control groups

were requested to think of a feature they were grateful for, this time belonging to the first classmate chosen in the sociogram as a negative social relationship (negative first choice). These writing tasks were supervised by researchers and then returned in an envelope to each child in the sixth and final meeting.

The sociogram was applied again at the end of the research (postintervention) and compared with the first.

For the control group, the application of the pre and postintervention questionnaires was the same as in the experimental group. Each meeting involved the reading of a popular children's story (e.g., Pinocchio, Sinbad the Sailor, The Steadfast Tin Soldier), followed by neutral activities related to the story read.

Results

The sociogram analysis before and after applying the intervention program showed that negative social relations significantly decreased in the experimental group ($t = 2.18$, $p < 0.05$), that is, at the end of the 6-week program the children chose fewer peers they did not wish to share their games with, compared to the number of peers selected before the applied intervention (pretest mean = 4.43, posttest mean = 2.45, percentage reduction in negative social relationships = 55.3%). However, nonsignificant differences were observed between pre and postnegative relationships in the control group ($t = 0.84$, $p > 0.05$).

In addition, the comparison of the postintervention negative social relationships between the experimental and control groups showed significant differences (experimental group mean = 2.45, control group mean = 5.13, $t = 2.78$, $p < 0.01$).

When comparing positive social relationships before and after the intervention, no significant differences were found in the experimental group ($p > 0.05$, $t = 0.10$) or in the control group ($t = 0.29$, $p > 0.05$). Moreover, no differences were observed when comparing positive social relationships between the experimental and control groups pre and post intervention ($t = 1, 17$, $p > 0.05$) (see Fig. 9.3).

In conclusion, this intervention reduced the number of negative social relationships between peers, contributing to the improvement of children's social networks.

General Discussion

The present studies show how the embodied experiences of cooperation and gratitude enacted during the positive interventions fostered social relationships, altruism, and physical well-being in children of primary school age. The findings demonstrate that the experience of working with others to attain shared goals and focusing on gratefulness positively modulated altruism and social interactions among peers, highlighting the great behavioural plasticity of children. Moreover, interventions involving cooperative playing not only increased positive relationships, but also contributed to a decrease in chronic stress levels. The positive outcomes of participating in the described interventions were assessed by means of quantitative methods, such as physiological parameters, sociometric measures, and tests of altruism, the use of which has not been thoroughly explored in children. Our findings tie in well with the hypothesis that altruism is an embodied and situated human resource, which can confer intrinsic benefits. Furthermore, results from all the studies mentioned indicate that positive transformations can be promoted through the enaction of the embodied social experience as proposed in the interventions described here.

On the one hand, we found that cooperative playing in combination with mind-body integration activities provided an opportunity for participants to enhance awareness of themselves and of others, possibly favouring the emergence of intrinsic altruism, beyond reciprocity and reputation. Following the intervention, altruistic attitudes, evaluated by children's sharing behaviour under anonymous conditions, increased in those children who participated in the intervention, whereas in the control group no such change was observed. Other studies also revealed that altruism was enhanced by cooperative play in children (Garaigordobil 2004, 2005) and that the experience of collaborating increased equitable sharing in preschool children (Hamann et al. 2011). Moreover, recent studies have shown that participation in a mindfulness-based prosocial training curriculum promoted self-regulation and prosocial behaviour in young children (Flook et al. 2015). In addition, a social and emotional learning program involving mindfulness and caring for others enhanced cognitive control, reduced stress, and favored well-being and prosociality in elementary school students (Schonert-Reichl et al. 2015).

The second case study further illustrates that activities involving cooperation and mind-body integration improved social relationships among peers. This positive outcome was accompanied by a reduction in chronic stress levels. In agreement with this, diverse investigations have revealed how empathic concern and compassion can help diminish stress levels (Brown et al. 2005; Kok and Fredrickson 2010; Pace et al. 2009, 2010, 2012). Several studies found that the quality and extent of social networks can influence the immune system (Cohen et al. 2003; Pressman et al. 2005); for example, social support and positive social interaction can reduce the incidence of virus infection and can enhance immune response (Coan et al. 2006; Cohen et al. 2003). In line with this, our findings support the existence of an intricate association between social connectedness and stress in the early stages of life. It is interesting to note that the intervention not only promoted an improvement in social and physiological parameters but also in relational attitudes. For example, changes were observed during the reflective instance when children shared their appreciation of the experience and listened to others. This perspective-taking instance fostered awareness of peers' perceptions, feelings, and needs, in addition to the self-perception of emotional states during the activities. This cognitive-based awareness favoured recognition of the consequences of their own actions. This embodied reflective moment, which contributed to the integration of affection and cognition, not only helped develop listening skills but also the cultivation of ethical know-how (to use Varela's term), which was also awakened by the actual experience itself. In the same vein, some authors have highlighted the importance of working on compassion and concern for others' well-being in children's healthy development and socialisation (Flook et al. 2015; Roeser and Eccles 2015; Taylor et al. 2015).

Gratitude was the main focus of the third case study. As a result of the intervention, negative social relationships decreased, whereas no differences were observed in the control group. The activities proposed during the intervention, therefore, such as reading and writing stories about positive qualities and characteristics to be thankful for, improved social relationships between children. The fact that this kind of intervention reduced negative interactions agrees with previous findings suggesting that social harmony can be promoted in schools (e.g., Lozada et al. 2014a, 2014b) and that gratitude can foster positivity and well-being, as also found in other studies (e.g., Bono et al. 2004; Emmons and Shelton 2002; Lyubomirsky 2008; McCullough et al. 2002; Seligman et al. 2005). It is worthy of note that in our study, negative social relationships diminished after the intervention but positive social relationships did not change (i.e., no changes were observed in the number of friends chosen to play with). That is, the program seems to have a greater impact on reducing exclusion among children than on increasing the number of peers included in the game, suggesting that the applied intervention was more effective in mitigating negative links between individuals than promoting new social bonds. This result could be associated with the type of activity proposed in this particular intervention. For example, thinking and writing a positive quality and a feature to be grateful for related to a classmate included in the list of peers selected to play with, did not lead to new friends being added to the list. However, the same activity related to a child not chosen as a playmate led to positive changes in the dynamics of rejection or exclusion of peers. This outcome seems reasonable given that the activity could contribute to reversing a negative perspective but not enhancing positive elections, since it probably reaffirmed preexisting relationships.

Interestingly, the embodied experiences which involved enacting cooperation and gratitude seem to have helped decrease self-centeredness in children, enabling them to connect with others, develop empathic concern, and appreciate what they receive from others. In other words, they became aware of others' positive attributes, were more conscious of the richness of social diversity and experienced the positive effects of giving, that is, they realised the happiness conferred by giving, not only receiving (Aknin et al. 2012; Lozada et al. 2011; Post 2011). This agrees well with the enactive theory which proposes that cognition emerges from participation and emphasises the key role of participatory sense making experiences, in which interaction plays more than a contextual role: it can promote and provide social cognition (De Jaegher et al. 2010; De Jaegher and Di Paolo 2007; Gallagher 2009).

In practical terms, when considering all the interventions carried out, we corroborated that these were easily replicable, given that most class teachers continued to perform the interventions during subsequent years with other grades. This suggests that they were confident about the beneficial effects and validity of this kind of intervention. The inclusion of these programs could be a valuable way of improving long-term welfare and it would be of interest for future research in this line to work with a greater diversity of ages, and different cultures.

In conclusion, the investigations presented here show that the interventions applied which sought to promote positive aspects in children, enabled them to relate to others from a new perspective, thus helping them improve social relationships between peers, enhancing empathic concern, and psychophysiological well-being. Our results emphasise the great flexibility and resilience of children when performing this type of embodied experience, which not only fosters empathy and prosocialness but also self-awareness. To our knowledge, this important topic has been little studied using the evaluation methods employed in the current work. Given that schools provide a stimulating environment that significantly influences children's development, the present findings highlight the benefits of applying these concrete ways of enhancing positivity in formal educational contexts, in which they could certainly contribute to enhancement of individual and social well-being.

References

Aknin, L. B., Hamlin, J. K., & Dunn, E. W. (2012). Giving leads to happiness in young children. *PLoS One, 7*(6), e39211. doi:10.1371/journal.pone.0039211.

Avinun, R., Israel, S., Shalev, I., Gritsenko, I., Bornstein, G., Ebstein, R. P., & Knafo, A. (2011). AVPR1A Variant associated with preschoolers' lower altruistic behavior. *PLoS One, 6*(9), e25274. doi:10.1371/journal.pone.0025274.

Bay-Hinitz, A., Peterson, R., & Quilitch, H. (1994). Cooperative games: A way to modify aggressive and cooperative behaviours in young children. *Journal of Applied Behavior Analysis, 279*, 435–446.

Bono, G., Emmons, R. A., & McCullough, M. E. (2004). Gratitude in practice and the practice of gratitude. In P. A. Linley & S. Joseph (Eds.), *Positive psychology in practice* (pp. 464–481). Hoboken: Wiley.

Brown, W. M., Consedine, N. S., & Magai, C. (2005). Altruism relates to health in an ethnically diverse sample of older adults. *Journal of Gerontology: Psychological Sciences, 60B*(3), 143–152.

Coan, J., Schaefer, H., & Davidson, R. (2006). Lending a hand: Social regulation of the neural response to threat. *Psychological Science, 17*, 1032–1039.

Cohen, S., & Janicki-Deverts, D. (2009). Can we improve our physical health by altering our social networks? *Perspectives on Psychological Science, 4*, 375–378.

Cohen, S., Doyle, W. J., Turner, R. B., Alper, C. M., & Skoner, D. P. (2003). Emotional style and susceptibility to the common cold. *Psychosomatic Medicine, 65*, 652–657.

De Jaegher, H., & Di Paolo, E. A. (2007). Participatory sense-making: An enactive approach to social cognition. *Phenomenology & the Cognitive Sciences, 6*(4), 485–507.

De Jaegher, H., Di Paolo, E. A., & Gallagher, S. (2010). Can social interaction constitute social cognition? *Trends in Cognitive Sciences, 14*(10), 441–447.

Di Paolo, E. A. (2005). Autopoiesis, adaptivity, teleology, agency. *Phenomenology & the Cognitive Sciences, 4*, 429–452. doi:10.1007/s11097-005-9002-y.

Di Paolo, E. A., & De Jaegher, H. (2012). The interactive brain hypothesis. *Frontiers in Human Neuroscience, 6*(163), 1–16.

Di Paolo, E. A., Rohde, M., & De Jaegher, H. (2010). Horizons for the enactive mind: Values, social interaction and play. In J. Stewart, O. Gapenne, & E. A. Di Paolo (Eds.), *Enaction: Towards a new paradigm of cognitive science* (pp. 33–87). Cambridge: MIT Press.

Eisenberg, N. (1982). *The development of prosocial behavior*. New York: Academic Press.

Eisenberg, N. (2002). Empathy-related emotional response, altruism and socialization. In R. J. Davison & A. Harrington (Eds.), *Visions of compassion* (pp. 131–164). New York: Oxford University Press.

Eisenberg, N., & Fabes, R. A. (1998). Prosocial development. In W. Damon & R. A. Fabes (Eds.), *Handbook of child psychology* (pp. 701–777). New York: Wiley.

Emmons, R. A., & Shelton, C. M. (2002). Gratitude and the science of positive psychology. In C. R. Snyder & S. J. Lopez (Eds.), *Handbook of positive psychology* (pp. 459–471). New York: Oxford University Press.

Fehr, E., & Fischbacher, U. (2003). The nature of human altruism. *Nature, 425*(6960), 785–791.

Fehr, E., Bernhard, H., & Rockenbach, B. (2008). Egalitarianism in young children. *Nature, 454*, 1079–1083.

Flook, L., Smalley, S. L., Kitil, M. J., Galia, B. M., Kaiser-Greenland, S., Locke, J., Ishijima, E., & Kasari, C. (2010). Effects of mindful awareness practices on executive functions in elementary school children. *Journal of Applied School Psychology, 26*, 70–95.

Flook, L., Goldberg, S. B., Pinger, L., & Davidson, R. J. (2015). Promoting prosocial behavior and self-regulatory skills in preschool children through a mindfulness-based kindness curriculum. *Developmental Psychology, 51*(1), 44–51.

Gallagher, S. (2009). Two problems of intersubjectivity. *Journal of Consciousness Studies, 16*, 298–308.
Garaigordobil, M. (2004). *Programa Juego 10-12 años. Juegos cooperativos y creativos para grupos de niños de 10 a 12 años*. Madrid: Pirámide.
Garaigordobil, M. (2005). *Programa Juego 6-8 años. Juegos cooperativos y creativos para grupos de niños de 6 a 8 años*. Madrid: Pirámide.
Garaigordobil, M., & Berrueco, L. (2007). Effects of an intervention program in children aged 5-6 years: Assessment of proactive change in behavioural and cognitive development factors. *Summa Psicologica, 4*(2), 3–19.
Gutiérrez, P. M. (1999). El sociograma como instrumento que desvela la complejidad. *Revista de Metodología de Ciencias Sociales, 2*, 129–151.
Hamann, K., Warneken, F., Greenberg, J. R., & Tomasello, M. (2011). Collaboration encourages equal sharing in children but not in chimpanzees. *Nature, 476*, 328–331.
Hamlin, J. K., Wynn, K., & Bloom, P. (2007). Social evaluation by preverbal infants. *Nature, 450*, 557–559.
Hamlin, J. K., Wynn, K., & Bloom, P. (2010). Three-month-olds show a negativity bias in their social evaluations. *Developmental Science, 13*(6), 923–929.
Held, R., & Hein, A. (1963). Movement-produced stimulation in the development of visually guided behavior. *Journal of Comparative & Physiological Psychology, 56*(5), 872–876.
Kok, B. E., & Fredrickson, B. L. (2010). Upward spirals of the heart: Autonomic flexibility, as indexed by vagal tone, reciprocally and prospectively predicts positive emotions and social connectedness. *Biological Psychology, 85*, 432–436.
Leighton, C. (1992). *El desarrollo social en los niños pequeños. Egocentrismo y altruismo*. Barcelona: Gedisa.
Lozada, M., D'Adamo, P., & Fuentes, M. (2011). Beneficial effects of human altruism. *Journal of Theoretical Biology, 289*, 12–16.
Lozada, M., Carro, N., D'Adamo, P., & Barclay, C. (2014a). Stress management in children: A pilot study in 7-9 year olds. *Journal of Developmental & Behavioral Pediatrics, 35*(2), 144–147.
Lozada, M., D'Adamo, P., & Carro, N. (2014b). Plasticity of altruistic behavior in children. *Journal of Moral Education, 43*(1), 75–88.
Lyubomirsky, S. (2008). *La ciencia de la felicidad*. Barcelona: Urano.
McCullough, M. E., Emmons, R. A., & Tsang, J. A. (2002). The grateful disposition: A conceptual and empirical topography. *Journal of Personality & Social Psychology, 82*(1), 112–127. doi:10.1037/0022-3514.82.1.112.
Moreno, J. L. (1972). *Fundamentos de la sociometría*. Buenos Aires: Paidós.
Pace, T. W., Negi, L. T., Adame, D. D., Cole, S. P., Sivilli, T. I., Brown, T. D., Issa, M. J., & Raison, C. L. (2009). Effect of compassion meditation on neuroendocrine, innate immune and behavioral responses to psychosocial stress. *Psychoneuroendocrinology, 34*(1), 87–98. doi:10.1016/j.psyneuen.2008.08.011.
Pace, T. W. W., Negi, L. T., Sivilli, T. I., Issa, M. J., Cole, S. P., Adame, D. D., & Raison, C. L. (2010). Innate immune, neuroendocrine and behavioral responses to psychosocial stress do not predict subsequent compassion meditation practice time. *Psychoneuroendocrinology, 35*(2), 310–315. doi:10.1016/j.psyneuen.2009.06.008.
Pace, T. W. W., Negi, L. T., Dodson-Lavelle, B., Ozawa-de Silva, B., Reddy, S. D., Cole, S. P., Danese, A., Craighead, L. W., & Raison, C. L. (2012). Engagement with cognitively-based compassion training is associated with reduced salivary C-reactive protein from before to after training in foster care program adolescents. *Psychoneuroendocrinology, 38*(2), 294–299. doi:10.1016/j.psyneuen.2012.05.019.
Park, N., Peterson, C., & Seligman, M. E. P. (2004). Strengths of character and well-being. *Journal of Social & Clinical Psychology, 23*(5), 603–619. doi:10.1521/jscp.23.5.603.50748.
Peterson, C. (2006). *A primer in positive psychology*. New York: Oxford University Press.
Post, S. G. (2011). It's good to be good: 2011 5th annual scientific report on health, happiness and helping others. *The International Journal of Person Centered Medicine, 1*(4), 814–829.

Pressman, S., Cohen, S., Miller, G. E., Barkin, A., Rabin, B. S., & Treanor, J. J. (2005). Loneliness, social network size, and immune response to influenza vaccination in college freshmen. *Health Psychology, 24*, 297–306.

Proctor, C., Tsukayama, E., Wood, A. M., Maltby, J., Eades, J. F., & Linley, P. A. (2011). Strengths Gym: The impact of a character strengths-based intervention on the life satisfaction and well-being of adolescents. *The Journal of Positive Psychology, 6*(5), 377–388. doi:10.1080/17439760.2011.594079.

Quinlan, D. M., Swain, N., & Vella-Brodrick, D. A. (2012). Character strengths interventions: Building on what we know for improved outcomes. *Journal of Happiness Studies, 13*(6), 1145–1163.

Roeser, R. W., & Eccles, J. S. (2015). Mindfulness and compassion in human development: Introduction to the special section. *Developmental Psychology, 51*(1), 1–6.

Schonert-Reichl, K. A., Oberle, E., Stewart Lawlor, M., Abbott, D., Thomson, K., Oberlander, T. F., & Diamond, A. (2015). Enhancing cognitive and social–emotional development through a simple-to-administer mindfulness-based school program for elementary school children: A randomized controlled trial. *Developmental Psychology, 51*(1), 52–66.

Seligman, M. E. P. (2011). *Flourish. A visionary new understanding of happiness and well-being*. New York: Atria Books.

Seligman, M. E. P., Steen, T. A., Park, N., & Peterson, C. (2005). Positive psychology progress: Empirical validation of interventions. *American psychologist, 60*(5), 410–421. doi:10.1037/0003-066X.60.5.

Seligman, M. E. P., Ernst, R. M., Gilham, J., Reivich, K., & Linkins, M. (2009). Positive education: Positive psychology and classroom interventions. *Oxford Review of Education, 35*(3), 293–311. doi:10.1080/03054980902934563.

Taylor, Z. E., Eisenberg, N., & Spinrad, T. L. (2015). Respiratory sinus arrhythmia, effortful control, and parenting as predictors of children's sympathy across early childhood. *Developmental Psychology, 51*(1), 17–25.

Varela, F. (1999). *Ethical know-how. Action, wisdom, and cognition*. Standford: Standford University Press.

Varela, F. (2001). *El fenómeno de la vida*. Santiago de Chile: Editorial Dolmen.

Varela, F., Thompson, E., & Rosch, E. (1992). *De cuerpo presente. Las ciencias cognitivas y la experiencia humana*. Barcelona: Gedisa.

Vygotsky, L. L. S. (1978). *Mind in society: The development of higher psychological processes*. Harvard: Harvard University Press.

Wall, R. B. (2005). Tai Chi and mindfulness-based stress reduction in a Boston public middle school. *Journal of Pediatric Health Care, 19*(4), 230–237.

Warneken, F., & Tomasello, M. (2006). Altruistic helping in human infants and young chimpanzees. *Science, 311*(3), 1301–1303.

Warneken, F., & Tomasello, M. (2008). Extrinsic rewards undermine altruistic tendencies in 20-month-olds. *Developmental Psychology, 44*(6), 1785–1788.

Warneken, F., & Tomasello, M. (2009). The roots of human altruism. *British Journal of Psychology, 100*, 455–471.

Warneken, F., Lohse, K., Melis, A., & Tomasello, M. (2011). Young children share the spoils after collaboration. *Psychological Science, 22*(2), 267–273.

Winnicott, D. W. (1979). De la dependencia a la independencia en el desarrollo del individuo. In D. W. Winnicott (Ed.), *Los procesos de maduración en el niño* (pp. 99–110). Barcelona: Editorial Laia.

Zahn-Waxler, C., Radke-Yarrow, M., Wagner, E., & Chapman, M. (1992). Development of concern for others. *Developmental Psychology, 28*(1), 126–136.

Chapter 10
Learning Healthy Relationships

Sue Roffey

Abstract Having positive, healthy relationships is one of the pillars of authentic well-being. All of us want to feel connected, valued, and have reliable alliance—people we can turn to when times are tough and who will also share the good times. Although many are doing well and shared humanity is still on the agenda, modern day society is experiencing a relationship crisis—family breakdown, high levels of bullying, narcissism, and self-interest, lack of empathy towards those in difficulty and unskilled interactions in many roles both at work and at home. Unless we actively intervene in education, children may learn unhealthy relationships from what they see and hear around them, including in the media. For the well-being of young people now and also for future generations we need to pay attention at a universal level to the two critical pillars of education: 'learning to be' and 'learning to live together'. This chapter outlines a philosophy and effective pedagogy for this learning based in the ASPIRE principles (agency, safety, positivity, inclusion, respect, and equality) alongside practical examples of how these might translate into the classroom for students of all ages. The 'twelve dimensions' of social and emotional learning that are briefly outlined here include the need for a congruent context and what this means within a school.

Abbreviations

ASPIRE	Agency, safety, positivity, inclusion, respect, and equality
CASEL	Collaborative for Academic, Social, and Emotional Learning
SEL	Social and emotional learning

S. Roffey (✉)
School of Education, Western Sydney University,
Locked Bag 1797, Penrith, NSW 2751, Australia
e-mail: S.Roffey@westernsydney.edu.au; Sue@sueroffey.com

C. Proctor (ed.), *Positive Psychology Interventions in Practice*,
DOI 10.1007/978-3-319-51787-2_10

Relationships and Well-Being

The quality of our relationships is now recognised as being critical for well-being at home, at work, and within our communities. Healthy relationships enhance a sense of connectedness, boost resilience, and give us reliable alliance. Sharing the good times with others often enhances positive experiences, and having emotional and practical support makes the worst of times more bearable. Children and young people therefore need to learn the social and emotional values and skills that will enable them to live well with others: communicate effectively, be a team-player, be compassionate and ethical, manage conflict, support, value and include others, and be confident in resisting peer pressure.

Relationships are there in all aspects of our lives and are on a continuum from our most intimate and long-term relationships to passing friendships, role specific relationships, those in our communities, and indeed those we have never met. How we perceive and position others who share our world, such as refugees, those from different cultures or another social milieu, make a difference to our expectations of the individuals we may come across, what we believe about them and how we treat them.

Relationships and Education

Although academic success opens doors and gives young people access to more choices, sustainable well-being does not lie in getting high test scores. You can be a successful A-plus student and live a miserable or shallow life if other things are not in place (Feinstein 2015). You can also have a meaningful and enjoyable existence without being a high-flyer at school.

Learning the values and practices of healthy relationships needs to be a core component of the educative process. Social and emotional knowledge and skills, however, cannot simply be taught in a didactic lesson format. Children learn how to relate by watching others and listening to how they speak to and about each other, the values they espouse, and how they demonstrate these. Their understanding comes from their own family members, teachers at school, the media and public figures on the television. Some of what they learn may be negative and unhelpful, especially in a culture that promotes individual success at the expense of collaboration and empathy.

This chapter covers both content and pedagogy in teaching relationships, and how this needs to be embedded within a whole school process. The pedagogy is summed up in the Circle Solutions approach (Roffey 2014) that helps to ensure that social and emotional learning (SEL) is a safe and positive experience for everyone, not 'therapeutic education' (Ecclestone and Hayes 2008). It is critical that SEL is an intervention for whole classes, as research indicates that teaching social skills in small groups to students who lack these does not lead to sustainable outcomes.

Once those individuals return to their usual classes, other children reinforce earlier behaviours, as their perceptions have not changed (Frederickson 1991). Having a universal approach also addresses the understanding and behaviours of those who look as if they are socially skilled but interact in ways that are self-serving or manipulative—this is demonstrated in some bullying behaviours.

The *twelve dimensions* that are briefly addressed in the latter part of this chapter build on the CASEL (Collaborative for Academic, Social, and Emotional Learning) framework of self-awareness, self-management, social awareness, relationship skills, and decision-making. They separate out some aspects for greater clarity, such as dealing with conflict and repairing relationships, but also broaden the concept to include the promotion of social justice, human rights, spirituality, and finding meaning. This framework also explores what contributes to a congruent educational setting for each of these dimensions.

An Appropriate Pedagogy for Relationship Education

According to the Delors Report (1996) there are four pillars of education, 'learning to know', 'learning to do', 'learning to be', and 'learning to live together'. Although you can teach the knowledge and skills that make up the core of the curriculum with an informative, instructional pedagogy, social and emotional learning requires a different and more subtle approach. Simply telling students how they 'should' be in the world and how to relate to others will have limited impact. They need a pedagogy that is experiential (doing things), interactive (doing things together), discursive (talking about what you are learning), reflective (thinking about what this means), and safe (not intrusive).

When children and young people have multiple opportunities to consider their own needs, how they want to be treated, and what makes them feel good about themselves and others, they begin to understand how they need to relate to others. When they work alongside peers who are not necessarily within their own social circle they make connections on what is shared rather than differences. When they try out alternative ways of being, and are asked to reflect both on what they feel and what they have learnt, they realise that they have choices, and what might be involved in making a 'good' choice. When they see their teachers model emotionally literate behaviour, they learn by watching and hearing as well as by doing. When they are given opportunities to practice the skills they have learnt these eventually become a way of being that goes beyond the theoretical.

The Importance of Process in Group Interactions

Circle Solutions is a value-based philosophy and pedagogy for practice in learning relationships. It builds on other similar interventions, such as the yarning circles in Aboriginal culture, learning circles, magic circles, quality circles, tribes and circle time. It has been developed not simply as a stand-alone intervention but as a tool for well-being and healthy relationships. In a school context students spend regular structured sessions with each other in a Circle format, but their learning relates to how they interact the rest of the time. The same framework can be used whenever there is a group process: in staff meetings, working with families, community consultations, policy and practice discussions, or student representative councils. It gives everyone a voice and addresses the often unspoken process issues that determine whether or not a gathering or meeting is constructive.

The facilitator is a full and equal participant in proceedings and engages in all discussions and activities. He or she is responsible for ensuring that the circle is run according to the foundational ASPIRE (i.e., agency, safety, positivity, inclusion, respect, equality) principles. Every Circle begins with a statement of the guidelines:

- What you have to say is important, so when you speak everyone else will listen to you—this means you also need to listen to others.
- You do not have to say anything if you don't want to—it is OK to just pass.
- There are no put-downs.

Participants are regularly mixed up so they talk and work with everyone. Although each person has a say, the focus is not simply on individual contributions but on exploring commonalities, devising ways forward, and group responsibility for outcomes. The emphasis is on strengths, solutions, and constructive dialogue.

The ASPIRE Principles

The ASPIRE principles for healthy relationships are: agency, safety, positivity, inclusion, respect, and equality. These summarise the common threads in the 17 chapters of *Positive relationships: Evidence based practice across the world* (Roffey 2012a). Here we give a brief overview of the definition and rationale for each of these and examples of how educators might engage students in putting these into practice.

Agency

Self-determination is a facet of authentic well-being. Having some control over what happens stops you feeling a victim of the actions of others (Deci and Ryan 2008). Agency is also about responsibility for taking action. It happens when a teacher uses their authority to empower students to make decisions rather than tell them what to do. When students are given opportunities to build an emotionally positive class environment with others they are more likely to adhere to agreements. Rather than having rules imposed they decide how they want to 'live together' and agree a set of guidelines. This can be done in stages or in one exercise, and can be applied in developmentally appropriate format for all ages.

Staged Approach

All students are mixed up, usually in a game. A simple one is 'silent statements' where participants: 'stand up and change places if… (e.g.) you had breakfast this morning', or '...you watched the match last night', or '...you have a younger sister'. Students then work in pairs with someone they were not originally sitting with. They discuss questions, such as *'what makes you feel good about coming to school'*, and are asked to come up with two statements they agree apply to both of them. Each person says one thing back to the whole circle and ideas are collated. A small group puts these ideas into class guidelines that summarise what people will do rather than not do. The following week the guidelines are put on the wall and students are asked to stand up and change places if they agree with each one as it is read out. Those who disagree are asked to work together to come up with something better. The agreed guidelines stay on the wall.

Single Game Approach

Students work in groups of four to devise a recipe for a safe and happy class. They think about the ingredients, how to put them in place and how they will know when the recipe is properly 'cooked'! What does a safe and happy class look like, feel like and sound like?

During the year, should issues arise that challenge the class being supportive of each other, students again look to the positive to find solutions that work for everyone.

Safety

There are many issues in children's lives that they need to reflect on, however to talk about highly personal matters in a universal setting may not only make people feel uncomfortable, but also breach confidentiality. Such concerns may need the support of an individual intervention, such as a counselling session. Participants in Circles, therefore, only ever discuss issues, not incidents. Discussing events that happen in the classroom or playground inevitably leads to naming, blaming, and shaming, which is not helpful. The following strategies are impersonal but address issues that matter:

- Using the third person in sentence completions rather than the first person—for example: 'Someone might be angry if…'.
- Pair shares—discussion about what partners have in common and giving feedback together: 'We agree that we both feel we belong when…'.
- Using stories to stimulate discussion, such as *William and the Worry Wart*.
- Games that encourage conversation on meanings—for example, groups making a statue (moving or still) that represents a certain emotion and then asking others to guess what this is.
- Symbols cards: these are laid out in the Circle, and students are asked to choose one that represents for them a particular quality, such as trust, gratitude, or optimism. They then discuss their choice with a partner or small group reminding them to only say what they feel comfortable with.
- Photos or other pictures are also excellent prompts for reflection on social and emotional values. There are many commercially produced cards (see section 'Resources' at the end of this chapter) that enable young people to talk about a wide variety of emotions, what might have happened for someone to feel that way, how different emotions are embodied and how we might express or change these. This can lead to rich, productive conversations that maintain distance and safety.
- Here is another example that can be used with young children:
  - **Sad Ted**: The circle facilitator introduces a Teddy and says he is very sad today. Children are asked to think about why he might be sad and then complete the sentence: *'Teddy might be sad because…'*. When the sentence has gone around the circle the facilitator points out that the children have shown that there are many reasons for being sad: *'We all feel sad sometimes. It is OK to feel like this'*. This activity 'normalises' difficult emotions and is a way of promoting resilience. In future Circles, children can be asked in small groups to think about how you might be able to tell someone is sad, what might cheer them up and what we could do in this class to help someone who is sad.

Trust is a strong relational value that is easily broken. Children often have to cope with adults not being reliable, promising what they do not deliver. It is important that children are given opportunities to reflect on this, but in impersonal, safe ways. Circle activities could include pairs discussing these statement stems and finding what they agree on:

– *'Being let down would make someone feel…'.*
– *'You know you can trust someone when…'.*

Safety is also supported by the application of choice—you do not have to speak if you don't want to. Experience indicates that people will speak when they feel safe, confident, and that they have something to contribute.

Positivity

Being both strengths and solution-focused, Circle Solutions is based on the burgeoning knowledge found in many branches of positive psychology. There are many ways Circles can help students identify, develop and find ways to use their own strengths and recognise these qualities in others. Dweck (2006) has highlighted the importance of helping children avoid a fixed mindset where they believe they either have a particular ability or not. When identifying strengths, therefore, it is more useful for participants to explore who they are 'becoming' and making choices about this. This promotes a 'growth mindset' and the possibility of change and optimism for the future.

It is easy for anyone to develop negative perspectives on others so students actively identifying the strengths in their classmates is a valuable exercise.

Perspective Glasses
The class teacher keeps a selection of cheap and cheerful spectacle frames in a box on the desk, the lenses having been removed. Each pair represents a strength, for example good listening, good sport, leadership, and so on. When a teacher notices that a student is demonstrating a particular strength they are allowed to wear those particular frames for the rest of the morning or afternoon. As they look through the glasses they identify other students who are showing the same strengths.

Acknowledgements
This is for a whole staff group. Participants attach a piece of paper with masking tape to each person's back. Using a medium sized felt pen they write anonymous statements about what they value about their colleagues. Each person ends up with ten statements and the activity is not complete until everyone has ten. Participants are then given time to read what has been written about them, reflect on how this makes them feel about themselves and their colleagues. They then make connections with what their students need. This is a powerful example of experiential learning.

Positive emotions promote an effective climate for learning: they not only enable students to focus but they also facilitate creativity and problem solving (Fredrickson 2009). Positive emotions include a sense of belonging, feeling valued, safe, comfortable, cared for, accepted, respected, and loved. Positive emotions are also experienced in moments of exuberance, excitement and shared humour. Laughter releases oxytocin into our bodies—the neurotransmitter that makes us feel good. This promotes connectedness and resilience. Shared humour in Circle sessions is one reason why students love them. They also respond positively to the playfulness that is embedded in many of the activities (Hromek and Roffey 2009).

All emotions are highly infectious—we have mirroring neurons in our brains that make us 'catch' what other people are feeling. A very simple activity is passing a smile around. Although this begins as a fixed smile by the time it has travelled around most people are smiling naturally.

Inclusion

Feeling that you belong is one of the most important factors in resilience and psychological well-being (Baumeister and Leary 1995). SEL cannot just be for the 'good' kids but is for everyone. Circles provide an opportunity for students to think about themselves differently but also change perspectives of each other.

The expectation is that everyone will work with everyone else. Participants are mixed up several times in a session so they are sitting next to a different person each time. This breaks up cliques, helps people get to know those they would not otherwise communicate with, and facilitates new understanding and perspectives. This happens most actively when pairs are looking for things they have in common, even if this is not anything of any depth.

Social Bingo

Each person is given a piece of paper containing up to nine squares. They have to find someone different for each square with whom they have a particular experience, interest, or preference in common: Suggestions are:

- Someone who likes the same food as you.
- Someone who has the same pet as you.
- Someone who has the same position as you in your family.
  Someone who has been to the same place as you—local or further afield.

It is the most vulnerable children in our communities who are most likely to be marginalised, suspended, and excluded from school. It is up to everyone, including other students to make sure that they feel they belong.

Walking in the Shoes of Others

The circle facilitator asks for a volunteer to role model a character. They are given one of following scenarios (or the teacher might make up another one) and asked to sit in the centre of the circle and read them out. They are asked to stay in character. The rest of the circle work in groups of three on the following questions:

- How will this person feel?
- How might you feel if this was you?
- How would you want to be happening?
- What three things could this group do to help this student feel included?
- What else might help?

The person acting the character remains in the Circle to answer any questions the groups might ask and then responds to the ideas that the groups come up with.

Scenarios:

My name is Banti—I do not always understand what I am asked to do because I only started to learn English a couple of years ago. When I make a mistake other students laugh and I feel stupid. I have decided not to speak in class and sometimes will not answer questions in case I get it wrong. This gets me into trouble with some teachers.

(continued)

My name is Charlie—I have only been in this class a few weeks. My mum and I used to live in another town but we had to leave to get away from my dad who broke my mum's arm. I am very angry with everything and also scared for my mum. Most people in this class have known each other a long time. When I try and join in they are not very friendly towards me. This makes me even angrier. Things are going from bad to worse.

My name is Savannah—I have a problem with my foot which means I walk lopsided and run slowly. I really like playing games but no one wants me in their team. I often spend playtimes on my own.

Some students may not have good role models for healthy relationships and others may be tolerated rather than loved. Young people who do not behave in acceptable ways may be given the message that things are better when they are not there. In Circles the aim is to meet the basic protective factors of connection, belief in the best of someone, and high expectations. This means that participation is always a choice but pupils need to abide by the guidelines. If they decide to leave they can always return so long as they demonstrate listening and respect. The first thing any adult needs to say is: *'you are important, we want you here, it is not the same without you'*. These are words that some young people rarely hear.

Respect

Respect is a value often cited in the mission statements of schools and other organisations, but not necessarily borne out in practice. Part of this is a problem with definition. It was not so long ago that 'respect' was accorded to role and position in society with the counter picture of 'respectful' meaning knowing one's place (Roffey 2005). This is no longer a commonly held definition. Egan (2002) explores what is meant by respectful practices and includes the following: the exhortation to do no harm, not rush to judgment, and not overpower a person's agenda with your own. Respect in this context is accorded as a human right, not awarded in response to power, attainment, or quality of character.

Respect is built into the Circle process by listening to each other—not interrupting, talking over or having private conversations—and not putting people down, either verbally or nonverbally. Respect is not just about listening but also in what is said *to* others and what is said *about* others. The social capital that builds trust and mutual support in any relationship, including within a whole organisation, is found in the micro-moments of high quality interactions (Dutton 2014). This includes greetings, acknowledgements, making requests rather than demands, showing interest, talking up strengths and sharing gentle humour. It also includes constructive conversations about others that do not make quick judgements.

The following activity has been developed to help young people realise how easy it is to decide what someone is like on limited, often surface information.

Envelope Game
This is suitable for students from middle primary through senior school. Small groups are given an envelope with a picture of an object on the front. The gender and age of the owner is the only information written on the envelope, for example:

- This bike belongs to a boy aged 12.
- This lunch-box belongs to a boy aged 6.
- This friendship bracelet belongs to a girl aged 10.

Groups are asked to think about the owner and what they might be like. They are then asked to take out five statements from the envelope one at a time and see whether each confirms or challenges their original thinking. Examples of statements are:

- He has a hearing impairment.
- He speaks three languages.
- The friend who gave her the bracelet is now friends with someone else and ignoring her.

Groups are asked to think about the challenges there might be in this person's life and what they have learnt from this activity.

Respect includes acknowledging others—not just by name but noticing what they have achieved and contributed. A very simple activity that is applicable to many ages is this sentence stem going around the Circle: *'I would like to thank you for…'*. Participants will need to have a moment or two to think about what they will say to the person sitting next to them.

Respect for cultural diversity is found in both verbal and nonverbal messages. When young people learn or work in institutions that do not represent people from their own community, do not find them represented in the media, and hear informal conversations that belittle their life-style or practices, it is unsurprising that they find it hard to show respect for the dominant culture. What is written on walls, in policy documents and newsletters, matters for whether communities feel acknowledged and respected, both in what is said and what is omitted.

Table 10.1 Twelve dimensions for content and context for learning relationships (Roffey 2010)

SEL dimension	Content	Context
Self-awareness • Being and becoming	Identification of values, beliefs, strengths, and goals	Clarity of school values, vision, priorities, and direction A focus on the well-being of the whole child
Emotional Awareness and Knowledge • Aetiology • Triggers • Embodiment • Social construction	Understanding the range of emotions and how they are experienced within the body Awareness of personal, social and cultural influences on feelings	Emotional 'tone' of the school, how this is demonstrated, and the influences on development
Emotional Skills • Regulation • Expression • Resilience	Dealing with and regulating negative emotion Acceptable expression of feelings within context Knowing what sustains emotional well-being and promotes resilience	Awareness of adult models of emotional literacy Communication of expectations Staff well-being and resilience
Shared Humanity • How do we position others in our world?	Appreciating uniqueness for self and others Valuing diversity Seeking what is shared	Celebration of diversity Actively addressing racism, sexism and homophobia Inclusive policies for students with special needs A sense of belonging and connectedness for all
Interpersonal Skills • Skills needed to establish and maintain positive relationships	Exploring the meaning and practice of relational values (e.g., kindness, care, helpfulness, warmth, respect, trust, support) Communication skills, especially listening Collaboration and cooperation	Facilitative teacher-student relationships. Student and staff voice Staff collegiality Collaborative pedagogies Positive communication practices Support systems
Situational Skills • Tuning into the emotional context.	Empathy Reading, interpreting and tuning into emotions in situations Not pre-judging Awareness of timing	Taking account of emotions in situations of challenge, change, failure and loss Flexibility and appropriate responsiveness in highly charged situations
Leadership	Goal setting Initiative Responsibility Confidence Dealing with peer pressure Opportunities to contribute	Communication of vision Acknowledging and trusting others; genuine consultation Staff ownership of initiatives 'Walking the talk' Avoiding a blame discourse
Promoting the Positive • Strengths and solutions approach	Optimism Gratitude Humour	Identifying and building strengths and solutions Positive behaviour policies Pedagogies for fun, meaning and engagement

(continued)

Table 10.1 (continued)

SEL dimension	Content	Context
Conflict and Confrontation • Dealing well with relational difficulties	Negotiation Compromise Appropriate assertiveness Problem-solving	Pre-empting potential conflict Appropriate use of authority De-escalating confrontation Addressing conflict actively Anti-bullying policies
Repair and Restoration • Mending damage in relationships and restoring community	Acknowledging hurt Acknowledging a range of responses in any given situation Willingness to compromise Responding to repair overtures Action to repair harm	Restorative approaches to behaviour Mistakes as part of learning Policies of re-integration for excluded students
Ethics and Integrity • Moral/human rights dimensions of SEL	Honesty Trustworthiness Consistency Ethical decision making Focus on human rights A philosophy for life	Core values in social justice Congruence between values, policies and practices Authenticity
Spirituality • Seeking meaning in life	Identity Mindfulness Perspective Congruence Environmental responsibility	Philosophy of education about the whole child in all dimensions and their contribution to humanity—not just their own success

Equality

When everyone has the opportunity to participate in activities and there is no individual competition, there is no hierarchy of winners and losers. The ability of a facilitator to participate fully and be on the same level as everyone else is a critical skill. It is the difference between being in charge of proceedings and being in control of people. Teachers have commented how much they have learnt about their students by joining in, and how being on the same level has often changed relationships within the whole class or group. Circles give *all* students an authentic voice, not just the natural leaders. Everyone has an opportunity to have their say, however briefly. Young people who have been silenced or have little control in their lives might shout to be heard, sometimes not just with words but also with challenging behaviours. When students are seen as disruptive we may shut these voices down. When pupils are not used to being taken seriously they can behave in silly ways at first. This soon stops when they know their turn will come to have their say.

We know that the more equality in a society the greater the well-being for all (Wilkinson and Pickett 2010) Therefore, alongside the important value of freedom is the equally important value of responsibility. Rights and responsibilities are two sides of the same coin. Working out what is fair can be complex but children need to learn how to balance their rights with the rights of others.

What is Fair?
Give small groups of students one of the following scenarios and ask them to discuss and suggest a solution. Share the outcomes with the Circle.

Scenario for Young Children:
Your friend has come over to play. He wants to stay inside and watch a cartoon. You want to go outside and play in the garden. How can you work this out so everyone is happy?

Scenario for Middle Primary Children:
You would love to have a dog. Your parents think that having a dog would be too much work and cost. What conversation might you have with your family?

Scenario for Senior Students:
Medical Associations want health warnings of foods with high sugar content as they damage health. The Food industry wants to sell as many products as they can and thinks that this would reduce sales. What are the issues here? What decision would you make and why?

Content and Context for Learning Relationships

Most people refer to the CASEL framework when discussing social and emotional learning (Weissberg et al. 2015). These are self-awareness, self-management, social awareness, relationship skills, and decision-making. The 12 dimensions given here (Table 10.1 and following) are simply a development from this, separating out some aspects for clarity and extending others to address issues of meaning and social justice. It also addresses a whole school context for congruence. This has come about through perceiving schools as ecologies (Roffey 2008, 2010). What happens in one part of the organisation impacts on others in a bi-directional, circular, and accumulative process. In order to address SEL effectively the whole school needs to be engaged in healthy relationships.

Twelve Dimensions of SEL

1. *Self-Awareness:* This is similar to the CASEL model with a focus on the identification of values and beliefs as well as strengths. People tend to act more on the basis of how they believe the world works and themselves in it than they do on evidence.

A school or any other organisation that values healthy relationships will ensure that 'learning to be' and 'learning to live together' have equal priority with 'learning to know' and 'learning to do' (Delors 1996).

2. *Emotional Awareness:* This is a pre-requisite to self-management. It addresses the biological and neurological aspects of emotion that are more hard-wired, but also involve cultural triggers. We are not all proud or embarrassed by the same things—they are culturally determined.

   There is now a strong body of evidence (Reyes et al. 2012) on the value of a positive emotional climate for optimal student engagement—promoting factors that enhance this makes sense for both learning and relational outcomes.

3. *Emotional Skills:* This is divided into: *emotional expression* – developing a language for emotion so that individuals can be articulate and more specific in describing how they feel, and *emotional regulation* – how to change what they feel in safe ways and promote factors that enhance resilience and emotional health.

   Staff well-being is aligned with student well-being (Roffey 2012b). When adults are feeling stressed and undervalued they are less likely to provide emotionally literate models to students.

4. *Shared Humanity:* High-level social skills can be manipulative and self-serving. This dimension actively values our unique individuality, but also seeks what people have in common. As human beings who share this world more unites us than divides us.

   In schools this dimension is mirrored in how diversity is valued. The APA report on Zero Tolerance policies (Skiba et al. 2006) shows that this can lead to authoritarian teacher-student relationships and concludes that schools need to promote a sense of belonging and connectedness across all the communities a school serves.

5. *Interpersonal Skills:* We do not have to be best friends with everyone, that is unrealistic, but knowing how to be friendly opens doorways to deeper relationships, and friendliness is a useful skill to have in many walks of life. Positive personal communication is a skill that some may be losing with the advent of social media and the busyness of everyday life. Students need opportunities to practice conversational skills, including active listening. Activities that require feedback from partners about what the other has said help hone these listening skills.

   Thousands of communications happen every day within a school and it is these that either promote high social capital or a toxic environment. How and what is communicated? Are positive comments routine or rare? Is the school a 'no put down zone' in the classrooms, staffroom, offices, and corridors and does this apply to everyone?

6. *Situational Skills:* This is where empathy lies. It is being able to have an understanding of someone else's situation, put yourself in their shoes, and imagine what that might mean. Situational skills are also related to the importance of timing in relationships—an issue that is rarely addressed and can be critical for a positive outcome.

What happens in a school to take account of the fact that some students (and staff) will be experiencing adversity? Are there support systems in place and are adults aware that validating the emotions of students can support more positive behaviours? (Roffey 2011)

7. *Leadership:* This dimension is where goal-setting, decision-making, and self-confidence lie. It is more about being a leader in your own life rather than being in charge of others.

   Within a whole school are those in authority aimed at controlling others or empowering them? What opportunities are there to give everyone a say in what happens? This is linked to the ASPIRE principle of agency.

8. *Promoting the Positive:* This dimension for SEL can be integrated across many others but is particularly focused on the relational factors that are known to promote resilience. This includes acknowledging positive qualities and bringing out the best in people—but also being able to have fun and laugh together.

   Students value teachers who make learning actively enjoyable. They like cooperative and project-based activities and the use of a wide range of technological approaches. What are the range of pedagogical frameworks available to enhance student engagement? And what happens to enhance collegial relationships?

9. *Conflict and Confrontation*: It is comparatively easy to establish a positive relationship but harder to manage when there are conflicts. This dimension explores skills of negotiation and compromise. Rather than being overwhelmed by relational differences students need to know there are options available when a confrontation arises. Individuals can either be submissive to the demands of another, be oppositional and aggressive, or state their position calmly and ask for what they want—being prepared to take account of someone else's position. Rather than positioning intransigence and inflexibility as 'being strong' it is 'appropriate assertiveness' that is defined here as a skill and a strength. Students learning about healthy relationships need opportunities to debate alternatives. They also need to consider whether self-respect lies in dominating others.

   Policies and practices across a school can limit conflict by establishing clear expectations for positive social behaviours. There are also skills involved in de-escalating confrontation that staff can learn and model to young people.

10. *Repair and Restoration:* None of us are perfect and we all make mistakes. Acknowledging this is critical, not only for relationships, but also for mental health. Aiming for perfection can leave individuals feeling constantly anxious about how they measure up.

    In schools, mistakes need to be accepted as part of learning, with an expectation that individuals will admit when things have gone wrong and be able to apologise for any hurt caused. Restorative approaches have much to offer, so long as they are embedded within a strong relational framework within a school.

11. *Ethics and Integrity:* This dimension aligns with the higher level strengths about who you choose to be in the world. It is based on the 'golden rule'—do as you would have others do to you—and includes behaving within a set of principles that honour this: being honest, reliable, consistent, and making deci-

sions that take into account the rights of others. Children from an early age understand the concept of fairness, but as young people grow and develop this dimension demands deep reflection on the complexities of ethical behaviour and what this means for personal integrity.

Many schools are now incorporating ethics education or philosophy for children into the curriculum. This dimension also challenges schools to explore the extent to which their policies address human rights.

12. *Spirituality and Meaning:* One of the pillars of authentic well-being (Seligman 2011) is having meaning and purpose in life. This dimension encourages young people to both appreciate the magic and mystery that is life itself, but also to see themselves as part of the bigger picture. Life is not just about acquisition and subjective well-being but about contributing and finding a meaningful purpose in existence. For some this will be linked to religion, to others protection of the environment—each individual needs to find what matters most to them.

    The purpose of a school is to educate the whole child, not just to achieve high academic success. This is particularly relevant for this dimension in ensuring that meaning is multi-faceted.

Summary

Hattie's (2009) meta-analysis of effective education highlights the centrality of the quality of the teacher-student relationship. Relationships within a school environment however, are multiple and ecological—the way teachers relate to each other impacts on relationships in the classroom (Roffey 2008). In an ecological framework learning and changes are bidirectional and teacher-student relationships may be changed by how peers are learning what is involved in healthy relationships. There is increasing evidence that social and emotional learning has a positive impact on inter-related outcomes (Durlak et al. 2011). This includes the development of prosocial behaviour leading to a happier classroom and increased student engagement. How this learning is facilitated and whether or not the context in which it is embedded is congruent also makes a difference to sustainable change (McCarthy and Roffey 2013).

What is now needed is a mixed method school evaluation of how the ASPIRE principles and the twelve dimensions make a difference over time to the levels of social capital across a school, the emotional climate in the classroom, social and emotional learning outcomes and the behaviour and engagement of individual students.

Resources

St Luke's Innovative Resources: http://www.innovativeresources.org.

References

Baumeister, R. F., & Leary, M. R. (1995). The need to belong: Desire for interpersonal attachments as a fundamental human motivation. *Psychological Bulletin, 117*(3), 497–529.

Deci, E. L., & Ryan, R. M. (2008). Self-determination theory: A macro-theory of human motivation, development, and health. *Canadian Psychology, 49*(3), 182–185.

Delors, J. (1996). *Learning: The treasure within*. Paris: International Commission on Education for the Twenty First Century, UNESCO.

Durlak, J. A., Dymnicki, A. B., Taylor, R. D., Schellinger, K. B., & Weissberg, R. P. (2011). The impact of enhancing students' social and emotional learning: A meta-analysis of school based universal interventions. *Child Development, 82*(1), 405–432.

Dutton, J. E. (2014). Build high quality connections. In J. E. Dutton & G. M. Spreitzer (Eds.), *How to be a positive leader: Small actions big impact*. San Francisco: Berrett-Khoeler.

Dweck, C. S. (2006). *Mindset: The new psychology of success*. New York: Random House.

Ecclestone, K., & Hayes, D. (2008). *The dangerous rise of therapeutic education*. London: Routledge.

Egan, G. (2002). *The skilled helper: A problem management and opportunity development approach to helping* (7th ed.). Pacific Grove, CA: Brooks/Cole.

Feinstein, L. (2015). *Social and emotional learning: Skills for life and work*. London: Early Intervention Foundation, UK Cabinet Office.

Frederickson, N. (1991). Children can be so cruel: Helping the rejected child. In G. Lindsay & A. Miller (Eds.), *Psychological Services for Primary Schools*. Harlow: Longman.

Fredrickson, B. (2009). *Positivity: Ground-breaking research to release your inner optimist and thrive*. Oxford: OneWorld.

Hattie, J. (2009). *Visible learning, a synthesis of over 800 meta-analyses relating to achievement*. London: Routledge.

Hromek, R., & Roffey, S. (2009). Games as a pedagogy for social and emotional learning. "Its fun and we learn things". *Simulation & Gaming, 40*(5), 626–644.

McCarthy, F., & Roffey, S. (2013). Circle Solutions: A philosophy and pedagogy for learning positive relationships. What promotes and inhibits sustainable outcomes? *The International Journal of Emotional Education, 5*(1), 36–55.

Reyes, M. R., Brackett, M. A., Rivers, S. E., White, M., & Salovey, P. (2012). Classroom emotional climate, student engagement and academic achievement. *Journal of Educational Psychology, 104*(3), 700–712.

Roffey, S. (2005). *Respect in practice: The challenge of emotional literacy in education*. Conference paper for the Australian Association for Research in Education. http://www.aare.edu.au/data/publications/2005/rof05356.pdf.

Roffey, S. (2008). Emotional literacy and the ecology of school wellbeing. *Educational and Child Psychology, 25*(2), 29–39.

Roffey, S. (2010). Content and context for learning relationships: A cohesive framework for individual and whole school development. *Educational & Child Psychology, 27*(1), 156–167.

Roffey, S. (2011). *Changing behaviour in school: Promoting positive relationships and wellbeing*. London: Sage.

Roffey, S. (Ed.). (2012a). *Positive relationships: Evidence based practice across the world*. Dordrecht: Springer.

Roffey, S. (2012b). Pupil wellbeing: Teacher wellbeing. Two sides of the same coin? *Educational and Child Psychology, 29*(4), 8–17.

Roffey, S. (2014). *Circle solutions for student wellbeing*. London: Sage.

Seligman, M. E. P. (2011). *Flourish: A new understanding of happiness and well-being – And how to achieve them*. New York: Free Press.

Skiba, R., Reynolds, C. R., Graham, S., Sheras, P., Close Conely, J., & Garcia-Vasquez, E. (2006). Are zero tolerance policies effective in the schools? An evidentiary review and recommendations. Zero Tolerance Task Force Report for the American Psychological Association.

Weissberg, R. P., Durlak, J. A., Domitrovich, C. E., & Gullotta, T. P. (2015). Social and emotional learning: Past, present, and future. In J. A. Durlak, C. E. Domitrovich, R. P. Weissberg, & T. P. Gullotta (Eds.), *Handbook of social and emotional learning: Research and practice* (pp. 3–19). New York: The Guilford Press.

Wilkinson, R., & Pickett, K. (2010). *The spirit level: Why equality is better for everyone*. London: Penguin Books.

Part III
Workplaces, Technology, and Communities

Chapter 11
Positive Psychology at Work: Research and Practice

Suzy Green, Olivia Evans, and Belinda Williams

Abstract This chapter aims to provide a broad review of the research and practice on positive psychology at work. We will also include reference to research and practice from the complementary field of positive organisational scholarship. We will commence the chapter with a brief introduction to four key psychological theories that are highly relevant to organisational applications of positive psychology work. Given there are many aspects of positive psychology relevant to the workplace and a full review is beyond the scope of this chapter, we have chosen to focus specifically on positive emotions, strengths, and resilience (mental toughness) as examples of three key areas that fall under the umbrella of positive psychology that are not only highly relevant in workplace settings, but are increasingly the primary focus of organisations pioneering in this field. We will conclude with implications for practice.

Keywords Positive psychology • Positive organisaitonal scholarship • Appreciative inquriy • Resilience • Mental toughness • Well-being

Abbreviations

AI	Appreciative inquiry
HQC	High quality connections

The original version of this chapter was revised. An erratum to this chapter can be found at DOI 10.1007/978-3-319-51787-2_16

S. Green (✉)
The Positivity Institute, Level 57, MLC Centre, 19-29 Martin Place, Sydney, NSW 2000, Australia
e-mail: suzy@thepositivityinstitute.com.au

O. Evans
The Career Guide, Melbourne, Australia
e-mail: olivia@thecareerguide.com.au

B. Williams
The Whole Being, Sydney, Australia
e-mail: b.murray.williams@gmail.com

C. Proctor (ed.), *Positive Psychology Interventions in Practice*,
DOI 10.1007/978-3-319-51787-2_11

IPOD	Innovation-inspired positive organisation development
MTQ-48	Mental toughness questionnaire-48
PERMA	Positive emotion, engagement, relationships, meaning, accomplishment
POB	Positive oganisational behaviour
POS	Positive oganisational scholarship
PP	Positive psychology
PPW	Positive psychology at work
SBO	Strengths-based organisation
SOAR	Strengths, opportunities, aspirations, results
STD	Self-determination theory
VUCA	Volatile, uncertain, complex, ambiguous

Introduction

> The only thing that is constant is change (Heraclitus, Greek Philosopher)

Whilst the opening quote has stood the test of time, in the twenty-first century it's become more meaningful than ever, particularly in regard to the world of work, which is changing at a feverish pace. 'Disruptors' include new technologies, innovations, and businesses themselves (e.g., Amazon, Alibaba, Airbnb, Uber). Some organisations have managed to adapt and respond with agility to such positive disturbances and associated challenges, however others have been forced out of business altogether.

For employees, there is immense pressure to '*adapt or die*' with many individuals experiencing significant stress and facing the reality of job loss, cost cutting, or retraining. Experts predict that 50% of occupations in organisations today will no longer exist by 2025 (CBRE 2014). So, in an increasingly volatile, uncertain, complex, and ambiguous environment (VUCA; Bawany 2015), individuals, teams, and organisations are looking for evidence-based approaches that can not only build resilience to survive, but enhance achievement, creativity, innovation, *and* well-being to thrive and gain competitive advantage.

What differentiates the organisations that flourish in this constantly evolving environment? Whilst currently small in number, an increasing proportion of organisations are turning their attention to the field of positive psychology (PP), as the science of optimal human functioning (Gable and Haidt 2005), to utilise evidence-based positive psychology interventions proven to enhance performance and well-being (Sin and Lyubomirsky 2009; Bolier et al. 2013). Similarly, there is increasing interest in the complementary field of positive organisational scholarship (POS) (Cameron et al. 2003). POS was developed to profile the extraordinary in organisations; the positive practices, attributes, and outcomes of the organisations themselves, and the positive organisational behaviours (POB) of their members (Cameron et al. 2011; Luthans et al. 2006).

In this vein, there are an increasing number of progressive organisations applying a 'positive deviance' approach to their organisational strategies, or an intentional and significant positive shift involving a range of deliberate interventions (Cameron et al. 2011; Mroz and Quinn 2009). However, because individual differences can vary so widely and organisations are complex, changes can be challenging to embed and measure across the board as positive or negative (Henry 2004; Lopez and Snyder 2003; Peterson 2006).

So while there may not be one 'silver bullet' to achieving positive psychology at work (PPW), there is growing evidence to suggest a multifaceted approach, across all levels of the organisation, and underpinned by cultural change, can be positively related to productive organisational outcomes (Froman 2010; Salanova et al. 2013). In this chapter we aim to provide an overview of the science and practice of PP and its application in the workplace (PPW), supported by examples of positive organisational scholarship. As scientist-practitioners, we will attempt to uncover the evidence base for the extraordinary positive mindsets, capabilities, activities, and honourable behaviours, and the positively deviant organisations that have experienced a range of benefits including enhanced engagement, collaboration, innovation, well-being, and productivity. We would argue that not only do organisations and individuals need the skills of PP and POS to perform and cope more effectively (i.e., increase resilience), but they also need PPW to evolve with confidence, determination, and hope.

Theoretical Underpinnings

> There is nothing so practical as a good theory (Kurt Lewin)

Whilst it may be argued that there are a number of theories that are relevant to PPW, we have chosen to explore briefly four key psychological theories we believe are of utmost relevance to organisations and with particularly actionable potential. These being, broaden and build theory (Fredrickson 1998), hope theory (Snyder 2000), self-determination theory (SDT) (Deci and Ryan 1985, 1991), and the positive emotion, engagement, relationships, meaning, and accomplishment model (PERMA; Seligman 2011). The practical application of these theories has proven to correlate with positive outcomes for organisations (and individual behaviours) including improved well-being, optimal performance, and growth (Froman 2010; Peterson 2006; Spreitzer and Sonenshein 2004).

We aim to provide a brief introduction to the four theories and a rationale as to their relevance in organisational settings. We will then aim to explore successful PPW organisational interventions specifically aimed at increasing positive emotions, strengths, and resilience at work. We will also profile the PPW practices of a number of successful organisations and finally consider implications for practice.

Broaden-and-Build Theory

Fredrickson's (1998, 2001) broaden-and-build theory of positive emotions purports that positive emotions, such as hope, joy, gratitude, and interest, *broaden* peoples' momentary thought-action repertoires and *build* long-lasting personal resources that are critical for individual well-being (Fredrickson 1998, 2004; Froman 2010; Kelloway et al. 2013; Mills et al. 2013). Fredrickson suggests these upward and outward spirals in positive emotion broadens attention, cognition, and action, enabling people to see new possibilities, bounce back from setbacks, connect with others, and reach full potential (Derryberry and Tucker 1992; Fredrickson 1998; Gasper and Clore 2002; Isen 1987; Johnson et al. 2010; Mills et al. 2013; Renninger 1992). In addition, they enable individuals to build skills and resources that have a long term impact on psychological and physical well-being (Kelloway et al. 2013; Mroz and Quinn 2009). Such functionality is of course in contrast to negative emotions' attention narrowing and body-mobilising effects that support quick, survival-promoting action (e.g., fight-or-flight).

In an organisational context, research suggests work groups with high positive to negative interactions from seemingly inconsequential interactions, such as a thank you note or a new productive collaboration, report valuable workplace outcomes, such as greater well-being, life satisfaction, creativity, productivity, resilience, and relate more positively with others (Foster and Lloyd 2007; Froman 2010; Kelloway et al. 2013; Vacharkulksemsuk and Frederickson 2013). For example, one study found that positive managers were more accurate and careful in strategic decisions and boosted their team's morale, resulting in more coordinated and effective activities (Fraser 2011). This relational aspect is particularly pertinent, as positive emotions can build relational capacity and resources, thereby providing a powerful tool for leaders and team members to foster relationships at work. Such positive affect spirals out from high performing teams, in line with emotional contagion (Barsade 2002), to client and community relationships also (Mills et al. 2013; Mroz and Quinn 2009; Spreitzer and Sonenshein 2004). Positive emotions and their application in the workplace will be more specifically reviewed later in this chapter.

Hope Theory

One particularly powerful positive emotion in organisations is hope, found to support and sustain the capacity of employee resilience (Froman 2010). Hope theory (Snyder 2000), however, is in contrast to other emotion-based hope theories (see Farran et al. 1995) and emphasises individual's perceptions of their capacities to: (1) clearly conceptualise goals (*goals*); (2) develop alternate routes to reach those goals (*pathways*); and (3) initiate and sustain the motivation for using those strategies (*agency*) (Green et al. 2006; Lopez et al. 2003; Rand 2009). Snyder (2000) claims that emotions are a by-product of goal-directed thought whereby positive emotions reflect perceived success in the pursuit of goals and negative emotions reflecting perceived failures. Snyder also acknowledges that there will be obstacles to almost any goal, high hopers can anticipate challenges and more readily generate alternate pathways (Luthans et al. 2006).

In organisations, research has found that high hopers report less burnout, are more optimistic, use knowledge to find better pathways to overcome obstacles, experience greater levels of well-being, organisational satisfaction and commitment, and perform better, particularly in challenging jobs (Bailey et al. 2007; Froman 2010; Peterson and Byron 2008). Hope also has the potential to buffer against the cost of mental illness at an individual and organisational level (e.g., through lost wages, medical costs, and disability claims), being increasingly relevant given the prevalence of depression in this setting as reflective of the wider community (Green et al. 2006; Lopez et al. 2003; Seligman and Csikszentmihalyi 2000; Seligman 2002).

All of the empirical evidence on hope, and its potential to increase well-being and optimal functioning, is dependent on whether hope is nurtured and developed (Peterson 2006). As such, leaders should be encouraged to evoke (and reinforce) hope in organisations (Lopez et al. 2003; Peterson and Byron 2008). For example, hope can be enhanced by encouraging individuals and teams to understand the power of hope by the creation of alternate plans, persevering despite obstacles, and developing key messages, visions, and goals shrouded in hope. The use of evidence-based coaching has also been shown to increase hope (Green et al. 2006; Grant et al. 2010). Thus, the use of executive coaching or broader workplace coaching in organisations may also be a highly effective way of building hopeful organisations.

Self-Determination Theory

Self-determination theory (SDT) is a motivational theory that proffers that people can optimise their functioning and growth when three related psychological needs are met; the need for competence, autonomy, and relatedness (Deci and Ryan 1985; Ryan and Deci 2000). Studies that led to the emergence of SDT included research on intrinsic motivation, that is, autonomously (or internally) motivated goals that are self-determined, and therefore authentic and self-concordant (Gagné and Deci 2005; King et al. 2004). The theory argues that when these needs are met, greater goal attainment, happiness, and well-being are achieved (King et al. 2004; Seligman and Csikszentmihalyi 2000; Sheldon and Elliot 1999). In contrast, controlled goals are externally motivated, introjected ('shoulds') and extrinsic, so not really in one's control and thus more readily associated with negative experiences, such as guilt, anxiety, and low goal attainment and psychological well-being (Brown and Ryan 2004; Gagné and Deci 2005).

It's recommended that organisations and their leaders become familiar with this theory and its practical implications. For example, leaders and their teams should be encouraged to set their own autonomous goals and identify their intrinsic motivation to do so. Targeted support should be given to those individuals that set or strive for goals that are extrinsically motivated (controlled goals). This might be done through one-on-one discussions or workplace coaching, to enhance motivation broadly for the task at hand or the job more broadly.

In terms of the three psychological needs (competence, autonomy, and relatedness), consideration can be given at the individual, team, or broader organisational perspective when looking to review how well these needs are currently being met or what could be done better to fulfil these needs. This might involve teaching SDT principles to leaders and staff more broadly and then supporting them to formulate changes that use those principles to create environments that facilitate greater satisfaction of these basic psychological needs. Deci et al. (2001) assessed satisfaction of employees' needs for competence, autonomy, and relatedness at work and found direct positive relations between the degree of need satisfaction and both work engagement and well-being on the job. Baard et al. (2004) found relations between satisfaction of these needs and employees' performance evaluations.

Examples of SDT at work that support autonomy, competence, and relatedness include technology giant Google, the multinational conglomerate, 3M (made famous for 'Scotch tape'), and the highly successful enterprise software company Atlassian. Each of these respective organisations have employed 'innovation times' where employees are allowed to spend time pursuing projects of personal interest. These projects clearly support the psychological need for autonomy, but can also provide employees with the opportunity to experience competence, particularly if they are working on a project that plays to their strengths and/or in teams that fulfil the psychological need of relatedness. The results speak for themselves and have resulted in products such as 'Gmail' and 'Google Maps' for Google and 'Post-It Notes' for 3M.

There is much an organisation can do to support fulfilment of the three psychological needs and a full review of the research and practical recommendations is beyond the scope of this chapter. However, structuring work to allow interdependence among employees and identification with work groups, as well as cultivating respect and concern for each employee, may have a positive effect on internalisation of autonomous motivation and work outcomes (van Knippenberg and van Schie 2000; Wall et al. 1986). A focus on the identification and usage of strengths in organisational settings also greatly supports the fulfilment of the need for competence and this will also be discussed later in this chapter.

PERMA

More recently, POS has placed a greater emphasis on the theory and measurement of employee wellbeing and flourishing (Kern et al. 2014). The PERMA model, developed by Seligman (2011), is a theoretical framework that represents the five essential elements of lasting well-being: positive emotion (P), engagement (E), relationships (R), meaning (M), and accomplishment (A) (Kern et al. 2014; Seligman

2011). The multidimensional nature of the PERMA model unpacks what constitutes well-being (instead of focusing on happiness alone) and therefore enables tailored approaches to improvement (Kern et al. 2014; Seligman 2011).

Organisational strategies to support and cultivate well-being might include setting goals, ensuring policies and practices are aligned to the PERMA principles, such as identifying and using talents and strengths at work, recognising people and events that give pleasure and bringing these to daily routines to evoke positive emotions, and creating opportunities for flow (Kern et al. 2014; Seligman 2011). Other strategies might include devoting time to building and maintaining relationships, determining the extent to which the organisation (and colleagues) are aligned to personal strengths, values, and beliefs, and devoting time and energy to accomplishing personal dreams (or pulling back if it's too much) (Seligman 2011).

A pilot evaluation of employee well-being at a large private school in Australia found that positive emotion, meaning, and accomplishment were most strongly related to health and life satisfaction, whereas engagement and relationships were most strongly related to job satisfaction and organisational commitment (Kern et al. 2014). In further support of this investment, a PricewaterhouseCoopers (2014) report commissioned by Beyondblue found that for every dollar spent on successfully implementing an appropriate 'mentally healthy workplace' action, such as well-being checks and coaching programs, there was on average \$2.30 in benefits to be gained by the organisation.

Interventions

In this section of the chapter we will provide evidence of successful PPW organisational interventions that specifically focus on the enhancement of positive emotions, strengths, and resilience (mental toughness) and include case study examples.

Positive Emotions

Whilst research on positive emotions has largely focused on assessing and promoting the beneficial impact to individual well-being, there is increasing interest in understanding the benefits of cultivating positive emotions, or more broadly speaking 'positivity' at work.

Fredrickson has provided foundational research on the role of positive emotions (e.g., hope, joy, gratitude, and interest) as the most important ingredient in the recipe for human flourishing, that is, living in the optimal range of human function (Fredrickson and Losada 2005).

It has been extensively documented that positive emotions, such as love and hope, have both protective benefits for cumulative stress, as they facilitate faster recovery from adverse events as well as having an amplifying effect on the

Table 11.1 Research on the impact of positive emotions on positive workplace outcomes

Outcome	Researchers
Positive behavior, attitude, retention, performance	Staw et al. (1994)
Job creativity—both as a precedent and antecedent	Amabile et al. (2005)
Job satisfaction and organizational commitment	Thorese et al. (2003)
Employee wellbeing, performance, reduced stress and burnout	Meyers et al. (2013)
Cognitive functioning, better decision making, and more effective interpersonal relationships among organisation members	Losada and Heaphy (2004) and Staw and Barsade (1993)
Helpful engagement with customers, attention and respectful behaviour	Sharot et al. (2007)

experience of positivity and well-being for the individual and surrounding community (Fredrickson 1998; Pressman and Cohen 2005). Alice Isen, a pioneer researcher in the study of positive emotions, focused on the beneficial cognitive impacts of positivity on individuals, finding that it facilitates cognitive flexibility (Isen et al. 1987), promotes intrinsic motivation (Isen 2003), boosts receptivity to new information (Estrada et al. 1997), and increases creativity to improve problem solving (Isen et al. 1987, 1991).

Research specifically into the role of emotions at work dates as far back as the 1930s to Hersey's (1932) study which looked at the role of positive emotions and their positive influence on efficiency. From this point there have been various theories and frameworks of organisational behaviour which have examined the role of positive emotions at work as a lever for effective performance, including but not limited to emotional intelligence (Goleman 1996), affective events theory (Weiss and Cropanzano 1996), positive organisational scholarship (Cameron et al. 2003) and Jane Dutton's (2014) work on high quality connections (HQCs).

With the popularisation of PP, research on the benefits and legitimacy of positive emotions in the workplace has flourished in the recent decade (Vacharkulksemsuk and Frederickson 2013). Research has found that experienced daily positive emotions at work mediated the relationship between one's job environment (e.g., autonomy, psychological climate of warmth and cooperation) and one's personal resources of optimism, self-efficacy, and self-esteem (Xanthopoulou et al. 2012). Furthermore, employees experiencing positive emotions are more helpful to customers, more creative, more attentive, and more respectful to one another (George 1998; Sharot et al. 2007) and the daily experience of positive emotions influences an individual's readiness to engage in particular organisationally beneficial behaviours (Weiss 2002).

Cameron et al. (2011) set about reviewing and consolidating the findings of research on positive emotions in organisational settings to date. The findings highlighted in Table 11.1, suggest that positive emotional well-being has a protective (buffering) as well as a promotive (amplifying) effect on positive individual behaviours (Fredrickson 1998; Seligman 2002; Staw et al. 1994; Tutu 1999).

This growing body of research has also led to the question, if the individual's well-being can benefit from an increase in the experience of positive emotion (and positivity more broadly), what are the benefits to systems, institutions, and workplaces, which rely on individuals to operate? POS researchers recognise that there is a smaller evidence base linking positive emotions to organisational effectiveness (Cameron et al. 2011). However, there is considerable research in organisational/industrial psychology that has provided substantial evidence for the link between positive individual behaviour (e.g., engagement, retention, organisational citizenship behaviour) and organisational outcomes (i.e., profitability, customer relationships, reduced turnover) (Harter et al. 2002, 2006; Salanova et al. 2005; Rotundo and Sackett 2002).

Case Study

There is a paucity of case studies documenting organisational focus on positive emotions, associated psychological well-being, and linking it directly to organisational effectiveness. This is not to say that there has been a lack of practical examples. One such example of an organisation that has been widely documented and stands out as an exemplary organisation, where employee well-being is a key performance strategy, is Google. Positive emotion and 'happiness' is a cornerstone of the Google culture, as there is a fundamental belief by the leadership team that it is critical to success. In line with the data driven nature of the company, their 'well-being strategy' has met the standard of rigorous data testing (Baldwin 2012). In addition, the Human Resources department is titled 'People Operations', as they view their people, just like their products, as an operational lever in the company's organisational effectiveness and outcomes (Pearce 2013; Kotler 2014). To this end, there are a number of ways in which Google has targeted the positive affect of their employees through positive practices including job structure, workplace design, and perks of which we will now explore.

Google has recognised that routine and repetitive work is a sure way to dull employee spirits through a failure to harness innate individual energy and potential. As previously mentioned, they offer employees up to 20% of the week as innovation time, to devote to projects of personal interest (although aligned with organisational priorities). By being given the opportunity to break free of requisite workplace routine, tasks, and duties, employees can engage with their strengths and interests, which Harzer and Ruch (2012, 2014) found to have a direct, positive impact on pleasure, engagement, and job satisfaction.

Workplace design is another key offering that makes up the Google employee value proposition and organisational strategy. Google is the well-documented pioneer of modern workplace design that offers employees freedom of choice in how they interact and utilise the environment. Not only do they provide playful spaces, such as cinemas, bowling alleys, and karaoke bars, but they also dedicate a significant proportion of their workplace to collaborative, activity-based zones versus conventional seating. They have adopted the hot-desking concept whereby employees have an individual locker and seating is not assigned. These initiatives provide opportunity for autonomy, adaptability, collaboration, and the spontaneous exchange of ideas, knowledge, personal interactions, and collaborative work. In doing so, individuals have enhanced opportunity to experience connectedness and positive emotions, which as we have outlined, lead to enhanced personal resources and positive organisational outcomes.

Similar to their workplace design, the elaborate perks enjoyed by Google employees well exceed the norm for typical blue chip organisations. Whilst this may not necessarily be a financially viable strategy for the vast majority of organisations and there isn't a definitive bundle of perks which are considered to be most effective in enhancing organisational outcomes, there is a lesson to be learnt for all organisations in valuing employee well-being and the individual's experience of the workplace. It points to a firm belief in the power of leveraging the individual's innate potential beyond a set point skill set, which is truly aligned with the philosophy of PP, focused on positive human functioning.

Undoubtedly, further focus on research is required to validate the positive signs of early research on the impact of positive affect on organisational outcomes. Furthermore, it will be important to look at ways to leverage employee affect in economical and accessible ways to ensure that the broad organisational community can benefit from evidence based findings.

Strengths

One of the most promising approaches to promoting positivity at work, and one that has gained substantial traction in recent years in research and application, is the identification and development of individual strengths (Park and Peterson 2009). Strengths are what we're naturally good at *and* enjoy doing, or patterns of thinking, feeling, or behaving that excite, engage, and energise, enabling performance at an optimal level (McQuaid and Lawn 2015). Research suggests that when we work from our strengths, it makes our goals easier to achieve, lowering stress levels, and improving well-being (McQuaid and Lawn 2015). Studies have found the more hours each day people use their strengths, the less likely they are to experience worry, stress, anger, sadness, or physical pain; and the more likely they are to have ample energy, feel well-rested, be happy, smile or laugh a lot, learn something interesting, and be treated with respect (Asplund 2012).

Peterson et al. (2010) found curiosity, zest, hope, gratitude, and spirituality to be the strengths most often associated with job satisfaction across a variety of occupations. Moreover, the possession of specific character strengths is also related to productive behaviours at work including effective leadership, increased productivity, and reduced turnover (Harzer and Ruch 2014). Research has also found that people who have the opportunity to do what they do best each day at work—even for just part of the day—are six times more engaged in their jobs (McQuaid and Lawn 2015). Further to this, in teams where most people are able to use their strengths regularly, staff turnover has been found to be lower, productivity to be higher, and customers to be more satisfied (McQuaid and Lawn 2015).

The Gallup Organisation has been championing the use of strengths in organisations for many years on the basic premise that 'to produce excellence, you must study excellence' (Clifton et al. 2002; Hodges and Clifton 2004). Over the last 30 or so years, millions of employees worldwide have been asked the question 'at work do you have the opportunity to do what you do best everyday?'. In their analysis, this single item is the strongest predictor of customer satisfaction, profit, productivity, turnover, and employee safety (Harter et al. 2002). Critically, less than 20% 'strongly agree'. Despite the majority of workplaces having traditionally focused on improving areas of weakness, this latest research suggests we optimise our experiences when we use our strengths (Froman 2010; Hodges and Clifton 2004; McQuaid and Lawn 2015; Spreitzer and Sonenshein 2004). As such, Buckingham and Clifton (2001) advocate for strengths-based organisations (SBO), or the systemisation of strengths (Mroz and Quinn 2009).

To truly systematise strengths, organisations can assist individuals to discover their strengths, and then embed strengths in organisational relationships, processes, and systems to improve their relationships and bring the best out in their teams (McQuaid and Lawn 2015). Some researchers advocate discovering strengths by simply paying attention to the activities people are good at and enjoy, however many researchers recommend using a valid and reliable strengths tool such as the VIA Survey, Gallup StrengthsFinder, or Realise2 (Buckingham 2007; Linley et al. 2010; Peterson and Seligman 2004; Rath 2007).

Whilst the cataloguing an assessment of strengths has been much of the focus to date, there is now a greater emphasis on strengths exploration and development. For example, Biswas-Diener et al. (2011) encourage people to find their 'golden mean' in strengths application, that is, to explore how to develop the right strengths, in the right amounts, in the right situations (without overplaying or underplaying them). Example interventions include strengths spotting, using strengths in new and novel ways, and strengths coaching (Rust et al. 2009).

The emerging research has also highlighted a significant role for organisational leaders and managers in supporting individuals and their strengths use at work (Park and Peterson 2009; Gallup 2013). For example, *2015 Strengths @ Work Survey* (McQuaid and VIA Institute 2015) found when managers had a meaningful discussion about employees' strengths, 78% of these employees reported feeling engaged and energised and 65% described themselves as 'flourishing' at work. Unfortunately, 68% of managers fail to have these conversations. Similarly, Gallup Research (2013) found that employees who feel ignored by their managers are twice as likely to be actively disengaged at work, while managers who focus on their employees' weaknesses cut active disengagement to 22% (indicating that even negative attention is better than no attention at all). In stark contrast, managers who focus on their employees' strengths cut active disengagement to 1%. The Corporate Leadership Council (2004) have also found that when managers focus on the weaknesses of an employee on average their performance declines by up to 27%, whereas when they focus on the strengths of an employee on average performance improves by up to

36%. Of course there is a time and place to address weaknesses and organisations and managers should also be mindful that developing strengths might not be appropriate for every employee in every circumstance (Biswas-Diener et al. 2011; Cooperrider and Godwin 2011; Linley et al. 2006).

Case Study

IBM is one organisation that has successfully shifted thinking, behaviours, improved performance, and received outstanding feedback through top-down 'strengths-based leadership' interventions.

The IBM Positive Leadership Program was established to provide senior leaders with the tools and resources to enhance their own leadership capability, personal resiliency and positive mindset, with subsequent positive impacts on their teams and the business. Executives completed the online VIA Survey and undertook exercises to help them identify, understand, and build their strengths. They also had the opportunity to take part in one-on-one coaching sessions. With similar goals in mind, IBM also ran a three part strengths-based leadership classroom series for all managers. In addition to the classroom content on strengths research, participants also completed the VIA Survey (Peterson and Park 2009; Peterson and Seligman 2004), received a tool kit with exercises to help them to continue to explore and build their signature strengths, and were invited to join a coaching call to hear how leaders had personally applied strengths at work both individually and with their teams. IBM also facilitated tailored strengths sessions at the team level for different business groups focused on providing an introduction to the principles of positive psychology, the strengths based approach to maximising human potential, and the opportunity to explore their individual strengths and how to use them to build performance and improve personal and team satisfaction (Retrieved from http://www.viacharacter.org).

Resilience

In addition to the use of positive emotions and strengths at work, resilience and 'mental toughness' (Clough et al. 2002) have been another PP focus for many organisations, particularly in the current climate. Work related stress is costing Australian industry more than $14.81 billion and financial impact to the bottom line has been cited as high as 45% of company operating costs (Medibank 2008). With resilience being defined as flexibility in response to changing situational demands, and the ability to bounce back from negative emotional experiences (Block and Kremen 1996), it is no surprise that in the increasingly demanding and dynamic world of business that this topic is rising to the fore as a key priority on the leadership agenda. Companies are struggling to create change amongst or buffer their employees from the unforgiving pressure that characterises the modern workplace so they are in search of ways to either recruit or develop their employees to safeguard performance outcomes and bottom line results. Wildavsky (1988), has highlighted this as a more effective strategy than one that seeks to control and defend against external circumstances. This approach is also akin to a common clinical psychology concept of focusing on internal locus of control, that is what one has the ability to influence.

Resilience in the workplace is not a new topic. It has received extensive attention and research, and been conceptualised at both the organisational (system) level as well as the individual (employee) level. A *resilient organisation* is seen to maintain a high level of performance even when environmental pressures mount, threats arise, and uncertainties deepen. It may even enhance performance as a result of the trauma: NASA has been cited as one such organisation (Boin and Schulman 2008).

With respect to *resilience of the individual*, the literature has built out the research and theoretical underpinnings in the form of mental toughness (Clough et al. 2002), grit (Duckworth et al. 2007), mindset (Dweck 2006), and hardiness (Kobasa 1979), just to name a few. The central tenant of these theories and approaches is their individuals have qualities within their personality, trait or mindset, which enable them to better manage (uncompromised) under stress and perform to the best of their abilities. That is, beyond ability and talent there are other developable aspects of an individual that organisations can tend to, to achieve positive outcomes for their organisation.

Mental toughness (Clough et al. 2002) is the most recent of these iterative theories of resilience and one that is gaining momentum in its application to the recruitment, top team assessment, succession planning, and development space within the workplace. The mental toughness model builds upon the 'three C' hardiness model (Kobasa 1979) to incorporate the central parameters of *control*, *commitment*, *challenge*, and *confidence*. A mentally tough individual has the ability to tolerate uncertainty, and to recognise and act on difficult decisions whilst being directly accountable. Mental toughness development programs are striking a chord within organisational settings, as pressure mounts and organisations are requiring more than technical expertise to get the job done. There is a growing recognition that eliciting, enabling, and supporting individuals to flourish will provide the necessary 'Teflon' coating in the ever-increasing dynamic, fast paced, and relentless environments of today's world.

The Mental Toughness Questionnarie-48 (MTQ-48; Clough et al. 2002), a scientific measure of mental toughness, provides useful feedback to individuals and organisations from which a developmental focus can be garnered and delivered. The development of mental toughness can be achieved through psychoeducation and training around positive thinking, visualisation, attentional control, anxiety control, goal setting, and biofeedback. An integral pillar of mental toughness development programs is the utilisation of individual coaching to support sustained implementation of learning and individual development needs. Research by Clough and his associates has reported remarkable positive predictive links between mental toughness and performance, well-being, transition management, and more aspirational, positive workplace behaviours—details of one such relevant case studies are outlined below.

Case Study

In the UK, one of the largest and most successful career guidance organisations, Greater Merseyside Connexion Partners, found that organisational changes were causing widespread uncertainty, stress, and anxiety, which in turn was impacting the leadership's ability to meet key goals and targets. It was acknowledged that little could be done to alleviate the pressures so they commissioned a leadership program ($n = 60$) focusing on mental toughness development with the aim of better equipping their leaders to navigate this work environment. The program took a two-pronged approach using facilitator led group workshops with follow up individual coaching. Each participant completed the MTQ-48 assessment pre and postprogram delivery, which facilitated participant insight, and at follow up reinforced the effectiveness of the cognitive and psychological strategies that they had implemented (Bethia et al. 2012). The program itself focused on educating the leadership around the mental toughness model and using the psychoeducation tools outlined above. A crucial element to the 'stickability' of the program learnings was the incorporation of individual coaching which enabled the participants to process the learning and develop useful strategies to apply in the context of their assessment results and individual work contexts. Remarkably, within 12 months the organisation had restored performance and was achieving or exceeding all of its goals and objectives. All managers reported being less stressed and better able to deal with stressors and challenges (Bethia et al. 2012).

Employee resilience is emerging as a key organisational resource amongst the more traditional concept of 'human resources'. The recognition of well-being beyond the physical and in addition to the absence of mental illness is gaining increasing momentum and recognition. Fortunately, there are a number of evidence-based frameworks available to support these organisational needs to identify and develop these resources whether as part of the recruitment, leadership development, or high potential assessment space. Whilst the research into the application of these constructs and programs within the workplace requires ongoing assessment in various styles of organisational settings, the initial results and indicators are promising. In the broader context of leveraging human potential for growth, performance and wellbeing, we look at ways to link together programs and positive workplace practices that recognise the power of the individual beyond a technician.

As we have seen, there are a number of PP theories and practices that are available to, and have been successfully applied in organisational settings. The remainder of this chapter will focus on *how* organisations can effectively integrate these PP applications into their operations in a sustainable way to attain a positively deviant culture, acknowledging the ever-present challenges and complexities, whilst achieving productive outcomes for the long-term.

Implications for Practice

Over the past 30 years there have been many organisations who have attempted to improve the efficiency of their operations and satisfaction of their workers by increasing their emphasis on positively deviant practices (Cameron et al. 2011; Henry 2004). More recently, as modern societies grapple with crises, social, and economic changes, organisations have introduced flexible and adaptive strategies and practices to meet business needs coupled with a renewed focus on the health of their employees and the organisation itself (Froman 2010; Salanova et al. 2013). These strategies and practices highlight that there are numerous ways to implement PPW, however attempts to do so can become piecemeal unless supported by an organisational change strategy aligned to the principles of PP and POS. There are however as many models of organisational change as there are practices.

Variations of McKinsey's 7S Model of organisational change (Waterman et al. 1980) have been used by countless organisations in efforts to systematise cultural change and how to effectively systematise a positively deviant culture is no different. Critical success factors in successful organisational change typically include strategy (e.g., visioning), structure (e.g., empowerment), leadership (e.g., instilling hope and 'walking the talk'), behaviours and capabilities (e.g., strengths identification and use), policies, systems, and processes (e.g., recruitment, promotion, reward, and technologies), and social support (e.g., coaching) (Froman 2010; Mills et al. 2013).

Appreciative inquiry (AI) is an approach, closely aligned to the aims and objectives of PP (Cooperrider and Srivastva 1987). AI has been increasingly used by organisations wanting to shift to a more positively deviant culture, by focusing generative efforts on positive aspects that already exist within the organisation, using 'what works' as the basis for cultivating whole-scale transformation (Froman 2010; Mills et al. 2013; Vacharkulksemsuk and Frederickson 2013). This has evolved to include innovation-inspired positive organisation development (IPOD; Cooperrider and Godwin 2011), a strengths based approach to organisational innovation and change, and a new business strategy method focused on strengths, opportunities, aspirations, and results (SOAR; Mills et al. 2013). These ideas of best and ideal can help shape meaningful paths for cultural change for leaders, groups and individual employees (Froman 2010).

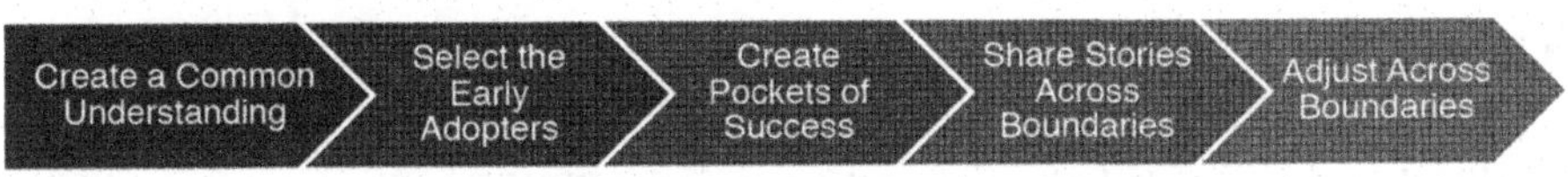

Fig. 11.1 Implementing POS in organisations (Mroz and Quinn 2009)

Mroz and Quinn's (2009) model for organisational change is another approach worth considering in the implementation of PPW and one that has previously been suggested as a model for organisational application of positive psychology in school settings (Leach and Green 2016). The model involves five stages: (1) *Create a Common Understanding*—this stage requires generating a broad understanding of the theories, techniques, language, symbols, and narratives of positive psychology and providing individuals with a chance to experience it and emotionally connect with it. There is also an opportunity to review existing good practice in the organisation that is already aligned to PPW. For some staff, it may not resonate, with others developing an intellectual understanding but still struggling to envision it in practice. There will be some individuals for whom it resonates deeply and who are motivated and energised to act and apply their learnings; (2) *Select Early Adopters*—these will be the individuals who (or individuals who form a team of champions) to embrace the principles and practices of positive psychology. They will be open to learning and coaching and willing to commit to written goals that will allow them to build on current good practice. They will also be focused on creating new ideas to make positive psychology meaningful at work, build their own positive emotions, and make positive connections to create a ripple effect in the organisation; (3) *Create Pockets of Success*—this is where risk-taking and experimentation is endorsed, encouraged, and delivered and early wins can be achieved. People are encouraged to work more to their strengths, develop action plans, support each other, make mistakes, feedback progress, and celebrate success; (4) *Sharing Across Boundaries*—sharing stories of success focused on how PPW adds value to existing good practice is shared more widely in the organisation. As success stories are celebrated and the wider benefits recognised others are more likely to be encouraged to replicate and adopt emerging good practice; and (5) *Adjust Across Boundaries*—success has been recreated and further realised and new approaches are being adopted throughout the organisation. Systems, policies, and practices are being adjusted to accommodate the shift. More often than not, mistakes will be made, relapse back to old patterns of behaviour will occur and some individuals will still not have buy-in and as a result may opt out. However, the message is clear from leadership that this is the future direction of the organisation (Fig. 11.1).

Research also supports the case for a multifaceted approach engaging individuals and groups at each level of the organisation to make positivity part of the corporate culture and more broadly (Salanova et al. 2013; Spreitzer and Sonenshein 2004). At this time however, we are unaware of any integrated model published in the PP or POS literature that connects PP, POS, and AI and further research is required to consider the benefits of such a model and approach.

Conclusion

Whilst there is overwhelming research support for PPW broadly speaking, with the large majority of support currently coming from research at the individual or group level, it's important to note that different PPW practices may be needed for different personalities, sectors, cultures, and contexts (Henry 2004). We need to avoid an over simplistic account of the complex interactions between basic human cognitive and motivational propensities and social context (Chirkov 2009).

In terms of organisational wide applications, involving longer term organisational change initiatives, we need to acknowledge that there have been many passing management fads stemming from the latest management book or what might be perceived to be working for competitors that aren't necessarily grounded in academic research (Henry 2004). We also know that the majority of organisational change efforts fail (Pascale 1999), however success is more likely if the change is collaboratively designed with a focus on organisational support for sustainability (Froman 2010; Henry 2004).

In addition, these movements toward more open, positive organisational cultures takes time, which can be difficult to maintain when competing against short-term organisational goals (Mroz and Quinn 2009). Moving an organisation toward a positive deviance is indeed a difficult undertaking particularly as there is often so much pressure to confirm to the 'norm'. It requires a number of individuals, clear on who they are and what they believe in, with continuous and sustained effort, and the right environment that supports it (Schaufeli and Salanova 2010). Two seemingly enduring challenges for organisations in pursuit of a 'positive' status have been the complexities inherent in systems, and difficulties in measuring success (Henry 2004; Spreitzer and Sonenshein 2004). More evidence is needed to prove PPW produces desirable changes in organisational effectiveness and validate precisely how these positive interventions translate to business outcomes (Cameron et al. 2011).

References

Amabile, T. M., Barsade, S. G., Mueller, J. S., & Staw, B. M. (2005). Affect and creativity at work. *Administrative Science Quarterly, 50*(3), 367–403.

Asplund, J. (2012). When Americans use their strengths more, they stress less. In *Gallup Business Journal* .Retrieved from http://www.gallup.com/poll/157679/americans-strengths-stress-less.aspx

Baard, P. P., Deci, E. L., & Ryan, R. M. (2004). Intrinsic need satisfaction: A motivational basis of performance and well-being in two work settings. *Journal of Applied Social Psychology, 34*, 2045–2068.

Bailey, T., Eng, W., Frisch, M., & Snyder, C. (2007). Hope and optimism as related to life satisfaction. *The Journal of Positive Psychology, 2*(3), 168–175.

Baldwin, H. (2012, July 24). Time off to innovate: Good idea or a waster of tech talent? *Computerworld.*

Barsade, S. G. (2002). The ripple effect: Emotional contagion and its influence on group behavior. *Administrative Science Quarterly, 47*, 644–675.

Bawany, S. (2015). *Leadership & quality of life: What does it take to be a quality of life change maker?* Retrieved from http://www.hr.com

Bethia, M. N., Rich, J., & Reeder, N. (2012). *Framework of outcomes for young people*. London: Department for Education, The Young Foundation.

Biswas-Diener, R., Kashdan, T. B., & Minhas, G. (2011). A dynamic approach to psychological strength development and intervention. *The Journal of Positive Psychology, 6*(2), 106–118.

Block, J., & Kremen, A. M. (1996). IQ and ego-resiliency: Conceptual and empirical connections and separateness. *Journal of Personality and Social Psychology, 70*, 349–361.

Boin, A., & Schulman, P. (2008). Assessing NASA's safety culture: The limits and possibilities of high-reliability theory. *Public Administration Review, 68*(6), 1050–1062.

Bolier, L., Haverman, M., Westerhof, G. J., Riper, H., Smit, F., & Bohlmeijer, E. (2013). Positive psychology interventions: A meta-analysis of randomized controlled studies. *BMC Public Health, 13*, 119–139.

Brown, K. W., & Ryan, R. M. (2004). Fostering healthy self-regulation from within and without: A self-determination theory perspective. In P. A. Linley & S. Joseph (Eds.), *Positive psychology in practice* (pp. 105–124). New Jersey: Wiley.

Buckingham, M. (2007). *The strengths engagement track: A benchmark study of 65 high performing teams.* Retrieved from http://www.tmbc.com/assets/sc/go/WhitePaper.pdf

Buckingham, M., & Clifton, D. (2001). *Now discover your strengths.* New York, NY: Simon & Schuster Adult Publishing Group.

Cameron, K., Dutton, J., Quinn, R., & Wrzesniewski, A. (2003). *Developing a discipline of positive organizational scholarship.* San Francisco: Berrett-Koehler Publisher.

Cameron, K., Mora, C., Leutscher, T., & Calarco, M. (2011). Effects of positive practices of organizational effectiveness. *The Journal of Applied Behavioural Science, 47*(3), 266–308.

CBRE. (2014). *Fast forward 2030: The future of work and the workplace.* .Retrieved from http://www.spc.ndhu.edu.tw/ezfiles/86/1086/attach/45/pta_38608_4387881_45874.pdf

Chirkov, V. I. (2009). A cross-cultural analysis of autonomy in education: A self-determination theory perspective. *Theory and Research in Education, 7*(2), 253–262.

Clifton, D. O., Anderson, E. C., & Schreiner, L. A. (2002). *Strengths quest: Discover and develop your strengths in academics, career, and beyond.* Washington, DC: The Gallup Organization.

Clough, P. J., Earle, K., & Sewell, D. (2002). Mental toughness: The concept and its measurement. In I. Cockerill (Ed.), *Solutions in sport psychology* (pp. 32–43). London: Thomson.

Cooperrider, D. L., & Godwin, L. (2011). Positive organization development: Innovation inspired change in a new economy and ecology of strengths. In G. M. Spreitzer & K. S. Cameron (Eds.), *The Oxford handbook of positive organizational scholarship, Oxford Library of Psychology.* New York, NY: Oxford University Press.

Cooperrider, D. L., & Srivastva, S. (1987). Appreciative inquiry in organizational life. In R. W. Woodman & W. A. Pasmore (Eds.), *Research in organizational change and development* (Vol. 1, pp. 129–169). Stamford, CT: JAI Press.

Corporate Leadership Council. (2004). *Driving performance and retention through employee engagement.* Washington, DC: Corporate Executive Board.

Deci, E. L., & Ryan, R. M. (1985). *Intrinsic motivation and self-determination in human behaviour.* New York: Plenum Press.

Deci, E. L., & Ryan, R. M. (1991). A motivational approach to self: Integration in personality. In R. Dienstbier (Ed.), *Nebraska symposium on motivation* (Vol. 38, pp. 237–288). Lincoln: University of Nebraska Press.

Deci, E. L., Ryan, R. M., Gagné, M., Leone, D. R., Usunov, J., & Kornazheva, B. P. (2001). Need satisfaction, motivation, and well-being in the work organizations of a former eastern bloc country: A cross-cultural study of self-determination. *Personality and Social Psychology Bulletin, 27*(8), 930–942.

Derryberry, D., & Tucker, D. M. (1992). Neural mechanisms of emotion. *Journal of Consulting and Clinical Psychology, 60*(3), 329–338.

Duckworth, A. L., Peterson, C., Matthews, M. D., & Kelly, D. R. (2007). Grit: Perseverance and passion for long-term goals. *Journal of Personality and Social Psychology, 92*(6), 1087–1101.

Dutton, J. E. (2014). Build high quality connections. In J. E. Dutton & G. M. Spreitzer (Eds.), *How to be a positive leader: Small changes, big impact.* San Francisco, CA: Bettett-Koehler Publishers.

Dweck, C. S. (2006). *Mindset: The new psychology of success.* New York: Random House.

Estrada, C. A., Isen, A. M., & Young, M. J. (1997). Positive affect facilitates integration of information and decreases anchoring in reasoning among physicians. *Organizational Behavior and Human Decision Processes, 72*(1), 117.

Farran, C. J., Herth, K. A., & Popivich, J. M. (1995). *Hope and hopelessness: Critical clinical constructs*. Thousand Oaks: Sage.

Foster, S., & Lloyd, P. (2007). Positive psychology principles applied to counseling psychology at the individual and group level. *Consulting Psychology Journal: Practice and Research, 59*, 30–40.

Fraser, A. (2011, May 12). Positivity in the workplace—How it translates to $$ for your business. *Business Chicks*.

Fredrickson, B. L. (1998). What good are positive emotions? *Review of General Psychology, 2*, 300–319.

Fredrickson, B. L. (2001). The role of positive emotions in positive psychology: The broaden-and-build theory of positive emotions. *American Psychologist, 56*, 218–226.

Fredrickson, B. L. (2004). Gratitude, like other positive emotions, broadens and builds. In R. A. Emmons & M. E. McCullough (Eds.), *The psychology of gratitude* (pp. 145–166). New York, NY: Oxford University Press.

Fredrickson, B. L., & Losada, M. F. (2005). Positive affect and the complex dynamics of human flourishing. *American Psychologist, 60*(7), 678–686.

Froman, L. (2010). Positive psychology in the workplace. *Journal of Adult Development, 17*, 59–69.

Gable, S. L., & Haidt, J. (2005). What (and why) is positive psychology? *Review of General Psychology, 9*, 103–110.

Gagné, M., & Deci, E. L. (2005). Self-determination theory and work motivation. *Journal of Organizational Behavior, 26*(4), 331–362.

Gallup. (2013). *State of the American workplace*. Retrieved from http://www.gallup.com/strategic-consulting/163007/state-american- workplace.aspx

Gasper, K., & Clore, G. L. (2002). Attending to the big picture: Mood and global versus local processing of visual information. *Psychological Science, 13*(1), 34–40.

George, J. M. (1998). Salesperson mood at work: Implications for helping customers. *Journal of Personal Selling and Sales Management, 18*, 23–30.

Goleman, D. (1996). *Emotional intelligence*. London: Bloomsbury.

Grant, A. M., Green, L., & Rynsaardt, J. (2010). Developmental coaching for high school teachers: Executive coaching goes to school. *Consulting Psychology Journal: Practice and Research, 62*(3), 151–168.

Green, S., Oades, L., & Grant, A. M. (2006). Cognitive-behavioral, solution-focused life coaching: Enhancing goal striving, well-being, and hope. *The Journal of Positive Psychology, 1*(3), 142–149.

Harter, J. K., Schmidt, F. L., & Hayes, T. L. (2002). Business-unit-level relationship between employee satisfaction, employee engagement, and business outcomes: A meta-analysis. *Journal of Applied Psychology, 87*, 268–279.

Harter, J. K., Schmidt, F. L., Kilham, E. A., & Asplund, J. W. (2006). *Q12 meta-analysis*. The Gallup Organisation.

Harzer, C., & Ruch, W. (2012). When the job is a calling: The role of applying one's signature strengths at work. *The Journal of Positive Psychology, 7*, 362–371.

Harzer, C., & Ruch, W. (2014). The role of character strengths for task performance, job dedication, interpersonal facilitation, and organizational support. *Human Performance, 27*(3), 183–205.

Henry, J. (2004). Positive and creative organization. In P. A. Linley & S. Joseph (Eds.), *Positive psychology in practice* (pp. 269–286). New Jersey: Wiley.

Hersey, R. B. (1932). Rates of production and emotional state. *Personnel Journal, 10*, 355–364.

Hodges, T. D., & Clifton, D. O. (2004). Strengths-based development in practice. In P. A. Linley & S. Joseph (Eds.), *Positive psychology in practice* (pp. 105–124). New Jersey: Wiley.

Isen, A. M. (1987). Positive affect, cognitive processes and social behaviour. In L. Berkowitz (Ed.), *Advances in experimental social psychology* (pp. 203–253). New York: Academic.

Isen, A. M. (2003). Positive affect as a source of human strength. In L. G. Aspinwall & U. M. Staudinger (Eds.), *A psychology of human strengths: Fundamental questions and future directions for a positive psychology* (pp. 179–195). Washington, DC: American Psychological Association.

Isen, A. M., Daubman, K. A., & Nowicki, G. P. (1987). Positive affect facilitates creative problem solving. *Journal of Personality and Social Psychology, 52*(6), 1122–1131.

Isen, A. M., Rosenzweig, A. S., & Young, M. J. (1991). The influence of positive affect on clinical problem solving. *Medical Decision Making: An International Journal of the Society for Medical Decision Making, 11*(3), 221.

Johnson, K. J., Waugh, C. E., & Fredrickson, B. L. (2010). Smile to see the forest: Facially expressed positive emotions broaden cognition. *Cognition and Emotion, 24*(2), 299–321.

Kelloway, E. K., Weigand, H., McKee, M. C., & Das, H. (2013). Positive leadership and employee well-being. *Journal of Leadership and Organizational Studies, 20*(1), 107–117.

Kern, M. L., Waters, L., Adler, A., & White, M. (2014). Assessing employee wellbeing in schools using a multi-faceted approach: Associations with physical health, life satisfaction, and professional thriving. *Psychology, 5*, 500–513.

King, L. A., Eells, J. E., & Burton, C. M. (2004). The good life, broadly and narrowly considered. In P. A. Linley & S. Joseph (Eds.), *Positive psychology in practice* (pp. 35–52). New Jersey: Wiley.

Kobasa, S. C. (1979). Stressful life events, personality, and health: An inquiry into hardiness. *Journal of Personality and Social Psychology, 37*, 1–11.

Kotler, S. (2014, May 6). Create a work environment that fosters flow. *Harvard Business Review*.

Leach, C., & Green, S. (2016). Integrating coaching and positive psychology in education. In C. van Nieuwerburgh (Ed.), *Coaching in professional contexts*. London: Sage Publications.

Linley, P. A., Joseph, S., Harrington, S., & Wood, A. M. (2006). Positive psychology: Past, present, and (possible) future. *The Journal of Positive Psychology, 1*(1), 3–16.

Linley, A., Willars, J., & Biswas-Diener, R. (2010). *The strengths book: What you can do, love to do, and find it hard to do—And why it matters*. Coventry: CAPP Press.

Lopez, S. J., & Snyder, C. R. (2003). The future of positive psychological assessment: Making a difference. In S. J. Lopez & C. R. Snyder (Eds.), *Positive psychological assessment—A handbook of models and measures* (pp. 461–468). Washington, DC: American Psychological Association.

Lopez, S. J., Snyder, C. R., & Pedrotti, J. T. (2003). Hope: Many definitions, many measures. In S. J. Lopez & C. R. Snyder (Eds.), *Positive psychological assessment—A handbook of models and measures* (pp. 91–107). Washington, DC: American Psychological Association.

Losada, M., & Heaphy, E. (2004). The role of positivity and connectivity in the performance of business teams: A nonlinear dynamics model. *American Behavioral Scientist, 47*(6), 740–765.

Luthans, F., Avey, J. B., Avolio, B. J., Norman, S. M., & Combs, G. M. (2006). Psychological capital development: Toward a micro-intervention. *Journal of Organizational Behaviour, 27*, 387–393.

McQuaid, M., & Lawn, E. (2015). *Your strengths blueprint: How to be engaged, energised, & happy at work*. San Bernandino, USA.

McQuaid, M., & VIA Institute. (2015). *The 2015 Strengths @ Work Survey*. Retrieved from http://www.michellemcquaid.com/strengthssurvey

Medibank. (2008). *Annual Report*. Retrieved from https://www.medibank.com.au/content/dam/medibank/About-Us/pdfs/MPL_Annual_Report_2008.pdf

Meyers, M. C., Van Woerkom, M., & Bakker, A. B. (2013). The added value of the positive: A literature review of positive psychology interventions in organizations. *European Journal of Work and Organizational Psychology, 22*(5), 618–632.

Mills, M. J., Fleck, C. R., & Kozikowski, A. (2013). Positive psychology at work: A conceptual review, state-of-practice assessment, and a look ahead. *Journal of Positive Psychology, 8*(2), 153–164.

Mroz, D., & Quinn, S. (2009). Positive organizational scholarship leaps into the world of work. In N. Garcea, S. Harrington, & P. A. Linley (Eds.), *Oxford handbook of positive psychology and work* (pp. 251–264). New York: Oxford University Press.

Park, N., & Peterson, C. (2009). Character strengths: Research and practice. *Journal of College and Character, 4*, 1–8.

Pascale, R. (1999). *Managing on the edge: How successful companies use conflict to stay ahead.* London: Viking.

Pearce, R. (2013, July 8). Hacking creativity: Making time for innovation. *Computerworld.*

Peterson, C. (2006). *A primer in positive psychology*. New York: Oxford University Press.

Peterson, S. J., & Byron, K. (2008). Exploring the role of hope in job performance: Results from four studies. *Journal of Organizational Behavior, 29*(6), 785–803.

Peterson, C., & Park, N. (2009). Classifying and measuring strengths of character. In S. J. Lopez & C. R. Snyder (Eds.), *Oxford handbook of positive psychology* (2nd ed., pp. 25–33). New York: Oxford University Press www.viacharacter.org.

Peterson, C., & Seligman, M. E. P. (2004). *Character strengths and virtues: A handbook and classification.* New York: Oxford University Press.

Peterson, C., Park, N., & Seligman, M. E. P. (2006). Greater strengths of character and recovery from illness. *The Journal of Positive Psychology, 1*, 7–26.

Peterson, C., Stephens, J. P., Park, N., Lee, F., & Seligman, M. E. P. (2010). Strengths of character and work. In P. A. Linley, S. Harrington, & N. Garcea (Eds.), *Oxford handbook of positive psychology and work* (pp. 221–231). New York: Oxford University Press.

Pressman, S. D., & Cohen, S. (2005). Does positive affect influence health? *Psychological Bulletin, 131*(6), 925–971.

PricewaterhouseCoopers. (2014). *Creating a mentally healthy workplace: Return on investment analysis.* Retrieved from https://www.headsup.org.au/docs/default-source/resources/bl1269-brochure---pwc-roi-analysis.pdf?sfvrsn=6

Rand, K. L. (2009). Hope and optimism: Latent structures and influences on grade expectancy and academic performance. *Journal of Personality, 77*(1), 231–260.

Rath, T. (2007). *Strengths finder 2.0.* New York, NY: Gallup Press.

Renninger, K. A. (1992). Individual interest and development: Implications for theory and practice. In K. A. Renninger, S. Hidi, & A. Krapp (Eds.), *The role of interest in learning and development* (pp. 361–395). Hillsdale, NJ: Erlbaum.

Rotundo, M., & Sackett, P. R. (2002). The relative importance of task, citizenship, and counterproductive performance to global ratings of job performance: A policy-capturing approach. *Journal of Applied Psychology, 87*, 66–80.

Rust, T., Diessner, R., & Reade, L. (2009). Strengths only or strengths and relative weaknesses? A preliminary study. *The Journal of Psychology, 143*(5), 465–476.

Ryan, R. M., & Deci, E. L. (2000). Self-determination theory and the facilitation of intrinsic motivation, social development, and well-being. *American Psychologist, 55*(1), 68–78.

Salanova, M., Agut, S., & Peiro, J. M. (2005). Linking organizational resources and work engagement to employee performance and customer loyalty: The mediation of service climate. *Journal of Applied Psychology, 90*(6), 1217–1227.

Salanova, M., Llorens, S., Acosta, H., & Torrente, P. (2013). Positive interventions in positive organisations. *Psychological Therapy, 31*(1), 101–113.

Schaufeli, W. B., & Salanova, M. (2010). *How to improve work engagement?* Cheltenham: Edward Elgar.

Seligman, M. E. P. (2002). *Authentic happiness: Using the new positive psychology to realize your potential for lasting fulfillment.* New York, NY: Free Press.

Seligman, M. E. P. (2011). *Flourish: A visionary new understanding of happiness and well-being.* New York, NY: Free Press.

Seligman, M. E. P., & Csikszentmihalyi, M. (2000). Positive psychology: An introduction. *American Psychologist, 55*, 5–14.
Sharot, T., Riccardi, A. M., Raio, C. M., & Phelps, E. A. (2007). Neural mechanisms mediating optimism bias. *Nature, 450*, 102–105.
Sheldon, K. M., & Elliot, A. J. (1999). Goal striving, need satisfaction, and longitudinal well-being: The self-concordance model. *Journal of Personality and Social Psychology, 76*(3), 482–497.
Sin, N. L., & Lyubomirsky, S. (2009). Enhancing well-being and alleviating depressive symptoms with positive psychology interventions: A practice-friendly meta-analysis. *Journal of Clinical Psychology, 65*, 467–487.
Snyder, C. R. (2000). *Handbook of hope: Theory, measures, and applications*. San Diego, CA: Academic Press.
Spreitzer, G. M., & Sonenshein, S. (2004). Toward the construct definition of positive deviance. *American Behavioral Scientist, 47*(6), 828–847.
Staw, B. M., & Barsade, S. G. (1993). Affect and managerial performance: A test of the sadder-but-wiser vs. happier-and-smarter hypothesis. *Administrative Science Quarterly, 38*(2), 304–331.
Staw, B. M., Sutton, R. I., & Pelled, S. H. (1994). Employee positive emotions and favorable outcomes at the workplace. *Organization Science, 5*, 51–71.
Thoresen, C. J., Kaplan, S. A., Barsky, A. P., Warren, C. R., & de Chermont, K. (2003). The affective underpinnings of job perceptions and attitudes: A meta-analytic review and integration. *Psychological Bulletin, 129*(6), 914–945.
Tutu, D. (1999). *No future without forgiveness*. New York: Doubleday.
Vacharkulksemsuk, F., & Frederickson, B. L. (2013). Looking back and glimpsing forward: The broaden-and-build theory of positive emotions as applied to organisations. *Advances in Positive Organizational Psychology, 1*, 45–60.
van Knippenberg, D., & van Schie, E. C. M. (2000). Foci and correlates of organisational identification. *Journal of Occupational and Organisational Psychology, 73*, 137–147.
Wall, T. D., Kemp, N. J., Jackson, P. R., & Clegg, C. W. (1986). Outcomes of autonomous workgroups: A long-term field experiment. *The Academy of Management Journal, 29*(2), 280–304.
Waterman, R. H., Peters, T. J., & Phillips, J. R. (1980). Structure is not organization. *Business Horizons, 23*(3), 14–26.
Weiss, H. M. (2002). Deconstructing job satisfaction: Separating evaluations, beliefs and affective experiences. *Human Resource Management Review, 12*(2), 173–194.
Weiss, H. M., & Cropanzano, R. (1996). Affective events theory: A theoretical discussion of the structure, causes and consequences of affective experiences at work. In B. M. Staw & L. L. Cummings (Eds.), *Research in organizational behavior: An annual series of analytical essays and critical reviews* (pp. 1–74). Greenwich, CT: JAI Press.
Wildavsky, A. (1988). *Searching for safety*. New Brunswick, NJ: Transaction Press.
Xanthopoulou, D., Bakker, A. B., Demerouti, E., & Schaufeli, W. B. (2012). A diary study on the happy worker: How job resources generate positive emotions and personal resources. *European Journal of Work and Organizational Psychology, 21*, 489–517.

Chapter 12
Applying Positive Organisational Scholarship to Produce Extraordinary Performance

Jandi Kelly and Kim Cameron

Abstract This chapter discusses the application of positive organisational scholarship (POS) and its impact on organisational performance. Specifically, we review how POS interventions implemented in two different businesses within the Prudential Financial Services Corporation led to extraordinarily successful performance in each business. We organise the various POS practices that were implemented into five themes, and we discuss how each positive practice was applied. Our purpose is to illustrate a few ways in which POS can be employed to enhance the performance of organisations.

Abbreviations

BHAG	Big harry audacious goals
BP	British petroleum
POS	Positive organisational scholarship
PRERS	Prudential real estate and relocation service
SMART	Specific, measureable, aligned, realistic, time-bound

What Is Positive Organisational Scholarship?

Positive organisational scholarship (POS) is concerned primarily with the study of especially positive outcomes, processes, and attributes of organisations and their members. POS does not represent a single theory, but it focuses on dynamics that are typically described by words such as excellence, thriving, flourishing, abundance, resilience, or virtuousness. 'Positive' refers to an affirmative bias and a focus on achieving the best of the human condition; 'organisational' refers to a focus on the processes and conditions in organisational contexts; and 'scholarship' refers to

J. Kelly (✉) • K. Cameron
Ross School of Education, University of Michigan, 500 S State, Ann Arbor, MI 48109, USA
e-mail: jandi@umich.edu; kim_cameron@umich.edu

C. Proctor (ed.), *Positive Psychology Interventions in Practice*,
DOI 10.1007/978-3-319-51787-2_12

empirically rigorous and theoretically based scientific procedures that ground the POS approach. The premise of POS research is that by understanding the drivers of positive practices in the workplace, organisations and individuals can create extraordinarily effective performance and achieve the best of the human condition (see Cameron et al. 2003; Cameron and Spreitzer 2012).

The Context

Prudential Retirement

In April 2004, Prudential Retirement acquired CIGNA Insurance Company's full-service retirement operations for $2.1 billion and appointed John Kim as CEO. The merger was described as like trying to merge the Red Sox and the Yankees. Two distinct cultures existed—one from New England and the other from the New York/New Jersey area. Both were very strong, very passionate, and very powerful. Business processes, human resources systems, and technological systems were understandably different. These differences translated into disparities in culture and language, which would need to be ameliorated before full integration could take place. The merger also presented challenges for employee recruitment and retention since job security was uncertain for all previous Prudential and CIGNA employees. The retirement business was in a highly competitive industry, and the survival of this newly formed firm was not at all assured (see Vanette and Cameron 2009).

Prudential Real Estate and Relocation

In the summer of 2009, as the financial markets were recovering from one of the worst recessions since the Great Depression, Jim Mallozzi was appointed as CEO of Prudential's Real Estate and Relocation Service (PRERS). The real estate business sells residential and commercial real estate franchises across North America. The relocation business helps individuals and families move locations throughout the world. It serves both U.S. Government employees and large corporations. At the time of Mallozzi's appointment, PRERS was facing a $70 million loss on top of a $140 million loss the year before. Morale both in the company and among customers was extremely low (see Cameron and Plews 2012).

In both companies, the CEOs—John Kim and Jim Mallozzi—purposely adopted POS as the preferred approach to their change efforts. What follows is a description of several of the most important interventions.

Intervention 1: Positive Energy

In order to create positive energy throughout the firm, one of Mallozzi's first steps as CEO was to shine a light on PRERS's assets and opportunities as opposed to weaknesses and roadblocks. He wanted to both challenge and support his employees in transcending traditional modes of deficit-based thinking. As an alternative, he described his goal as creating an atmosphere that empowered staff to generate solutions and achieve unprecedented industry milestones. He encouraged employees to 'identify what we have rather than focusing on what we don't have'.

Value-Added Feedback Exercise

One way Mallozzi strove to enhance positive energy, was through personal feedback exercises. For example, one activity prompted employees to take a minute each to tell three different colleagues three things they noticed about their unique value-adding contributions or the ways in which they demonstrated leadership strengths. Unlike typical feedback activities that focus on areas for improvement, a positive approach unveils intrinsic and often underappreciated staff attributes. Drawing attention to positive assets and behaviours not only garnered PRERS employees' attention but also contributed notably to the level of positive energy among team members.

Reflected Best-Self Exercise

Both Kim and Mallozzi focused on leveraging the unique strengths of their leadership teams and on enhancing positive energy. For example, they used the *reflected best-self exercise* to capture and highlight staff members' talents and capabilities[1]. This strategy involves having each senior team member solicit written anecdotes from at least 20 friends, coworkers, and family members in response to a question such as: '*When you have seen me make a special or valuable contribution, what distinctive strengths did I display?*' or '*When you have seen me display my best, what unique value did I create?*' These individuals each received up to 60 behavioural descriptions of when they displayed their best selves. Participants were then guided through a process to create a 'best-self portrait', which highlighted often-overlooked strengths and personal resources. Most importantly, it uncovered ways in which leaders could contribute additional value to their teams, units, and the larger organisation.

[1]Accessing the reflected best-self process and developing best-self portraits among individuals are available at: http://positiveorgs.bus.umich.edu/cpo-tools/reflected-best-self-exercise-2nd-edition/

Positive Energy Networks

Research suggests that individuals can be characterised as 'positive' or 'negative' energisers (Owens et al. 2016). Positive energisers cultivate vitality and esteem, leave others uplifted and energised, and bring life to the organisation and its members. In contrast, negative energisers deplete feelings of positivity and enthusiasm in others. Unlike inherent preferences or attributes, such as charisma or extroversion, positive energising is a learned behaviour. Organisations can therefore foster and leverage such behaviours by empowering positive energisers to boost both personal productivity and accelerate the contributions of those around them. One of the most effective mechanisms these CEOs implemented to enhance performance, was to identify and empower positive energisers.

Both firms implemented a positive energy mapping process. In PRERS, for example, several thousand employees participated in an assessment of positive energy. Using a 7-point Likert scale, individuals were asked to rate the extent to which they were positively energised by others in their business units. Twenty-six of the most energising people throughout the company were then brought together at corporate headquarters and charged with infusing the new culture and values into the rest of the company in only 60 days. Without the CEO present in the room, this group established a strategy to accomplish this daunting assignment. The result was that, in a 2-month period, 93% of PRERS 2000 employees had been 'infected' with a new culture and with positive energy. One outcome was that employee engagement scores increased in 9 out of 10 categories. This group continued to collaborate over time and established a self-sustaining effort to incorporate fresh POS principles into PRERS daily practices.

Intervention 2: Everest Goals

Both Prudential leaders also adopted the POS practice of establishing Everest goals (Cameron 2012). The concept of an *Everest Goal* is based on the idea that climbing Mt. Everest is among the most challenging activities most people can imagine. It requires supreme planning, training, effort, teamwork, and personal mastery. The physical, mental, and emotional strength required to climb Mt. Everest exceeds the capacity of must human beings by a wide margin. Everest goals share similar attributes—they represent the peak, the culmination, the supreme achievement that individuals can imagine. They signify accomplishment well-beyond ordinary success.

In addition to being SMART goals (that is, Specific, Measureable, Aligned, Realistic, Time-bound), Everest goals possess five additional attributes: (1) Everest goals are focused on attaining positive deviance—extraordinary, spectacular achievement; (2) Everest goals represent 'goods of first intent'—they possess profound and inherent meaningfulness; (3) Everest goals focus on affirmative orientation—strengths rather than weaknesses and opportunities rather than threats; (4)

Everest goals represent a positive contribution—not just problem solving or getting rid of obstacles; (5) Everest goals create and foster sustainable positive energy—no extra incentive is needed to pursue the goal.

The Power of Five Exercise

One Everest goal established by Mallozzi was to transform client relationships. To make progress toward reaching this objective, Mallozzi engaged his leadership team in the *Power of Five Exercise*, which consisted of three requirements. First, each team member identified five new client prospects. The challenge was to creatively maximise company resources to acquire these firms as clients. Second, employees were challenged to 'wow' five existing clients. When asked what wow meant, Mallozzi suggested that they ask the clients what it would take to wow them. Third, employees were empowered to fire five clients who were exuding negative energy and draining the company's vitality. The goal was to stop counting clients, but instead, to cultivate clients that count.

The results exceeded expectations. One client on the verge of leaving the firm became one of PRERS's greatest advocates due to employees' sincere efforts to learn about and support this customer's core values and objectives. Another client with whom PRERS's severed ties moved on to exhaust a competitor's energy while PRERSs dedicated the energy it saved to more fruitful undertakings.

Reformulating an Everest Goal

Prudential Retirement had established a corporate goal that leaders thought represented an ultimate achievement. The goal was to acquire $10 billion in assets by the year 2010. This goal was not unlike many other corporate goals that Jim Collins (2001) labelled BHAGs (big harry audacious goals). For most firms, these represent an ultimate stretch, or a dreamed-for achievement. The trouble is, employees in the mailroom, in the accounting department, or on the sales force are not motivated by such goals. Ensuring the top brass get rich or the company expands financially is not intrinsically motivating for lower-level employees. These kinds of goals—albeit representing extraordinary performance—have little personal meaning. After learning about the concept of Everest goals, the company reformulated its target to better represent the attributes of Everest goals—that is, inherent meaning, sustainable positive energy, goods of first intent, and so forth. The goal was changed to establishing secure retirements for 10 million people by the year 2010.

This may not seem like much of a change, but now the mailroom clerk, the accountant, or the salesperson understood that if they did their jobs well, their own grandmother would never have to worry about financial security during old age. The stress of retirement would be removed for people they cared about and people who were important in their lives. The goal took on personal meaning and represented an inherently valuable outcome. The result of this motivating goal was that Prudential Retirement became the largest and most successful unit in the entire corporation (see Vanette and Cameron 2009).

Intervention 3: Reciprocity Networks

Reciprocity Network Exercise

One POS practice of notable impact was the creation of a reciprocity network[2]. In this exercise, individuals identify a need, a problem, or a request for assistance. They write the request on a Post-It Note and then take 30 s to explain it to their colleagues in a group setting. Colleagues, in turn, write down resources they may have, people they may know, or assistance that can be provided to address as many requests within their ability. The intent is to create a network of resources and connections based on reciprocal exchange that would never have been recognised otherwise.

In PRERS, the top 30 leaders in the firm joined Mallozzi in writing down current problems on Post-It Notes that they were struggling to solve. One example highlights the impact that is associated with this exercise. The General Counsel, sceptical that anyone headquartered in the USA could possibly assist him, shared that he was tasked with the necessity of hiring legal counsel for the French office in Paris. By the time the reciprocity network exercise was completed, the General Counsel received four solid connections of competent legal counsel who could be available to take this new position in Paris.

A variation on this exercise was implemented several months later at the annual convention with 2500 real estate agents from across the county. In his first keynote as CEO, Mallozzi engaged the crowd in a large-scale reciprocity network activity. In the midst of his speech, Mallozzi asked each audience member to take out their handheld devices and text or email one great business idea to a website on the screen. The ideas were targeted at how to acquire a new customer or how to keep a customer for life. Over the next 36 h, participants generated over 2200 ideas—900 of which were unique—and the whole list of ideas was shared, in turn, with everyone who had made a contribution. This success prompted the launch of PRERS online network *NextWork*—what's next and what works—as a space for all PRERS community members to share best practices and mentor one another on a continual basis.

Although distinct in scope, these various renditions of this exercise illustrate the power of reciprocity and the often-untapped potential of inviting others to contribute in positive ways.

---

[2] Information about reciprocity networks and the technology to implement the process can be found at: http://www.humaxnetworks.com

Change Teams

In each of the two firms, CEOs created 'change teams' to serve as a source of positive energy and to accelerate the change process. In Prudential Retirement, for example, six members of the change team were selected from among the top 100 senior executives. These individuals were released from many of their responsibilities and commissioned to lead the culture change and turnaround efforts. This change team not only advocated POS principles in their own functional areas and across business units, but they organised coaching sessions, seminars, and open forums to regularly discuss questions, concerns, and successes company-wide. The team even produced a video demonstrating the impact of POS on improved customer service.

The change team paid special attention to employees who demonstrated interest in POS. Doing so created a *pull,* rather than a *push*, strategy and multiplied their impact—their efforts created visibility for themselves, as well as tangible evidence that they were making a difference. The change team organised at least two POS seminars annually in different geographic locations to expose all Prudential Retirement employees POS practices. Furthermore, as POS became more institutionalised, the team served as an advisory board to Human Resources and provided feedback on ways to sustain forward momentum in disseminating positive practices and positive leadership. These efforts subsequently led to the creation of mini-change teams throughout the organisation to foster and facilitate POS practices at local levels.

Intervention 4: Measuring the Positive

Assessing High Not Just Low

Like most companies, PRERS conducted client satisfaction surveys consisting of Likert scales ranging from 1 (low) to 5 (outstanding). In the past, PRERS leadership was preoccupied with expunging scores in the 1–3 range. As a result of refocusing their culture on positive practices, PRERS changed this approach to emphasise the successes that lead to scores at the outstanding end of the scale. This shift, however, was not always easy for some units to implement. When visiting the French office, for example, Mallozzi asked employees how they might achieve '5 s'. The French PRERS staff explained that they had never measured anything above a '3'. They were so consumed with addressing the problems—the '1 s' and '2 s'—that no one could recall a rating of 5.

Mallozzi encouraged the team to brainstorm moments when the French office had experienced organisational excellence and had actually achieved 5-level performance. Almost immediately, an employee recalled that over the past several weeks, French PRERS staff had stationed themselves at the Charles De Gaulle Airport around-the-clock to greet relocated clients from Japan's recent earthquake and tsunami. The employee described the event in this way:

> They had to leave all their goods behind them. They have no place to live. They are being forced back into this country. We were there greeting them at the airport, helping them find a place to live, giving them bottled water as they got off the plane, helping them get back into France as quickly as we could. No other company is doing that. We are the only ones out there doing it on behalf of our clients.

This simple exercise of measuring and concentrating on the positive helped the French PRERS team realise an overlooked act of positive deviance that not only warranted celebration, but served as a source of motivational renewal.

Client Scores

In their efforts to reinvent their cultures, both CEOs encouraged line managers to conduct multiple small experiments to achieve positive deviance related to customer relationships. These efforts supplemented larger corporate development projects, which can take years to measure. Units experimented with different approaches to delighting customers and 'wowing' clients, and they assessed not only *who*, but *what* and *how*, successes were achieved. The intent was to share practices and positive achievements in order to replicate these efforts. Measurements focused on how to achieve extraordinary success rather than how to overcome or resolve problems.

As client satisfaction measures increased, celebrations and recognition ceremonies were regular occurrences. After 18 months of experiments, trial and error initiatives, and small wins, this focus on assessing and sharing positive practices resulted in client services scores reaching historic highs. Some units even achieved 100% satisfaction with the most demanding clients.

Intervention 5: Implementing Positivity and Virtuousness

An Abundance Culture

Developing an abundance culture means that an organisation engenders and is guided by virtuous practices. That is, compassionate support for one another, optimism, inspiration, forgiveness, integrity, generosity, respect, and gratitude are all aspects of the type of culture labelled 'abundance'. Research has confirmed that organisations that develop an abundance culture are significantly more effective than other organisations (Cameron et al. 2004). Virtuous practices have a major impact not only on employees and customers, but also on actual bottom line performance including profitability, productivity, and customer retention (Cameron et al. 2011). One manager recalled that three recent hires ultimately joined Prudential because of the way people talked about the abundance culture, the POS perspective, and the manner in which business was conducted.

As these two Prudential businesses moved toward a more well developed abundance culture, current and prospective clients began to notice. Clients began to view the improved cultural environment and high levels of staff engagement as key differentiators of the company. One example of this development was the transformation of a senior manager's historically tense relationship with a client. After learning about POS, the senior manager consciously strove to take a positive approach to all interactions with the customer. In turn, the client shared more about his life and markedly strengthened his tie with Prudential and several personal and professional relationships. Commitment to a life-long relationship resulted. In a separate case, a client relationship manager had described Prudential's efforts to create an abundance culture to better meet customers' needs to a potential client. Prudential's mindset to 'focus on the good' caught the prospect's interest and resulted in his company adding Prudential Retirement to its short list of service providers.

Virtuous Practices

In PRERS, intentional steps were taken to implement extraordinarily positive and virtuous behaviours. For example, when visiting the company's London offices, Mallozzi got to know some representatives at a European client, British Petroleum (BP). He shared how Prudential was using POS initiatives to change the company culture, and he invited BP to engage in these efforts. Several weeks later, the Deep Water Horizon oil spill occurred in the Gulf of Mexico. The disaster was one of largest environmental spills in history and resulted in the loss of 11 lives. BP was the target of the negative headlines surrounding the event, and leaders at BP were blasted in the USA and throughout the global press.

Mallozzi approached his European contacts to explain that he understood BP was relocating a number of employees to the Gulf region in order to address the crisis. Drawing upon the abundance culture of PRERS, Mallozzi offered relocation services free of charge to BP for the duration of the crises. When BP asked why PRERS would make such an offer, Mallozzi explained:

> [W]e all have a responsibility for what's going on in the Gulf. We all need to try to help in ways large and small. This is the best way that I can think of to help you. It's a sincere offer. If you'd like to take us up on it, great, if you don't, that's fine. I certainly understand.

BP executives indicated that most phone calls from other firms were threats of lawsuits, and PRERS offer was the only offer for complimentary assistance. Several months later, BP issued a request-for-proposal for a new vendor for corporate relocations. PRERs was specifically invited to be one of the participants. Mallozzi summarised the lesson as: 'It's okay to help others and not expect anything in return. When we do that, fabulous things can happen'.

Setting the Tone in Meetings

Several micro-interventions were implemented throughout the company, including ongoing staff meeting changes. Leaders began to open meetings by highlighting recent team successes, and employees were invited to share business accomplishments, reflections on flourishing professional relationships, and achievements in their personal lives. One manager shared how POS principles motivated her to hold family meetings during which each member shared characteristics he or she most admired and valued about one another. A second employee kept a 'gratitude journal' of insights, such as her toddler's positive sentiments of his teacher and her interactions with co-workers that brought a sense of meaning and purpose to her work. She shared these observations with her child's teacher and colleagues, which created a positive feedback loop and enhanced these relationships.

Results

In the end, POS practices enabled Prudential Retirement to successfully assimilate two very different companies while maintaining 95% of their client base, boosting employees' satisfaction scores, decreasing turnover, and growing earnings by about 20% annually on a compound rate. Prudential Retirement became the corporation's largest business unit. Moreover, when John Kim moved on to become president of New York Life Insurance Company, the abundance culture and virtuous practices stayed in place at Prudential.

A formal assessment indicated that that Prudential Retirement had improved on 35 of 38 positive practices after just 1 year of its POS change initiative. Statistical analyses revealed that POS practices significantly affected Prudential Retirement's climate, voluntarily turnover, and financial performance. Specifically, POS practices positively impacted the work environment (e.g., employee morale), managerial effectiveness (e.g., relationships between bosses and subordinates), and employee retention (e.g., intent of employees to leave) within the firm at the $p < 0.01$ level. Business units with higher scores on positive practices experienced a better work environment, more effective relationships with management, and greater numbers of employees intending to stay with the firm. Positive practices also had a stronger impact on actual voluntary employee turnover than did the standard morale and climate scores commonly used in organisations. A third analysis indicated that the correlation between positive practice scores for each business unit within Prudential Retirement and six aggregated measures of financial performance (i.e., average assets, sales, customer account retention, cash flow, revenues, and expenses) was significant at the $p > 0.0001$ level.

In Prudential Real Estate and Relocation Service, the firm improved from a $70 million loss to a $20 million profit in the first 12 months, and the company achieved two times its expected business plan. Profits more than doubled from what insiders expected. PRERS was awarded the 2010 JD Power Award for Service in its Real Estate Franchise business in addition to three Trippel Survey awards for outstanding client service in its Relocation Company. Customer satisfaction scores improved in 9 out of 12 categories, even though Mallozzi was initially aspiring for 8 out of 12. Improvement occurred in 9 out of 10 categories in the employee engagement survey, and Mallozzi received 110 written pages of comments in the annual employee engagement survey. Approximately 60% were comments about the positive changes in the company. (Employee comments are usually complaints or criticisms.) The company scored in first quartile status in the employee survey for the first time in years. Two years after Mallozzi became CEO, PRERS stock price was higher than Prudential Financial Service's stock value overall.

The intent of this chapter has been to describe several of the practical applications that have emerged from positive organisational scholarship as a field of study. Some of these practices can be labelled and described with specificity, but some are more nuanced and emerged from the adoption of a way of thinking, a set of cultural assumptions, and an approach to positive leadership. Prudential leaders were creative in identifying ways to make an abundance culture come alive and to make POS applicable. The bottom line results they achieved are a good indication their success.

References

Cameron, K. S. (2012). *Positive leadership: Strategies for extraordinary performance*. San Francisco: Berrett-Koehler.

Cameron, K. S., & Plews, E. (2012). Positive leadership in action: Applications of POS by Jim Mallozzi. *Organizational Dynamics, 41*, 99–105.

Cameron, K. S., & Spreitzer, G. M. (2012). *Oxford handbook of positive organizational scholarship*. New York: Oxford University Press.

Cameron, K. S., Dutton, J. E., & Quinn, R. E. (2003). *Positive organizational scholarship*. San Francisco: Berrett Koehler.

Cameron, K. S., Bright, D., & Caza, A. (2004). Exploring the relationships between organizational virtuousness and performance. *American Behavioral Scientist, 47*, 766–790.

Cameron, K. S., Mora, C., Leutscher, T., & Calarco, M. (2011). Effects of positive practices on organizational effectiveness. *Journal of Applied Behavioral Science, 47*, 266–308.

Collins, J. (2001). *Good the great*. New York: Harper.

Owens, B. P., Baker, W. E., Sumpter, D. M., & Cameron, K. S. (2016). Relational energy at work: Implications for job engagement and job performance. *Journal of Applied Psychology, 101*, 35–49.

Vanette, D., & Cameron, K. S. (2009). Implementing positive organizational scholarship at prudential. Ross School of Business, William Davidson Institute, University of Michigan.

Chapter 13
Positive Technologies for Improving Health and Well-Being

Cristina Botella, Rosa Maria Banos, and Veronica Guillen

Abstract In the last 20 years there have been two important developments of great importance to the field of psychological treatments. On the one hand, this meant the movement of positive psychology, and on the other, the introduction of information and communication technologies (ICT) to improve the daily clinical practice. In this paper a new field of study that attempts to strengthen ties and build bridges between them is introduced: Positive Technologies. This perspective seeks to promote the use of technology to foster personal growth and the development of human virtues and strengths, thus contributing to social and cultural development. In this chapter, we present four positive technologies: (1) 'EMMA's World', a virtual reality system developed for the treatment of stress-related disorders. It can provide to the user meaningful virtual environments capable of activating and enhancing the emotional processing of the event experienced, and fostering a more positive projection toward the future. As a positive technology, it can be classified at the eudaimonic level; (2) 'EARTH of Well-Being', a virtual reality application designed to induce positive emotions in a controlled way and reinforce psychological resources, covering the hedonic and eudaimonic levels; (3) 'Smiling is Fun', a positive technology intervention designed to generate coping resources and foster psychological well-being at both at the hedonic and eudaimonic levels; and (4) 'BUTLER', which aims to contribute to improve the quality of life of the elderly. It includes the most popular Internet services integrated into a single platform, adapting its characteristics to the

C. Botella (✉)
Department of Basic Psychology, Clinical and Psychobiology, Jaume I University, Av. Vicente Sos Banyat s/n, 12071 Castellon, Spain
e-mail: botella@uji.es

R.M. Banos
Department of Personality, Evaluation and Psychological Treatment, University of Valencia, Av. De Blasco Ibáñez, 13, 46010 Valencia, Spain
e-mail: banos@uv.es

V. Guillen
Department of Personality, Evaluation and Psychological Treatment, University of Valencia, Av. De Blasco Ibáñez, 13, 46010 Valencia, Spain

Centro Clínico Previ, Calle Grabador Esteve, 12, 46004 Valencia, Spain
e-mail: vguillenbotella@gmail.com

C. Proctor (ed.), *Positive Psychology Interventions in Practice*,
DOI 10.1007/978-3-319-51787-2_13

needs of the elderly population. It is designed to cover the three levels of positive technologies: hedonic, eudaimonic, and social interaction. All these applications are presented and the different possibilities and advantages that this perspective may involve are analysed.

Abbreviations

AG	Augmented reality
EMA	Ecological momentary assessment
EMI	Ecological momentary interventions
ICT	Information and communication technologies
PP	Positive psychology
PPI	Positive psychological intervention
PT	Positive technologies
PTSD	Posttraumatic stress disorder
VR	Virtual reality

Introduction

Psychology has begun to accept subjective well-being as a relevant object of study that deals directly with the exploration of human strengths and the factors that contribute to happiness. Although this topic has been present in psychology (and philosophy) in one-way or another for a long time, its establishment as a specific aim of scientific study is attributed to positive psychology (PP; Seligman and Csikszentmihalyi 2000).

Although the main purpose of PP is to foster well-being, it also focuses on reducing distress, which, although related, is not the same thing. PP seeks to make psychology a more 'balanced' discipline, considering both the sources and the difficulties of psychological health. For this purpose, psychologists have tools that not only help to mitigate suffering, but also promote well-being (Tarragona 2010). Based on these approaches, several positive psychological interventions (PPIs) have been developed in recent years.

PPIs can be defined as interventions or intentional activities aimed at cultivating positive feelings, cognitions, and behaviours (Sin and Lyubomirsky 2009). Most PPIs consist of simple and brief exercises or activities that can be implemented in one's daily routine, where commitment and practice become key elements in their effectiveness (Sheldon and Lyubomirsky 2006). From the initial establishment of PP's objectives to the present, evidence has shown the effectiveness of these interventions for enhancing well-being and alleviating depressive symptomatology, as illustrated by the metaanalyses carried out by Sin and Lyubomirsky (2009) and Bolier et al. (2013).

From their origins, PPIs have taken advantage of the benefits offered by the information and communication technologies (ICTs). In fact, the meta-analysis by Bolier et al. (2013) concluded that the main modality of the PPIs analysed uses a self-applied format, sometimes with clinical, face-to-face support, but mostly delivered online.

ICTs can help us to design and deliver psychological interventions, making them more attractive and flexible. In addition, ICTs make it possible to reach a population that otherwise would not have access to this type of intervention (Andrews et al. 2010). The current technological advances in healthcare not only offer a new way to deliver treatment, but they also open up new possibilities for assessment and intervention. For instance, the current available sensorisation systems via mobile technologies allow the constant monitoring of an intervention or the individual's environment with a degree of ecological validity that had not previously been achieved in psychology. Other examples of ICTs' potential can be found in other technologies, such as virtual reality (VR) or augmented reality (AR), which offer increasingly high quality and low cost simulations of environments and situations, making them powerful tools for therapeutic change. Another example would be videogames, which are also presented as innovative learning methods aimed at improving the motivational and adherence components, variables of enormous relevance in treatment effectiveness and efficiency. Due to these possibilities offered by ICTs, many developed countries are considering basing their health solutions on them.

Taking into account the growing relationship between ICTs and PPIs, and the increasing literature on PPIs delivered through technologies, it is not surprising the growing interest for this intersection. Recently, Botella et al. (2012) and Riva et al. (2012) suggested the term 'positive technologies' (PTs) to refer to the scientific and applied approach to studying the use of technology to improve the quality of personal experiences. This perspective seeks to promote the use of technology to foster personal growth and the development of human virtues and strengths, thus contributing to social and cultural development.

Botella et al. (2012) and Riva et al. (2012), also established a classification for PTs, based on conceptualisations of subjective, psychological, and social well-being. According to these authors, each of these levels has critical variables (hedonic (emotion regulation), eudaimonic (flow and presence), and social (collective intentions and social connections) levels) that can be used to guide the design of technological applications whose purpose is to influence different aspects of well-being. Examples of hedonic PTs would be those that induce a positive and enjoyable experience, such as a VR environment of joy induction. Eudaimonic PTs include technologies that help people to achieve experiences focused on the search for a full and meaningful life. Social PTs include technologies that support and enhance communication among individuals, groups, and organisations.

In this chapter, we present some of the PTs designed by our research team that have been employed in the clinical psychology field for the treatment of various disorders, but also with the objective of promoting the well-being and happiness.

Positive Technologies

EMMA: Engaging Media for Mental Health Applications

EMMA's World is a VR system that was initially developed for the treatment of stress-related disorders, especially posttraumatic stress disorder (PTSD), the adjustment disorders, and complicated grief. These disorders all involve the occurrence of an event that has a negative, strong, and important impact on the life of the person experiencing it, along with the emergence of clinically significant cognitive, emotional, and behavioural symptoms after experiencing these events. So far, the VR systems used to treat these disorders, especially PTSD, have used VR as a strategy for exposure to the traumatic event. To do so, they represent a scenario or series of scenarios related to a specific problem or fact (e.g., Difede and Hoffman 2002). However, these scenarios can rarely be used to treat other problems different from those for which they were designed. This limitation is particularly important, due to the large quantity and variety of traumatic and/or stressful events that can lead to the development of these problems. In addition, none of the VR systems designed had used VR for both exposure and the implementation of tools and PPIs within the framework of PP. From this perspective, and considering EMMA's World as a PT, it can be classified at the eudaimonic level.

EMMA's World is an application capable of adapting to the specific needs of each case, providing meaningful virtual environments capable of activating and enhancing the emotional processing of the event experienced, promoting the acceptance of the problem as part of life, and fostering a more positive projection toward the future. Instead of building 'realistic' scenarios, this system combines different visual and auditory elements in order to evoke the meanings and emotions associated with the negative event in a symbolic way. Therefore, EMMA's World allows the creation and customisation of virtual environments that can be modified in real time, and where it is possible to introduce customised multimedia elements (photos, music, texts, videos, or narratives by the users).

EMMA's room simulates an open architectural structure (without walls), where it is possible to observe the surrounding landscape. This room contains the following tools: (1) a database, a large movable screen with different elements that the person can manipulate (designed objects in 3D, photos, music and sounds, colours and slogans, or proverbs). The system also makes it possible to introduce elements provided by the patients themselves into this database, such as photos or music; (2) pedestals or platforms, which form the structure where the chosen elements are placed, with the possibility of mixing and associating the elements in different ways; (3) an inventory, a small viewfinder located at the top right of the screen that serves to carry the elements from the database to the platforms and, from there, to the *Book of Life* where they can be stored; (4) the Book of Life, a virtual book that contains an index and a series of pages where patients can write the chapters of their lives. Patients divide the story of the stressful event into chapters, and the elements processed and elaborated during the therapy are stored. The Book of Life helps

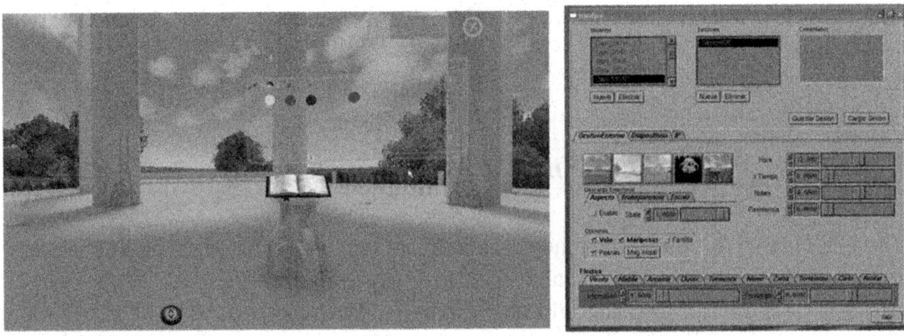

Fig. 13.1 The EMMA's room and the system

patients to recall, analyse, and elaborate the events, and it allows them to write and rewrite (with words and the database elements) the emotional experiences associated with the situations and project their own future; (5) the 'emotional processor', an artefact that emerges from the ground when activated. It is the place where the elements related to the painful experience do not have the power to emotionally disturb the patient anymore, and the actions taken with these elements seek to symbolise this transformation.

The EMMA environments make up another important part of the system. They are composed of five different predefined landscapes or scenarios that patients can choose (see Fig. 13.1): a desert, an island, a threatening forest, a snow-covered town, and a meadow. Initially, each landscape was designed to evoke different emotions. The landscapes can be selected and modified in real time in order to foster mood and the induction of emotions and reflect the changes in affect that a patient can experience during the session. Changes can be made in the environmental conditions (e.g., wind, rain, snow, fog, a storm, an earthquake, or vines growing) or the time representation (e.g., varying the time of the day or the speed of time), and these changes can be represented with different levels of intensity.

Along with developing the system, we also worked on designing treatment protocols for both the treatment and the use of this tool (Botella et al. 2008). Patients are told that EMMA's World is a place where they can express their problems, thoughts, and feelings, and it is designed to help and support them. Once patients are immersed in the scenarios, the therapist asks the patients to relate their memories of the disturbing experiences in present time, with as many details as possible, while reflecting the experience through the virtual environment at the same time. The selected elements that patients have chosen and worked on during the sessions are stored in The Book of Life, which is designed to help patients to bring order to their lives, represent how they solve emotional and behavioural problems while facing the disturbing elements of their experience, and store these changes.

Several studies carried out by our research group have shown the usefulness and efficacy of EMMA's World for the treatment of stress-related disorders (e.g., Baños et al. 2009, 2011). We believe that EMMA's World is an important step in VR applications in the field of psychological treatments, allowing therapists to work with patients in 'virtual worlds' and 'real worlds' that fit the specific needs of each patient at different moments.

EARTH of Well-Being: Emotional Activities Related to Health

The EARTH system was designed as a self-guided intervention to induce positive emotions in a controlled way and reinforce psychological resources through PP strategies. As a PT, EARTH could be classified at both the hedonic and eudaimonic levels. It was initially developed for the Mars-500 project to investigate the health and capacity for work of a crew, while simulating the conditions of an interplanetary manned flight (Botella et al. 2016a). Subsequently, it was adapted for the general population and other groups, such as cancer patients, with the aim of promoting different aspects of positive affect and hedonic and eudaimonic well-being for a variety of people. This platform consists of three modules of activities: Park of Well-Being, Well-Being Through Nature, and The Book of Life.

The *Park of Well-Being* offers the opportunity to learn and experience positive emotions through two virtual environments, one to experience joy and the other to experience calm and relaxation. Both virtual environments simulate a park in a city, and the light, sounds, and content of the exercises were adapted to the specific target emotion (joy or relaxation). Places in the park correspond to five exercises that include self-statements, choosing pictures for self-statements, listening to music, watching scenes from movies, and recalling an autobiographical emotional experience. Every resource is a key element in the emotional induction procedures (see Fig. 13.2).

Well-Being Through Nature includes two virtual environments consisting of nature landscapes that are also especially designed to produce joy and relaxation in patients. Each environment in the system trains participants in different psychological techniques that help to achieve correct emotional regulation. In the joy environment, participants are trained in reminiscing about pleasant memories that were part of their lives, and they exercise their conscious attention by observing nature and learning to concentrate and pay attention to every little detail. In the relaxing environment, participants practice slow breathing and other attentional aspects that help them to contemplate and appreciate the peace and calm that nature can provide.

The *Book of Life* is a personal diary consisting of several chapters. Each chapter proposes an exercise, and participants can write and incorporate different multimedia resources such as pictures, music, and videos. The Book of Life includes 16 exercises, each containing a main instruction and a series of questions aimed at guiding the users and facilitating their memory activation. Each exercise trains the patients in different aspects of a specific positive autobiographical memory, focusing on important psychological strengths such as optimism, hope, and self-esteem. It is important for participants to be engaged and involved in each activity. They also need to write down every detail that comes to mind and choose a picture, music, and/or movie that helps them to represent the story.

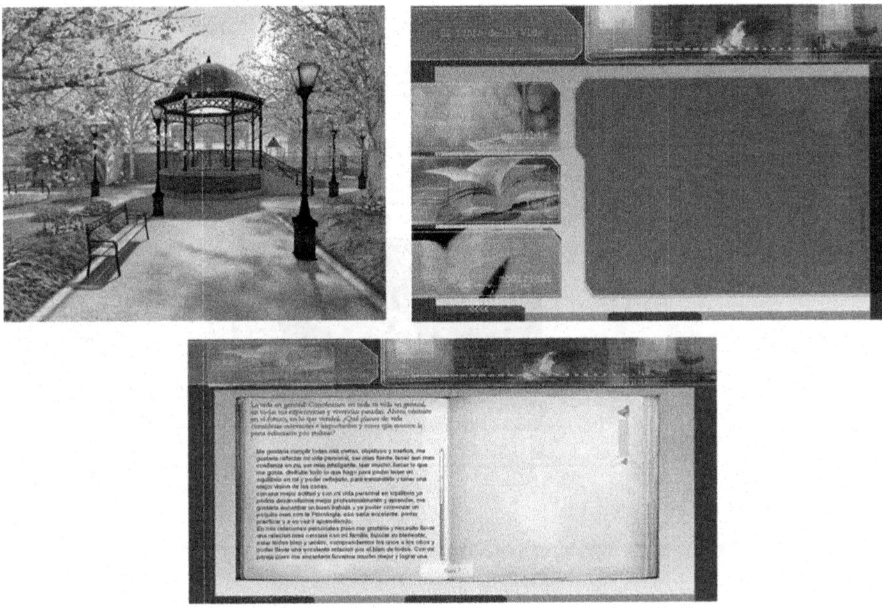

Fig. 13.2 The Park of Well-Being and The Book of Life in the EARTH system

All the strategies included in EARTH are based on theories of well-being, in terms of positive emotions (e.g., Diener 1984), optimal functioning, and psychological health (e.g., Ryff 1989). Instead of focusing only on one strategy to improve well-being and personal resources, the EARTH system offers several techniques and tasks, as some authors have suggested that the use of a variety of positive intervention techniques could be useful for maintaining and enhancing their effects (Parks et al. 2012).

EARTH has been validated in different populations: students (Baños et al. 2014), people with adjustment disorders (Andreu-Mateu et al. 2012), the elderly (Baños et al. 2012), and cancer patients (Baños et al. 2013). Outcomes suggest that EARTH is capable of promoting subjective well-being, not only in the general population in a controlled setting, but also in participants with a psychological or medical condition.

Smiling Is Fun

Smiling is Fun is a PT designed to generate coping resources and foster psychological well-being, and it is included at both the hedonic and eudaimonic levels. It is an Internet-based, multimedia (videos, images, cartoons, etc.), self-administered programme designed to reduce the incidence of psychological disorders with mild or moderate severity and high prevalence rates (such as depression, anxiety, and adjustment disorders), attend to people at high risk in stressful situations

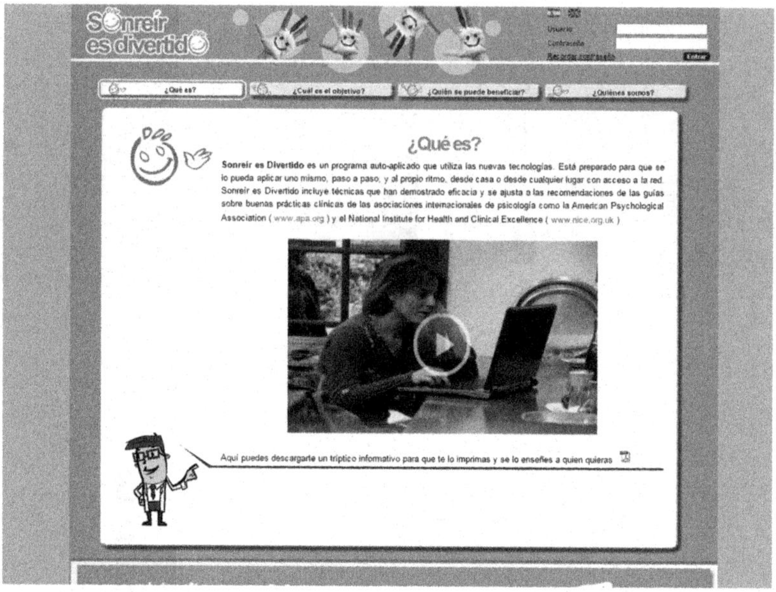

Fig. 13.3 The Internet-based self-administered programme Smiling is Fun

(prevention), or reduce the severity in people who already present clinical symptoms (treatment). In sum, Smiling is Fun teaches different adaptive ways to face and overcome the problems addressed. It is a protocoled intervention programme that is easy to disseminate and useful from a cost-benefit point of view. It is a self-help programme to be applied from home or any location with Internet access at the preferred or needed rhythm, and it includes techniques with demonstrated efficacy (e.g., behavioural activation, cognitive restructuring) and a series of PP strategies (e.g., mood induction procedures, fostering optimism and acceptance, learning to identify and maintain the good moments, etc. (see Fig. 13.3). In addition, self-assessment is important throughout the programme, as the current clinical guidelines indicate that 'what we know about ourselves can help us'. Smiling is Fun has three basic elements:

1. An initial assessment protocol aimed at providing the users with information about their current situation with regard to stress, depression, and coping capacity.
2. A structured protocol intervention, organised in sequential modules, where patients advance through the programme as they learn and practice the techniques offered in each module.
3. A protocol of continuous assessment, module by module. The users can access this information whenever they like. Thus, the programme provides immediate feedback about the users' progress. This assessment continues in the follow-up to obtain information about long-term effectiveness.

When designing Smiling is Fun, psychological aspects, such as the achievement of trust, rapport, and empathy, were taken into account. These are key aspects in this context. With this aim in mind, Smiling is Fun provides information about the research group that developed the programme, the problems, situations, and potential users of the programme, the logic on which the intervention is based, the confidentiality of the data, and tips about how to use the programme.

The modules are sequential and include texts, cartoons, and videos. Each module has a specific purpose and includes exercises designed to help the user to learn various psychological techniques. The programme is designed to last between 6 and 10 weeks, and it includes:

- *M1. Motivation for Change:* Users are asked to think about whether they really want to change, and consider the advantages and disadvantages of changing. They are told that change depends on them, and the importance of being motivated to learn all the skills included in the programme is highlighted.
- *M2. Understanding the Emotional Problems:* The objective is for the person to adopt a new attitude: to understand problems and difficulties as part of daily life and see them as an opportunity to learn and grow.
- *M3. Learning to Move on:* It teaches the importance of being active in 'moving on' and being involved in life. It emphasises that abandoning activities when there is psychological distress is not beneficial and only makes problems worse. Hence, being active is recommended.
- *M4. Learning to be Flexible:* It explains how irrational thoughts contribute to keeping the person trapped in a vicious cycle of distress, negative mood, and inactivity. It shows the importance of increasing one's flexibility in interpreting situations and learning to generate several alternatives in the same situation.
- *M5. Learning to Enjoy:* It teaches the importance of the emotions, both negative and positive. On the one hand, negative emotions help us to detect and escape from danger and, therefore, are crucial for short-term adaptation. On the other hand, positive emotions also play an important role in development, as they are useful for broadening our intellectual, physical, and social resources. Several methods are presented to generate positive experiences, and involvement in meaningful activities and contact with other people are recommended.
- *M6. Learning to Live: The Importance of Values and Goals:* It shows the difference between having positive experiences that only represent moments of momentary pleasure and achieving psychological well-being. Skills are developed to deal with problems without denying or avoiding them, and this module emphasises the importance of establishing goals based on the user's own values, in order to achieve psychological well-being.
- *M7. Living and Learning:* It explains that life is a constant learning process. All life experiences can be useful, and it is important to 'learn to learn' from them, in order to improve our sense of self-efficacy. Life is a process of continuous learning, change, and personal growth.
- *M8. From now on, What Else…?* It highlights that the end of this programme is only the beginning of each person's path. Smiling is Fun provides tools and

techniques to continue and strengthen what has been learned, but it points out that the user sets the path.

Smiling is Fun uses three complementary transversal tools that accompany the user throughout the intervention process: (1) *Activity Report*, which provides feedback to users, showing that their mood and well-being are related to the activities performed, and the benefits of being active; (2) *The Calendar*, which provides information about homework and tasks already achieved, reminding the user about those still outstanding and allowing users to know where they are throughout the programme; and (3) '*How am I?*', which offers a set of graphs and feedback to chart the user's progress on the level of activity, psychological distress (anxiety and sadness), and the intensity of positive emotionality (active, enthusiastic, energetic, with vitality) and negative mood (angry, fearful, stressed, tense, moody, etc.). These graphs represent the data that people give about anxiety, mood state, and positive and negative affect on the *Activity Report* when they finish each module.

Smiling is Fun has been tested in a risk-specific population, that is, long-term unemployed men, and it has obtained good results (Botella et al. 2016b). Studies have also examined the differential efficacy of the programme for the prevention and treatment of mild or moderate emotional disorders, with or without the support of the clinician (Mira 2014). Data indicate that participants improve when the programme is applied with clinical support (a brief weekly phone call—maximum length of 5 min—where no clinical aspects are analysed) and without clinical support, that is, using only the resources the programme provides (feedback graphs, emails, SMS reminders). Results have shown that positive affect and the accomplishment of activities are related to the improvement, and this improvement is maintained at the 1-year follow-up. Furthermore, Smiling is Fun has been highly rated by the participants. These results indicate that this PT may be useful to help other populations in the future; therefore, it may contribute to achieving important benefits from both psychological and cost-benefit perspectives.

BUTLER: To Improve Well-Being and Enhance Human Interactions

Computers may provide a great opportunity to be in contact with others and establish social networks that help to relieve the isolation and loneliness of many elderly people. The use of Internet and email can help to improve the quality of life of the elderly, connecting them to the outside world and facilitating contact with their families and society in general. Undoubtedly, the benefits of bridging the digital divide are innumerable, but it is necessary for users to be capable of using ICTs in order to enjoy them.

To help to bridge this gap, we developed a PT called BUTLER that covers the three levels of PTs: hedonic, eudaimonic, and social interaction. It is a system that includes the most popular Internet services integrated into a single platform, adapting its characteristics to the needs of the elderly population. Users can use email, videoconference, and blogs, and they can visualise digital images, listen to audio files, broaden their social network by finding new users with similar interests, and surf the Internet (see Fig. 13.4). BUTLER aims to contribute to improving the quality of life of the elderly, enhancing communication and providing training in positive emotions and mindfulness. The system addresses three profiles of users: elderly people, professional health agents, and relatives or friends of the elderly person, with two application levels: *Leisure* and *Clinical.*

All of the available resources in the BUTLER system have been designed to be self-administered, but it also contains an avatar, represented by an elderly butler who supports the user with audio and text instructions and provides positive reinforcement, such as: '*You are doing really great*' or '*I see that you can already type letters on the Internet; let's go a bit further*'.

BUTLER-Leisure

It is an open platform that facilitates the user's enjoyment of ICTs and enhances the social connection between the elderly and other people:

Videoconferencing and E-mail It allows the user to communicate with relatives, friends and other users of the BUTLER network by writing e-mails or starting a videoconference.

The Book of Life It works as a blog where users can write and include multimedia elements (images, texts, and melodies) that can be stored with the help of an assistant. The users can use all these elements to write in The Book of Life, send photographs in e-mails, or just listen to or watch their favourite songs and images. The aim of this tool is to improve communication and enhance social relationships in elderly people, as it allows them share their life memories with other users, relatives, or friends. In addition, it is possible to decide which pages of the book can be read by other people, and which ones are private.

Friends The objective is to promote the creation of a virtual community in order to broaden the support network of the elderly. The system shows the photograph of each user of the BUTLER network and a small description of his/her profile. The system compares different profiles by affinity (city of residence, place where they were born, hobbies and interests, etc.), and it offers a list of users that could be of interest to the user. The user can choose to send an invitation to another user to start a relationship, share The Book of Life, or add him or her to the address book.

Internet This application provides access to the Internet through Google. With this option, control over the design of the webpages external to BUTLER is lost; therefore, a button has been added that the user can click to return to BUTLER.

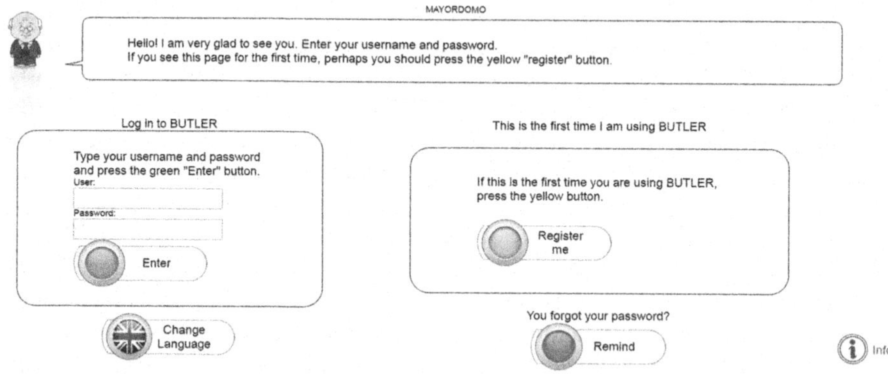

Fig. 13.4 Logging into the BUTLER system

BUTLER-Clinical

This application is not open to everyone, and it is designed to improve the mood state of the elderly and enhance their personal resources. It includes the following tools:

Assessment The aim of this application is to detect symptoms of anxiety and depression in users. It includes a decision algorithm that allows BUTLER to react in real time to the user's clinical needs. At the beginning of each session, the avatar performs an exploration through a series of scales. If a mood state within a normal range is detected, the system offers all the recreational resources; if any alteration in the mood state is detected (anxiety, depression, physical distress), the system carries out a more detailed exploration and, depending on the result, only offers the most suitable resources for the user's mood state. Furthermore, a warning is sent to the responsible caregiver (formal or informal), depending on the severity of the outcome.

Virtual Worlds to Generate Positive Emotions This tool includes two virtual environments that simulate natural settings (one for joy and one for relaxation) and present various visual and auditory stimuli that immerse the users in a positive emotional atmosphere to produce changes in their moods. These virtual environments include several strategies designed to produce transient emotional states in a controlled manner (Velten's induction procedure, Lang's pictures, music, and films) (Botella et al. 2009). Although the landscape is the same for both virtual environments, the voice that guides the walk, the colours used, the sounds, and the narratives have been adapted according to the emotion that each environment (joy and relaxation) tries to evoke. In the *Relaxing Environment,* the narrative invites the user to use slow breathing; in *Mindfulness*, it asks them to pay full attention to all the environmental sounds. In the *Joyful Environment,* the narrative invites users to enjoy the day and all the surrounding nature. In addition, the system trains users to recall joyful autobiographical memories, focusing on the details and reliving pleasant sensations. All of this is accompanied by a joyful melody.

BUTLER has been tested, confirming that this system is well-accepted by users, both in terms of its usefulness in improving the well-being of the elderly and in terms of its usability (Botella et al. 2009; Castilla et al. 2013). Furthermore, the system has already shown its capacity to improve users' mood states because the level of satisfaction, joy, relaxation, and general mood state significantly increased in all the sessions (Baños et al. 2012; Etchemendy et al. 2011). Therefore, BUTLER could be considered a PT that is capable of enhancing all the hedonic and eudaimonic levels of well-being by encouraging contact and social relationships in the elderly.

Discussion

In this chapter, we have presented some of the PTs developed by our research group, in order to illustrate the contribution they can make to improving health, quality of life, and well-being in different populations. In all of them, following the principles of positive psychology, the objective is not only to repair or reduce what is damaged or works badly in each person; instead, the objective is to enhance what is working well or produce new conditions for functioning that protect people, preventing the appearance of problems (Seligman and Csikszentmihalyi 2000). The purpose is to enhance positive emotions, coping resources, or strengths in the users. In addition, in each case, we have presented the available evidence supporting its effectiveness. This point is especially important because many of the applications based on ICTs developed in recent years have not been validated (Tomlinson et al. 2013). Undoubtedly, all these new applications have an enormous potential to improve the health of citizens and play an important role in future healthcare systems, making care more accessible and reducing barriers to getting help (Kazdin and Blase 2011; Simon and Ludman 2009). However, it is necessary to provide data to offer people evidence-based applications. Fortunately, there is already a clear awareness of these shortcomings, and some studies have tried to attract attention to this problem and offer a series of recommendations (Bakker et al. 2016). Research in this field is expected to provide evidence-based PTs in the near future.

Moreover, these new applications are increasingly based on devices such as smartphones. Users feel very comfortable using self-help materials that can easily be downloaded on familiar devices such as smartphones, and the strategies of EMAs (Ecological Momentary Assessment) and EMIs (Ecological Momentary Interventions) play an important role (García-Palacios et al. 2014). EMAs permit the participant to report on behaviour, emotions, and behaviour in natural settings and close in time to experience; EMIs are treatments delivered to the participant during their everyday lives in natural settings. For reasons of space, we could not address them here, but it will also be necessary to work on transferring all or part of these PTs to mobile devices that can be used by users anywhere and anytime.

Similarly, in the future we expect to see the combined use of different ICTs (e.g., sensors, Internet, VR and AR, mobiles, etc.) and innovative strategies, such as *Serious Games*. These combinations will lead to new PTs developed to provide users with coping resources or new capabilities. Therefore, the advantages of incorporating the end-users during the entire process should be taken into account (user-centred design PTs). These developments suggest the possibility of reaching a multitude of people, with the members of these populations spreading these PTs to other potential users, trying not only to improve themselves, but also to help others.

The future presents a spectacular possibility for helping to prevent or solve certain pressing health problems, such as the rejection of vaccinations or strategies to protect people from the zika virus or HIV, or propose or disseminate basic strategies for providing training in health habits in certain third-world countries (e.g., applications to produce resilience, or specific Serious Games related to how to feed or bathe my baby; serious games related to the need to respect girls).

It would be possible to create a large repository of PTs based on serious games, to which the whole world could have access, in order to improve both mental and physical health, and help people to be better trained to help themselves or others.

References

Andreu-Mateu, S., Botella, C., Quero, S., Guillén, V., & Baños, R. (2012). La utilización de la realidad virtual y estrategias de psicología positiva en el tratamiento de los trastornos adaptativos. *Behavioral Psychology/Psicología Conductual, 20*(2), 323–348.

Andrews, G., Cuijpers, P., Craske, M. G., McEvoy, P., & Titov, N. (2010). Computer therapy for the anxiety and depressive disorders is effective, acceptable and practical health care: A meta-analysis. *PloS One, 5*(10), e13196.

Bakker, D., Kazantzis, N., Rickwood, D., & Rickard, N. (2016). Mental health Smartphone apps: Review and evidence-based recommendations for future developments. *JMIR Mental Health, 3*(1), e7.

Baños, R. M., Botella, C., Guillen, V., García-Palacios, A., Quero, S., Bretón, J. M., & Alcañiz, M. (2009). An adaptive display to treat stress-related disorders: The EMMA's world. *British Journal of Guidance and Counselling, 37*(3), 347–356.

Baños, R. M., Guillen, V., Quero, S., García-Palacios, A., Alcañiz, M., & Botella, C. (2011). A virtual reality system for the treatment of stress-related disorders: A preliminary analysis of efficacy compared to a standard cognitive behavioural program. *The International Journal of Human-Computer Studies, 69*(9), 602–613.

Baños, R. M., Etchemendy, E., Castilla, D., García-Palacios, A., Quero, S., & Botella, C. (2012). Positive mood induction procedures for virtual environments designed for elderly people. *Interacting with Computers, 24*(3), 131–138.

Baños, R. M., Espinoza, M., García-Palacios, A., Cervera, J. M., Esquerdo, G., Barrajón, E., & Botella, C. (2013). A positive psychological intervention using virtual reality for patients with advanced cancer in a hospital setting: A pilot study to assess feasibility. *Supportive Care in Cancer, 21*, 263–270.

Baños, R., Etchemendy, E., Farfallini, L., García-Palacios, A., Quero, S., & Botella, C. (2014) EARTH of well-being system: A pilot study of an information and communication technology-based positive psychology intervention. *The Journal of Positive Psychology, 6*(9), 482–488.

Bolier, L., Haverman, M., Westerhof, G. J., Riper, H., Smit, F., & Bohlmeijer, E. (2013). Positive psychology interventions: A meta-analysis of randomized controlled studies. *BMC Public Health, 13*(1), 1.

Botella, C., Baños, R. M., & Guillén, V. (2008). Una propuesta de tratamiento para los trastornos adaptativos: Creciendo en la adversidad. [A proposed treatment for adjustment disorders: Growing up in adversity]. In C. Vázquez & G. Hervás (Eds.), *Psicología Positiva Aplicada* (pp. 129–154). Bilbao: Desclée de Brouwer.

Botella, C., Gallego, M. J., García-Palacios, A., Baños, R. M., Quero, S., & Alcañiz, M. (2009). The acceptability of an Internet-based self-help treatment for fear of public speaking. *British Journal of Guidance and Counselling, 37*(3), 297–312.

Botella, C., Riva, G., Gaggioli, A., Wiederhold, B. K., Alcaniz, M., & Banos, R. M. (2012). The present and future of positive technologies. *Cyberpsychology, Behavior, & Social Networking, 15*(2), 78–84.

Botella, C., Baños, R. M., Etchemendy, E., García-Palacios, A., & Alcañiz, M. (2016a). Psychological countermeasures in manned space missions: "EARTH" system for the Mars-500 project. *Computers in Human Behavior, 55*, 898–908. doi:10.1016/j.chb.2015.10.010.

Botella, C., Baños, R. M., Etchemendy, E., García-Palacios, A., & Alcañiz, M. (2016). Psychological countermeasures in manned space missions: "EARTH" system for the mars-500 project. *Computers in Human Behavior, 55*, 898–908. doi:10.1016/j.chb.2015.10.010.

Botella, C., Mira, A., Moragrega, I., García-Palacios, A., Bretón-López, J., Castilla, D., Riera, A., Soler, C., Molinari, G., Quero, S., Guillén, V., Miralles, I., Nebot, S., Serrano, B., Majoe, D., Alcañiz, M., & Baños, R. M. (2016b). An Internet-based program for depression using activity and physiological sensors: Efficacy, expectations, satisfaction and ease of use. *Neuropsychiatric Disease and Treatment, 12*, 393–406. doi:10.2147/NDT.S93315.

Botella, C., Serrano, B., Baños, R., & García-Palacios, A. (2016c). Virtual reality exposure-based therapy for the treatment of posttraumatic stress disorder. A review of its efficacy, the adequacy of the treatment protocol, and its acceptability. *Neuropsychiatric Disease and Treatment, 15*, 2533–2545.

Castilla, D., García-Palacios, A., Bretón, J. M., Miralles, I., Baños, R. M., Etchemendy, E., Farfallini, L., & Botella, C. (2013). Process of design and usability evaluation of a telepsychology web and virtual reality system for the elderly: BUTLER. *International Journal of Human-Computer Studies, 71*(3), 350–362.

Diener, E. (1984). Subjective well-being. *Psychological Bulletin, 95*, 542–575.

Difede, J., & Hoffman, H. (2002). Virtual reality exposure therapy for World Trade Center Post Traumatic Stress Disorder. *Cyberpsychology and Behavior, 5*(6), 529–535.

Etchemendy, E., Baños, R. M., Botella, C., Castilla, C., Alcañiz, M., Rasal, P., & Farfallini, L. (2011). An e-health platform for the elderly population: The BUTLER system. *Computers and Education, 56*(1), 275–279.

García-Palacios, A., Herrero, R., Belmonte, M. A., Castilla, D., Guixeres, J., Molinari, G., Baños, R. M., & Botella, C. (2014). Ecological momentary assessment for chronic pain in fibromyalgia using a smartphone: A randomized crossover study. *European Journal of Pain, 18*(6), 862–872. doi:10.1002/j.1532-2149.2013.00425.x.

Kazdin, A. E., & Blase, S. L. (2011). Rebooting psychotherapy research and practice to reduce the burden of mental illness. *Perspectives on Psychological Science, 6*(1), 21–37.

Mira, A. (2014). *Eficacia diferencial de un programa de intervención autoaplicado a través de Internet para la prevención y el tratamiento de la depresión leve o moderada con apoyo y sin apoyo por parte del terapeuta* (Doctoral dissertation). Universitat Jaume I, Castellón de la Plana (Spain). ISSN: 978-84-697-1980-0. http://hdl.handle.net/10803/284396

Parks, A. C., Della Porta, M. D., Pierce, R. S., Zilca, R., & Lyubomirsky, S. (2012). Pursuing happiness in everyday life: The characteristics and behaviors of online happiness seekers. *Emotion, 12*(6), 1222–1234.

Riva, G., Banos, R. M., Botella, C., Wiederhold, B. K., & Gaggioli, A. (2012). Positive technology: Using interactive technologies to promote positive functioning. *Cyberpsychology, Behavior, & Social Networking, 15*(2), 69–77.

Ryff, C. (1989). Happiness is everything, or is it? Explorations on the meaning of psychological well-being. *Journal of Personality and Social Psychology, 57*, 1069–1081.

Seligman, M. E. P., & Csikszentmihalyi, M. (2000). Positive psychology: An introduction. *American Psychologist, 55*(1), 5–14.

Sheldon, K. M., & Lyubomirsky, S. (2006). How to increase and sustain positive emotion: The effects of expressing gratitude and visualizing best possible selves. *The Journal of Positive Psychology, 1*(2), 73–82.

Simon, G. E., & Ludman, E. J. (2009). It's time for disruptive innovation in psychotherapy. *Lancet, 374*(9690), 594–595.

Sin, N. L., & Lyubomirsky, S. (2009). Enhancing well-being and alleviating depressive symptoms with positive psychology interventions: A practice-friendly meta-analysis. *Journal of Clinical Psychology, 65*(5), 467–487.

Tarragona, M. (2010). Psicología positiva y psicoterapia. In A. Castro Solano (Ed.), *Fundamentos de Psicología Positiva*. Paidós: Buenos Aires.

Tomlinson, M., Rotheram-Borus, M. J., Swartz, L., & Tsai, A. C. (2013). Scaling up mHealth: Where is the evidence? *PLoS Medicine, 10*(2), e1001382.

Chapter 14
How Design Can (Not) Support Human Flourishing

Anna E. Pohlmeyer

Abstract What role does the design of products, services, and the built environment have on people's psychological well-being? This chapter introduces the emerging field of Positive Design, which studies the mechanisms and manifestations of design that stimulates human flourishing. After a brief account of research on Positive Psychology Interventions, this chapter examines the possibilities and limitations of design for well-being. It is argued that especially the enablement of pleasurable and meaningful experiences and activities in daily life is a promising approach. Four Positive Design examples related to *taking notice* and *savouring* are provided in order to illustrate new forms of Positive Psychology Interventions. These examples range from designs whose explicit core function is the promotion of well-being to common, everyday products that foster determinants of well-being as an additional effect. A number of challenges that Positive Psychology Interventions in practice currently face and the potential benefits of Positive Design are considered. In particular, this chapter discusses the strengths of Positive Design in terms of reach, adherence, and person-context-activity-fit.

Abbreviations

BIT Behavioural intervention technologies
PPI Positive psychology interventions

Introduction

In his book '*Flourish*', Martin Seligman (2011) expressed an ambitious goal for the field of positive psychology: by the year 2051, 51% of the world's population should be flourishing. With this aim in mind, new questions for the field have naturally

A.E. Pohlmeyer (✉)
Department of Industrial Design, Delft University of Technology,
Landbergstraat 15, 2628 CE Delft, The Netherlands
e-mail: A.E.Pohlmeyer@tudelft.nl

C. Proctor (ed.), *Positive Psychology Interventions in Practice*,
DOI 10.1007/978-3-319-51787-2_14

arisen: How can the knowledge gained in positive psychology be shared with people from all walks of life, worldwide? How can empirical evidence on what makes people happy be translated into effective real-world applications? It is clear that a genuine pursuit of Seligman's goal ought to be collaborative and multi-disciplinary in character. Fortunately, concrete efforts of this nature have already begun: new insights have escaped the physical and communicative constraints of labs and scientific publications and found their way into classrooms, board meetings, coaching sessions, public policy agendas, as well as web-based and mobile applications (Bolier and Abello 2014; Calvo and Peters 2014; Linley and Joseph 2004). To support human flourishing worldwide, every means available should be applied. Notwithstanding promising initiatives, including examples of eHealth, reach and adherence of existing solutions remain limited (e.g., Christensen et al. 2006, 2009; Mohr et al. 2013; Ludden et al. 2015). This chapter introduces a new subfield of positive psychology that holds the potential to substantively contribute to Seligman's vision: *positive design*.

Positive design investigates how designs[1] can stimulate human flourishing (Desmet and Pohlmeyer 2013; Pohlmeyer 2012). Research questions include '*What influence does the designed environment have on people's well-being?*' or '*How should products, services, and systems be designed to maximise their potential to foster well-being?*' and '*In what ways can design support positive changes in behaviour?*' Shaping and testing new applications of positive psychology findings within everyday situations is pivotal to these questions; translating lab interventions into daily interactions means that the impact of positive psychology will reach more people in a wider variety of situations. Furthermore, context-sensitive designs can support a good fit with a person's lifestyle, which will make it easier to initiate and sustain the practice of happiness-enhancing activities (Lyubomirsky 2007). Paul Dolan (2014) concisely defined happiness as '*experiences of pleasure and purpose over time*' (p. 3), which closely relates to the core understanding of positive design: to mediate, create, and support meaningful and pleasurable experiences (over time). In addition to designing for pleasure in the present, the positive design framework by Desmet and Pohlmeyer (2013) proposes that in order to foster a feeling of purpose, design can also encourage people to live in accordance with their personal values, and commit to ideally self-concordant goals (Sheldon and Elliot 1999) which supports a life of personal significance. In addition to satisfying subjective desires, positive design also takes a moral stance, by specifically stimulating human virtues (Pohlmeyer and Desmet 2017), and thereby taking the impact one has on the world into account. In sum, positive design is a possibility-driven approach that deliberately stimulates human flourishing through design.

After a brief introduction to research on positive psychology interventions, this chapter examines the possibilities and limitations of how design can support human well-being. Four positive design examples are provided which will illustrate possi-

[1] The term 'design' is used here in a broad sense: it encompasses all forms of tangible and intangible artifacts (e.g., products, services, (digital) systems, visual communications, built environment) that have been created by designers for people.

ble directions of application. Finally, a number of challenges that positive psychology interventions in practice currently face and the potential benefits of positive design are considered.

Is It Actually Possible to Become Happier? And if So, How?

Is it possible to get happy? Or get happier? Some scepticism about the potential to increase one's level of happiness has arisen in light of twin studies (Lykken and Tellegen 1996) that revealed that happiness is, at least to a certain extent, genetically determined. Furthermore, other researchers have suggested that despite increases (and decreases) in happiness levels in the short term, people will eventually return to a baseline level of happiness in the long run (Brickman and Campbell 1971). According to this line of thinking, any attempt to somehow permanently change one's happiness level is doomed to fail, or the equivalent of running on a kind of 'hedonic treadmill' (Brickman and Campbell 1971) that goes nowhere despite great effort and the apparent movement of the treadmill itself.

Fortunately, positive psychology researchers have exciting and encouraging news: it is, after all, possible to become lastingly happier (Diener et al. 2006; Boehm and Lyubomirsky 2009; Seligman et al. 2005). While acknowledging a genetic set range as a determinant of happiness, as well as the challenge of adaptation processes, it has been shown that happiness can be lastingly increased through positive intentional activities (Lyubomirsky et al. 2005). We are neither destined to remain unhappy—should we happen to be rather pessimistic, grumpy, or insecure—nor is happiness only found in the realisation of 'ideal circumstances'. Instead, happiness is a *process* that one can influence with one's daily actions.

Rather than merely assessing our potential for change, a wealth of knowledge and evidence-based strategies dealing with *how* to increase well-being has emerged in the form of positive psychology interventions (PPIs) (Lyubomirsky 2007; Bolier et al. 2013; Seligman et al. 2005; Sin and Lyubomirsky 2009). PPIs have been defined as 'treatment methods or intentional activities that aim to cultivate positive feelings, behaviors, or cognitions' (Sin and Lyubomirsky 2009, p. 468), which, in turn, enhance people's happiness. Some prominent interventions that have been shown to be effective are gratitude letters (Lyubomirsky et al. 2011; Seligman et al. 2005), counting one's blessings (Emmons and McCullough 2003; Lyubomirsky et al. 2005), savouring life's joys (Bryant and Veroff 2007; Quoidbach et al. 2010), practicing random acts of kindness (Lyubomirsky et al. 2005), and using one's strengths in a new way (Seligman et al. 2005). Also, overall, two meta-analyses including 51 (Sin and Lyubomirsky 2009) and 39 (Bolier et al. 2013) randomised controlled intervention studies, respectively, have shown that PPIs can increase well-being and reduce depressive symptoms.

Such interventions open up a promising avenue toward practically empowering people to help themselves (and one another) to flourish, which is at the heart of Positive Psychology (Seligman 2011). Building on the success of evidence-based strategies, 'the next stage of research requires implementing these strategies in ways to support their use in real-world contexts' (Schueller and Parks 2014, p. 145). As one possible approach, this chapter proposes that design can intentionally support PPIs. For this, it is important to differentiate between the static material value of design on the one hand, and the variable experiential value it provides on the other.

Limitations and Opportunities of Design for Happiness

Unfortunately, people seem to hold dear many myths about where to find happiness that are not necessarily in line with scientific evidence (Lyubomirsky 2013). An overemphasis on enhancing external status, becoming rich, or generally living in affluence in a consumption-driven society, are examples of modern happiness delusions. This focus on material value implies that design can have only a limited impact on people's long-lasting happiness. After detailing two central reservations regarding design for well-being, different ways in which design *can* support well-being after all will be described.

Several studies have documented a relative well-being effect created by experiences and activities versus material goods and changes in circumstances, respectively (Lyubomirsky et al. 2005; Nicolao et al. 2009; Carter and Gilovich 2014; Patterson and Biswas-Diener 2012). For instance, Lyubomirsky et al. (2005) showed that only a small portion of inter-individual differences in happiness can be explained by our demographic and material circumstances (e.g., marriage, income, age, and culture), whereas a substantial influence on well-being can be obtained through performing positive intentional activities such as nurturing relationships, cultivating optimism, and taking care of one's body (Lyubomirsky 2007). One reason that accounts for the relatively low impact of circumstantial changes is the phenomenon of *hedonic adaptation* (Frederick and Loewenstein 1999; Lyubomirsky 2011). No matter how much a bride is overwhelmed with positive emotions on her wedding day or how exciting it is to finally own a car, people eventually get used to these changes, and the initial (positive) affective responses decrease, potentially to a point where one takes the change for granted. Hedonic adaptation processes have been observed in relation to all kinds of changes, including winning the lottery (Brickman et al. 1978), getting a pay raise (Di Tella et al. 2010), getting married (Lucas et al. 2003), and changing jobs (Boswell et al. 2005). The upside of adaptation is that we also adjust to negative changes like accidents, rejections, and losses, and that adaptation followed by rising aspirations is a key driver of personal growth and development (Lyubomirsky 2011). However, adaptation to positive changes poses a serious challenge to increasing overall happiness levels. Although the level and intensity of positive emotions appears to flatten after all kinds of changes, it has been found to happen particularly fast after changes in material circumstances and possessions, in contrast to after changes in activities and experiences (Patterson and Biswas-Diener 2012). The sustainable happiness model (Lyubomirsky et al. 2005) consequently advises investing in positive intentional activities, and how life is lived, rather than in attempts to change circumstances.

In a similar vein, research has shown that when experiential purchases are compared to material ones, the former engender greater well-being effects in participants, who also feel that the money spent on experiences was more wisely invested (van Boven 2005). These findings led to the so-called 'experience recommendation': if you want to increase your happiness level, invest in experiences rather than material possessions (Nicolao et al. 2009). There are many reasons for the superiority of experiences over material objects (see Carter and Gilovich 2014, for an overview). For instance, people are less likely to directly compare different kinds of experiences (e.g., a seeing a concert, travelling, eating out) than they are to compare material objects (e.g., cars, televisions, couches), because our experiences are unique to each of us. Another reason why experiences have a stronger link to people's subjective well-being is associated with the meaning they have for one's self-image. If I were to describe myself, I would try to give an impression of my character, how I typically behave, and perhaps also how I dealt with a critical situation. This information would give you (and myself) a much better picture of who I am than an inventory list of my possessions would. A third reason why the impact of experiences is relatively profound in terms of happiness, is that their performance usually involves other people and is thus usually social in nature. Research has shown time and again that social connections and relatedness are essential for human beings to flourish (Seligman 2011; Huppert and So 2013).

The findings above underscore the value of using positive activities as a way to lastingly increase one's well-being. At the same time, one might be sceptical about whether design and consumer products can lead to sustainable increases in happiness at all. I would, however, like to argue that designed artefacts do have the potential to markedly support people's efforts to increase and maintain their happiness levels. Importantly, I do so without trying to nullify the above recommendations—on the contrary, I will argue in support of them: Design for well-being can play a pivotal role in facilitating activities and enabling experiences.

On August 7th, 1974, Philippe Petit fulfilled a dream he had cherished for many years. On that day, he dared to do something illegal, unprecedented, and truly beautiful: he walked (and danced) for nearly an hour on a wire that he and his companions had affixed between the Twin Towers of New York's World Trade Center, fully aware that he could be arrested (see James Harsh's 2008 documentary '*Man on Wire*'). Now, while his balancing act certainly required remarkable physical agility and the courageous mind of an enthusiast, the experience would not have been possible without one key element: that very ordinary wire. The physical properties of the wire and the rigging made the whole spectacle possible. Hence, the *design enabled an experience* that was singularly pleasurable and meaningful to its user. While walking on a tightrope between two skyscrapers is obviously an extreme example, there are countless everyday activities and experiences that are facilitated or even made possible in the first place by design. Think about telecommunication technologies that bring friends and families closer together, or consider sporting equipment like bicycles, skis, and sailboats, or social network platforms that connect people who did not know each other beforehand.

Positive design is a matter of perspective. Should an object derive its value from its material worth or from what it enables us to do? In a laboratory study, a wire would undoubtedly not have scored particularly high on a well-being scale. Yet the experience of walking in the sky meant the world to Philippe Petit. The potential of design to enable experiences has been largely neglected in the studies above: the strict dichotomy between experiences and material goods observed was effective in uncovering general differences in relative well-being effects, but overlooked the potential 'means to an end'—happiness, that even mundane design can present. Recently, Guevarra and Howell (2015), as well as the work we have been doing in our own lab, has found that 'experience enablers', such as sporting equipment and musical instruments, turn out to have rather similar effects on need fulfilment and well-being as experiences do. Both have a greater impact on people's happiness than 'purely' material acquisitions. These findings highlight that design can be far richer and more meaningful than the simple appreciation of its material properties, and that it can, in fact contribute to happiness, if designed and perceived as an experience enabler, that is with a clear emphasis on its intangible rather than its material value.

In addition to enabling experiences, there are at least two further ways that designs might serve as resources for well-being: (1) as *symbolic* representations of someone or something meaningful, for example a wedding ring, and (2) as *support* for desirable behaviours, for example planners and feedback loops (Pohlmeyer 2012). As to the former, we all have something we consider precious, not because it has resale value, but because it means something to us personally. It might be irreplaceable like a stuffed toy that has been at your side since you learned how to walk, it might be the brooch inherited from a deceased grandma, or it might be a Buddha statue that represents deeply felt spiritual beliefs. All of these objects illustrate examples of meaning attached to an object (Csikszentmihalyi and Rochberg-Halton 1981; Fournier and Richins 1991; Casais et al. 2015). Such physical representations remind us of what, or who, is important to us. Yang (2015) ascertained that sentimental value can decelerate hedonic adaptation to objects, and that while feature-related utility wears off over time, sentimental value does not.

Finally, design can also *support* positive endeavours, without directly enabling experiences. Famously, Benjamin Franklin used a 'virtue table' to track his weekly progress toward a consistently virtuous life. The table itself did not enable specific experiences or behaviour, yet it is said to have supported his commitment to the goal. A more widely used, recent example of this kind of perspective is activity trackers, which monitor physical activity via wearable or portable sensors and tracking software. It is, however, important to note that design is not merely a matter of technology, but of a user-centred, context-sensitive orchestration of interactions. In addition to providing users with relevant information and feedback in a timely fashion, design can prompt the initiation of a favourable, for example happiness-enhancing, behaviour, help users plan and make decisions (e.g., by suggesting choice alternatives), commit to goals, and recover from relapses.

In sum, there are multiple ways that design can stimulate well-being. As shown, the most promising impact on well-being can be expected if designs are used as facilitators of experiences and activities, and not as sources of well-being itself (Pohlmeyer 2012; see Kasser 2002 for an overview of the negative relationship between materialism and well-being). By mediating and creating pleasurable and meaningful experiences that enhance happiness, design stimulates PPIs in practice.

Two main possibility-driven approaches in this regard can be differentiated, that Calvo and Peters (2014) have called 'active' and 'dedicated', respectively.

- *Active*: the (re)design of interactions that are part of existing devices or services. In addition to its core function, determinants of well-being are actively stimulated by the design, for example, an alarm clock designed in such a way that the wake up sound is a personal message by one's grandchildren as a sign of relatedness.
- *Dedicated*: a design whose core function is the promotion of well-being, for example, *Tiny Task* (Ruitenberg and Desmet 2012): colourful key chain tokens suggest small, original, and fun experiences to engage in, each of which relates directly to one of the 12 happiness-enhancing strategies suggested by Lyubomirsky (2007).

Both approaches have their strong points, and should be pursued with equal vigour. While dedicated designs might show a greater increase in well-being, active designs might be used more frequently, and by a greater audience, and thus have a greater reach.

In the following, a selection of design examples[2] will be used to illustrate challenges relative to PPIs in practice, and the benefits that positive design might provide.

Four Design Examples: Taking Notice and Savouring

A considerable amount of theoretical and empirical work has been published on the benefits of taking notice, savouring, and gratitude, for example, 'counting one's blessings' (Bryant and Veroff 2007; Emmons and McCullough 2003; Seligman et al. 2005). Consequently, diary-like journals and digital apps are recommended as they offer users the chance to turn reflecting on positive events into a daily ritual. However, despite their low threshold of engagement, not everyone is fond of putting thoughts into words, and some might find it difficult to establish such rituals.

Memoriam Tea, designed by Max Tak, subtly transforms the existing practice of making and drinking a cup of tea into a ritual opportunity to reflect upon a positive achievement or quality. Specifically, Memoriam Tea takes advantage of the brief, everyday moment while the tea is steeping to stimulate positive thinking. The typical interaction of tea brewing was redesigned in such a way that teabags are wound around a wooden stick; once unwound, the stick is placed across the cup, and serves as a tea bag holder. A half-completed sentence is engraved on the stick that invites the user to reflect on achievements and positive events while the tea is releasing its aroma (see Fig. 14.1). Sentence examples include '*three good things that happened today…*', '*I feel proud of…*', *and* '*…are skills that I have*'. Although Memoriam Tea is similar to classic PPIs, it actually exemplifies an 'active' design for well-being,

[2] The four examples are design concepts developed under my supervision by students taking the course called 'Exploring Interactions', as part of TU Delft's 'Design for Interaction' Master's degree program.

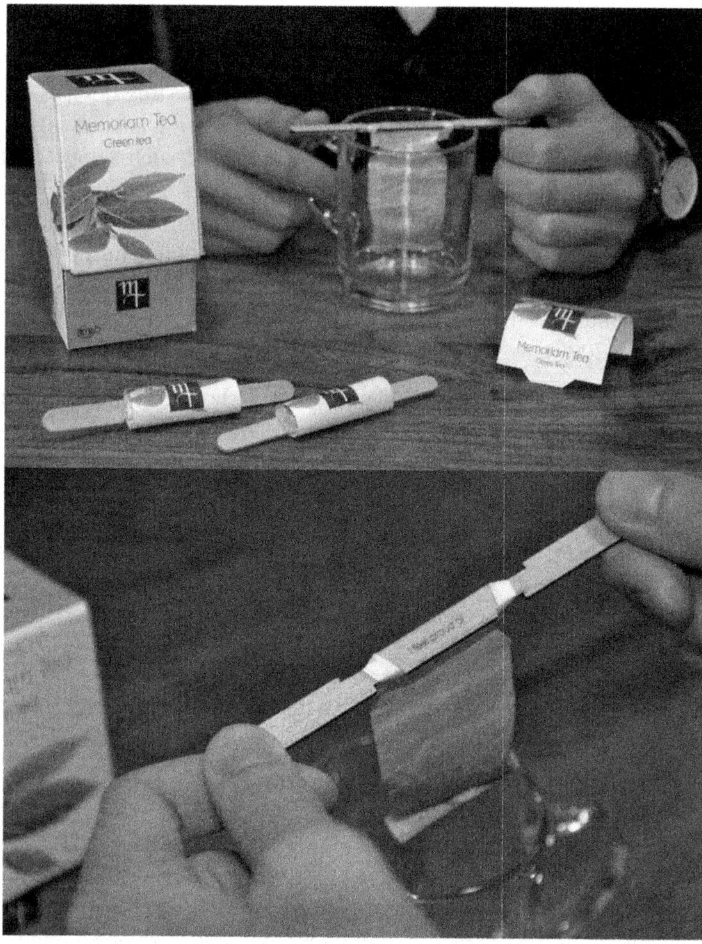

Fig. 14.1 Memoriam Tea (reprinted with permission)

where the main function is still the tea bag, but the re-design has added a well-being component. This was a conscious choice made during the design process, in order to reach people who might be hesitant to acquire products that are dedicated to boosting happiness, but might be open to a cup of tea.

An example of a 'dedicated' design for well-being is the smartphone application *Huddle*, designed by Frank Stemerding. Interestingly, despite being a dedicated design, Huddle also has the potential to reach an audience beyond 'happiness seekers' (Bergsma 2008; Parks et al. 2012), because it has been tailored to suit the personal interests of a target demographic: amateur sport teams. While such teams might bond strongly on the field, this feeling can abruptly end once members leave the clubhouse. After losing a match, players might tend to perceive everything as negative, although there might have been several high points during the game. A

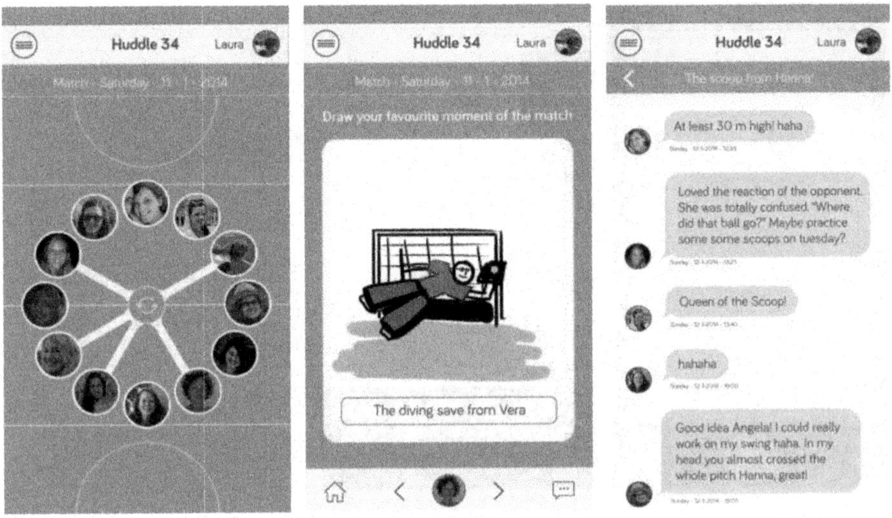
Huddle 34
Laura
Huddle 34
Laura
Draw your favourite moment of the match
The diving save from Vera
Huddle 34
Laura
At least 30 m high! haha
Loved the reaction of the opponent. She was totally confused. "Where did that ball go?" Maybe practice some some scoops on tuesday?
Queen of the Scoop!
hahaha
Good idea Angela! I could really work on my swing haha. In my head you almost crossed the whole pitch Hanna, great!

Fig. 14.2 Huddle (reprinted with permission)

huddle is the circular formation of a team to agree on a joint strategy and to motivate each other. The Huddle app (see Fig. 14.2) adopts this metaphor by inviting players to savour the things that went well during a session, and prolong the feeling of connectedness. The principle is quite simple: after a training session or a match, an administrator posts a question or assignment, for example '*Draw your favourite moment of the match*', *or* '*Give a team member a compliment*'. Teammates join the huddle by posting a reply. Importantly, users can only see (and comment on) others' responses if they have also contributed. It is thus a voluntary task driven by curiosity rather than obligation. After all, the task suggested should not be perceived as an inconvenient chore. This app supports the attendance to, reliving, sharing and thereby the prolongation of positive moments. In other words, it is an application dedicated to savouring, which has been shown to increase well-being and counteract hedonic adaptation (Bryant and Veroff 2007; Lyubomirsky 2011).

When you walk your typical route back home after a long day at work, do you still take notice of the small details in your surroundings? *Explordinary*, designed by Julia Mattaar, is a Smartphone application that allures people into (again) becoming aware of their immediate environment, by giving theme-related photo assignments to users on their way home. A theme could be, for example: '*Find something green*' (see Fig. 14.3). The user's focus is drawn to features in the surrounding area that he or she might normally not notice. After taking and posting a picture with a smartphone, users can then see pictures that others took on the same route, related to the same theme. This sharpens the eye even more to look around attentively. After a fixed number of completed assignments, users can order a selection of their favourite pictures as postcards. Familiar surroundings are instantly transformed into pieces of amateur artwork that can be collected or shared with others. Surprisingly, exploring the ordinary can turn it into something extraordinary.

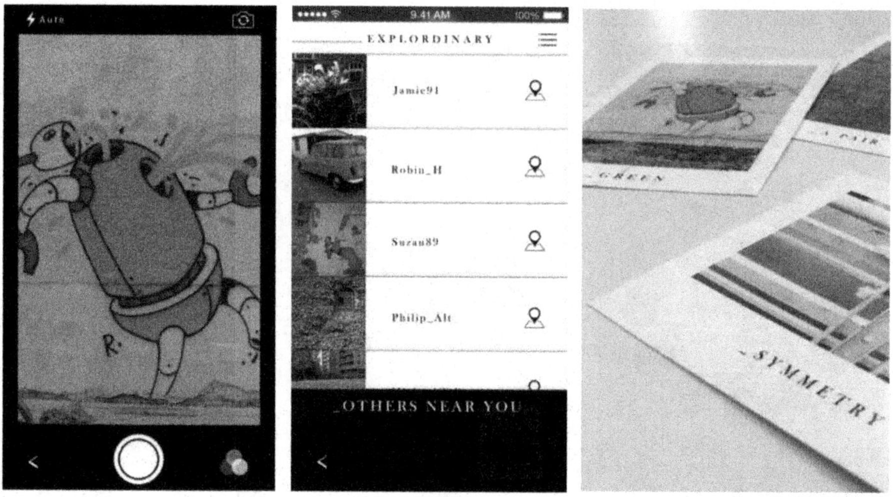

Fig. 14.3 Explordinary (reprinted with permission)

Oftentimes, design seeks to optimise (personal) processes by increasing efficiency. However, one effective savouring technique explicitly focuses on being in the present moment (Quoidbach et al. 2010; 'absorption' in Bryant and Veroff 2007), which can be a challenge at times, considering the hectic pace many people have chosen to maintain. *TeaShell*, designed by Lisa van de Merwe, is a counterexample of design that strives for maximum efficiency: due to the shape and absence of a handle (as shown in Fig. 14.4), TeaShell is a mug that must be held with both hands to ensure balance. It is also rather inconvenient to use while standing or walking, as both hands are fixed in the centre. Moreover, when holding the mug, the hands appear to be cherishing something precious. These features invite the user to focus on the moment of drinking tea, and physically hinder multi-tasking, for example making a phone call. The goal of this project was to stimulate a moment of mindfulness and absorption in the present. Ultimately, this is achieved by kindly forcing users to pay attention to the warm beverage in front of them—and nothing else. Imagine the impact positive psychology will have if more everyday items were designed with well-being-relevant principles in mind.

Challenges of Positive Psychology Interventions and Added Value of Design

Ultimately, the aim to gain a better understanding of what constitutes psychological well-being is not an end in itself, but the sound, scientific foundation to help as many individuals and communities as possible to thrive (Seligman 2011). To achieve this goal, positive psychologists stress the potential to extend knowledge applicable

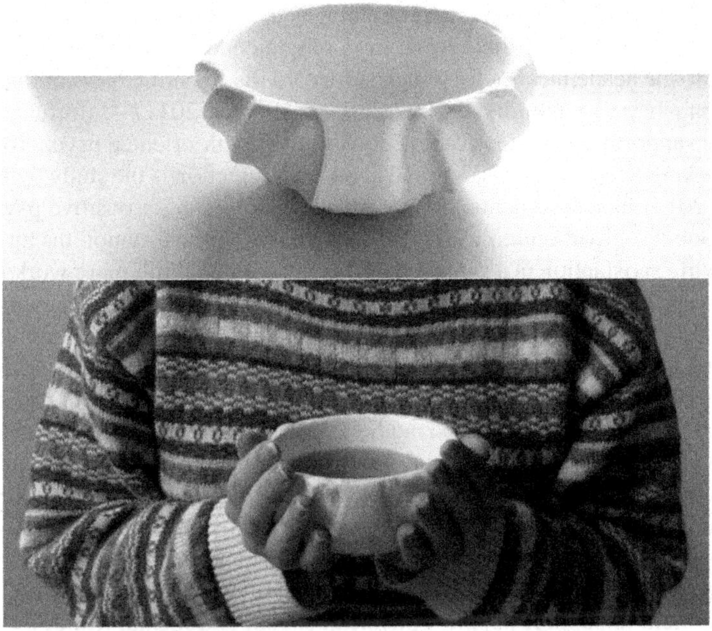

Fig. 14.4 TeaShell (reprinted with permission)

in the context of *self-help* to also include populations who might otherwise not receive care, that is, expanding a therapist-centred care model to encompass self-administration and prevention (Mohr et al. 2013; Schueller et al. 2013; Schueller and Parks 2014). Yet the reach of, motivation for, and adherence to PPIs remains limited. In the following sections, these challenges will be considered, alongside the overall importance of achieving a good fit with personal preferences and lifestyles. Opportunities that positive design can create will be explored.

Reach

For the effectiveness of PPIs to truly unfold, they have to actually weave themselves into people's lives. So in order for them to have any impact at all, they have to be both useful…and actually *used*. While their utility has been demonstrated in numerous studies (Bolier et al. 2013; Sin and Lyubomirsky 2009), the resulting knowledge and tools have yet to reach people as a minimum prerequisite. Of course, if these interventions do find their way into the everyday, another hurdle is to elicit users' willingness to adopt and adhere to these new practices.

Original and engaging PPIs, made available outside the context of professional guidance, can enlarge the number and diversity of people that can be reached. One prevalent means of self-administered training is the self-help book. Many renowned scientists have published their work in books intended for the general public, in addition to the academic articles which safeguard the scientific basis of their recommendations (e.g., Lyubomirsky 2007, 2013; Seligman 2011). Unfortunately, hard evidence supporting the effectiveness of reading growth-oriented psychology books is still lacking (Bergsma 2008). A first step in this direction is the study by Parks and Szanto (2013) that documents the effectiveness of reading a positive psychology-based book (i.e., Lyubomirsky 2007) to improve depressive symptoms and slightly improve life satisfaction in a sample of college freshmen. Still, more work is needed in this respect. Some of the benefits offered by so-called 'bibliotherapy' are its affordability (compared to guided therapy), its fairly low threshold of engagement (including a greater degree of privacy), and the fact that it is far more accessible to the general public than scientific journals. Yet, it appears that despite this potential, the genre attracts only a limited audience. For instance, the readership of the monthly '*Psychology Magazine*', presumably representative of this segment of the population, is predominantly female and well-educated (see Bergsma 2008).

A second promising means of disseminating (knowledge of) PPIs exists in the domains of positive technology (Riva et al. 2012) and positive computing (Calvo and Peters 2014; Sander 2011). Behavioural intervention technologies (BITs) are an emerging field to support people's physical, social, and mental health by administering evidence-based interventions through technologies, such as smart mobile devices, the web (including social media), virtual reality, and sensors (Mohr et al. 2013). An example of an online PPI, that is BIT, is the iPhone application *Live Happy,* developed by Signal Patterns and Sonja Lyubomirsky. The app is based on Lyubomirsky's book '*The How of Happiness*' (2007), and includes exercises for a variety of positive activities, for example, it suggests capturing a moment with the phone's camera to savour it and establish a savouring album. In theory, BITs have enormously compelling potential in terms of reach, accessibility, and integration into everyday life. Moreover, Bolier and Abello's (2014) review of randomised controlled studies of online PPIs demonstrated that these can also enhance subjective psychological well-being and reduce depressive symptoms in the short and long term. Given the omnipresence of technology in many societies, BITs seem to have the remarkable capacity to increase well-being in a scalable, sustainable, and cost-effective way (Bolier and Abello 2014; Sander 2011; Schueller et al. 2013).

In practice, however, there remains a discrepancy between the encouraging potential of BITs on the one hand, and on the other, not only their real-world reach, but also the adoption of and adherence to what they propose (Mohr et al. 2013). Similar to self-help books, many online solutions are sought by only a distinct user group—for instance, some studies have reported audiences of predominantly higher-educated women (see Ludden et al. 2015 for an overview). Moreover, despite widespread availability, not everyone has access to the necessary technologies, is able to use them, for example due to a lack of technology literacy, or feels comfortable using technology for the purpose of a PPI, for example due to privacy concerns

(Mohr et al. 2013). Hence, in some cases, BITs might even introduce barriers. Although internet access around the world is spreading by the minute, and especially digital natives can be expected to embrace and integrate the digital into all areas of life, it is still worth considering additional channels of dissemination and application of PPIs in practice.

As explained, although ordinary books and technology may be highly promising vectors for PPIs, they typically appeal to specific user groups, for example 'readers', or those with access to and expertise with technology. Moreover, initial data suggests that people who actively seek ways to work on their happiness might also not be 'representative for all mankind', but can rather be assigned to one of two clusters: 'distressed', that is people with heightened depressive symptoms, and 'non-distressed', that is people who are neither remarkably happy, nor show signs of clinical depression (Parks et al. 2012). One solution for greater reach is certainly a combination of different approaches, for example education, coaching, and technologies. Positive design holds the promise of being a key contributor in this equation, as it can offer additional means of interactions that might speak to, and get through to, more people than regular books and BITs do. The Huddle app, for example, does not specifically target happiness-seekers, but rather amateur sport teams. Yet it supports the positive activity of savouring. Furthermore, design has already entered most households and public places worldwide through ordinary commodities (available to millions of people) including solutions for mobility, health care, and telecommunication. Imagine what might happen if concomitant practices and products (e.g., how we interact with others in traffic or stay in touch with loved ones far away) were (re)designed in such a way that they not only make our lives easier and faster, but actually create opportunities for us to flourish. As demonstrated by TeaShell, products as simple as a teacup can be redesigned with well-being principles in mind. If more designs deliberately took well-being effects into account by emphasising positive emotion regulation (Pohlmeyer 2014), eliciting a combination of pleasure, personal significance, and virtue (Desmet and Pohlmeyer 2013), or addressing psychological needs like competence, relatedness, and autonomy (Ryan and Deci 2000) as suggested by Hassenzahl et al. (2013), more and more people could be reached in the real world and, importantly, also in a preventative manner (see Jimenez et al. 2015 for an overview of different design approaches).

Happiness-seekers tend to engage in multiple positive activities at one time (Parks et al. 2012), which may be more effective than engaging in only one activity (Sin and Lyubomirsky 2009). Yet, much happiness-related research focuses on studying the effectiveness of a single intervention at a time (Bolier et al. 2013). Fortunately, happiness-enhancing activities mediated through design can be introduced in a multitude of ways, on a variety of occasions, as well as in specific combination. This can reach more people and increase variety, which can in turn reduce hedonic adaptation (Lyubomirsky 2011) and thereby ideally also lead to an activity being maintained.

Adherence to New Behaviours, and Maintaining Them

Despite the (temporarily) rosy outlook that positive activities may foster, no one said that to act accordingly, moreover, in a self-guided manner was going to be easy—sustained individual effort and commitment are essential to an intervention's effectiveness in stimulating human flourishing (Lyubomirsky et al. 2011; Sin and Lyubomirsky 2009). Unfortunately, several studies of (online) PPIs have seen low compliance and high dropout rates (Christensen et al. 2006, 2009; Farvolden et al. 2005; Ludden et al. 2015; Kelders et al. 2012). For instance, Farvolden et al. (2005) observed an alarmingly high attrition rate while testing a freely available, web-based programme for panic disorder and agoraphobia: only 1% of over 1100 registered users completed the full 12-week program. Preventative programmes that focus on the promotion of well-being do not have the outward urgency that treatment-oriented programmes do. Uptake and adherence is thus expected to be a challenge of comparable relevance also in PPIs for prevention. A recurring theme that may be partially responsible for the observed high attrition rates is low motivation and engagement (Mohr et al. 2013; Morris and Picard 2014; Schueller and Parks 2014). While motivation can be expected to be high when starting a new activity, it is at risk of decline over time. The challenge is thus to sustain user motivation for longer periods.

It comes as no surprise that dropout rates from open access sites are distinctly higher than dropout rates from randomised controlled trials (Christensen et al. 2009). One limitation of findings based on experimental research that should therefore be taken into consideration is the imperfect resemblance of motivational factors in real-world and scientific settings: without the dedication and potential incentive that participating in a research study entails, people might not be sufficiently committed in everyday life.

When the aim is to sustain health benefits and feelings of happiness, reduced long-term engagement underscores a real need for interdisciplinary collaboration when designing for behaviour change: engineers can, for instance, write valuable algorithms for data collection and feedback, or build mobile and/or web-based platforms, for example, for social sharing. Yet, a considerate design is still needed to keep users motivated, engaged, committed, and interested. For this, designers build on findings from the behavioural and social sciences with regards to motivation, volition, and habit formation. They translate these into design strategies, and manifest solutions in their final form and context.

Increasingly, researchers in the field realise that meticulous attention needs to be paid to the design of PPIs and BITs (e.g., Bolier and Abello 2014; Mohr et al. 2013; Morris and Picard 2014; Schueller et al. 2013). How a system is designed will affect how (and whether) it is understood, accepted, and used by people. Established design principles of interface design, user experience design (ISO 2010), and persuasive technologies (Fogg 2003), are valuable starting points to make PPIs and BITs easy to use and engaging, which can positively affect adherence (Kelders et al. 2012). At the same time, a profound comprehension of user context and the identification of design principles that foster behavioural change for well-being (Jimenez et al. 2015) is needed to conceptualise (novel) interactions that are relevant, appropriate, and effective for people in their everyday lives.

Fogg (2003) proposes that three elements are needed at the same time for behaviour to occur: a trigger, motivation, and ability. If a person is not motivated at all, he or she will not act. Likewise, if the person lacks the necessary skills, despite possibly being motivated, the behaviour will also not manifest. Finally, an external or internal trigger elicits a behaviour, for example the smell of a freshly baked cake draws me to the kitchen for a snack. All three elements can be supported through design. Design can actively support execution and skill building (*ability* and self-efficacy beliefs), it can add incentives, for example through optimal challenges, social collaboration or competition, and personal relevance, as well as lower the threshold of engagement (*motivation*), and it can be the *trigger* itself, give sensibly-timed cues, or be integrated to existing practices that in turn serve as triggers.

In contrast to a 'one size fits all' solution, Ludden et al. (2015) propose personalisation, the use of metaphors, and ambient information as valuable design strategies, and emphasise positive affect elicited by the designed solution to increase adherence. Desmet and Pohlmeyer (2013) also discuss the potential of pleasure-evoking design, not only as a direct approach to increasing happiness, but also as an instrument of motivation to stimulate well-being effects in the long-term. Simply put, design can make positive activities fun and personally relevant so that they feel less like a chore. The effort of initiating an activity is thereby perceived as less strenuous. If, as a consequence, a user is more engaged with a positive activity over a longer period of time, delayed well-being effects can come about. Short-term pleasure and the ease of the individual exercises is one of the crucial mechanisms of Tiny Task to reach long-term well-being (Ruitenberg and Desmet 2012).

Maintaining an activity through positive affect can also be achieved by linking the activity to something rewarding. While Huddle and Memoriam Tea celebrate the good, that is personal achievements, Explordinary celebrates the everyday. The primary motivation to engage with Explordinary is not necessarily to become more attentive, but to have fun, meet the challenges of a photographer, and take pride in the details one discovers and shares. Furthermore, linking a positive activity to an existing practice, or embedding it within that practice as in Memoriam Tea and TeaShell, can sustain positive activities, since the practice itself already occurs 'naturally'.

Although adherence is particularly crucial for medical programmes with a progressing syllabus, PPIs do not automatically have to be full programmes that run over the course of several weeks. Small, positive activities can also effectively increase well-being (Lyubomirsky and Layous 2013). People prefer to engage in multiple activities in parallel, rather than sticking to one single intervention (Parks et al. 2012), and this preference can be supported by multiple small activities mediated through everyday design. Lyubomirsky and Layous (2013) suggest that positive activities increase happiness to the extent that they stimulate positive thoughts, feelings, behaviour, and psychological need satisfaction. There are compelling examples of how designed artefacts can create meaningful experiences of even mundane practices by stimulating psychological needs, such as autonomy, competence, and relatedness (Hassenzahl et al. 2013). Do you feel connected when watching TV; do you feel autonomous when using public transport; do you feel competent when cleaning your room? If the answer is no, the future might have exciting prospects for you.

Person-Context-Activity-Fit

It is important to note that not all positive activities are an optimal fit for everyone. Fortunately, there are numerous activities to choose from—the point is to engage in the ones that suit you best. A good fit takes personal strengths, weaknesses, goals, needs, and lifestyle into account (Lyubomirsky 2007). The greatest happiness impact can be expected from activities that feel natural, are enjoyable, and are related to self-concordant goals and beliefs (Lyubomirsky 2007; Sheldon and Elliot 1999). Furthermore, different features of the activity, for example variety, dosage, and of the person, for example self-efficacy beliefs (whether one believes that one is able to do the activity), as well as the interaction between these all impact the resultant well-being effects (Lyubomirsky and Layous 2013).

The implementation of PPIs in the real world thus necessitates a careful understanding of the context itself, the individuals pursuing the activity, and their lifestyles, in order to determine how an intervention can be tailored accordingly. Mapping a user's context and understanding their underlying needs and values is a strength of a user-centred design approach (e.g., Sleeswijk Visser et al. 2005). Activities can be selected and/or optimised for specific contexts and user groups. For instance, reminders might only be sent when the situation allows, for example not during an opera visit. However, the opposite is also possible: a context can be tailored to and integrate positive activities, as shown with TeaShell. In addition, activities can be made more enjoyable, and abstract recommendations can be translated into concrete interactions, which lower the threshold of initiation.

Furthermore, design can provide an appropriate (possibly physical) medium for interventions. In laboratory experiments, interventions are mainly communicated via instructions. For instance, participants of an intervention group might be asked to count blessings (vs. hassles) for a couple of weeks (Emmons and McCullough 2003; Lyubomirsky et al. 2005). One way to disseminate results is simply to report their effectiveness, for example on websites or in self-help books, and to invite people to do the same. Information and instructions are, however, not necessarily sufficient, and might therefore not be the best options.

In line with this, Shawn Archor (2010) pointed out a crucial paradox of human behaviour: 'common sense is not common action' (p. 146). So even if we all agree that it would be better for our happiness if we, for instance, learn to forgive, it is easier said than done. Similarly, a 2012 survey (Kaplan 2012) with over 2000 participants illustrated a 'gratitude gap', which illustrated the difference between the perceived value of experiencing gratitude on the one hand, and demonstrating gratitude on the other: while 90% considered themselves to be grateful people, only 52% of female and 44% of male respondents outwardly expressed gratitude on a regular basis. Hence, despite strong beliefs about the benefit and value of positive activities, self-guided behaviour change does not necessarily come easily. Positive design proposes supplemental interactions as means to communicate and facilitate positive activities. It can trigger, recommend, enable, enhance as well as represent relevant experiences and moves beyond the cognitive and verbal to the tangible, multi-sensory, and interactive.

Tiny Task (Ruitenberg and Desmet 2012) is a good illustration of added value through tangibility. The key chain tokens not only provide instructions; they are also reminders of the experience that one has committed to, that is every time one uses the key, he/she is reminded to plan or do the assignment right away. This also extends to the social realm—friends might ask what the token is about. And once a task is completed, the token serves as a piece of memorabilia for the user to reminisce over, or as a prompt to share the story with others. Even more, the token itself (and thereby the task) can be passed on during a social encounter. Hence, giving a positive activity a tangible representation stimulates adherence as well as a snowball-effect of dissemination.

By materialising the findings of positive psychology, explicit well-being intentions might even become obsolete. For instance, as shown in the examples above, amateur sports players might simply enjoy reflecting on a match in a playful way with their peers, without necessarily having decided to 'work on their happiness'. Likewise, instead of reading about the advantages of counting one's blessings, of being absorbed in the moment, of taking notice, design solutions serve as prompts that encourage the behaviour in situ. Positive design provides opportunities to engage in pleasurable and meaningful experiences, both explicitly *and* implicitly.

When implementing PPIs in real-world contexts, positive design can easily and effectively make use of the fact that design is already part of today's real-world context. It would be a missed opportunity (and a shirked responsibility) if designed products, services, systems, and environments that surround us were not refocused using the lens of well-being.

Conclusion

Positive psychologists have developed a wealth of evidence-based interventions and strategies that boost hopes that perhaps Seligman's (2011) vision that the majority of people are flourishing can come true. In addition to parallel approaches, the ways design can support this goal range from reducing sources of discomfort and ill-being to crafting digital and physical solutions that intentionally promote well-being.

Design can optimise the design of existing BITs and PPIs. Additionally, it can introduce (and facilitate) new, 'dedicated' design interventions, or embed well-being principles into products and services used as part of everyday practices that have a different core functionality, that is 'active design'.

As a result, PPIs can become increasingly and seamlessly integrated into our lives. People would be able to opt for well-being solutions everywhere—in the privacy of their homes, at work, online, in exchange with others, and even in public spaces. Such reach, creating new means with which to act and interact, as well as offering a sensitive fit to the respective context, all demonstrate the clear benefits of positive design for PPIs in practice. Ideally, more people will be reached, on more occasions, and in such a way that positive activities will be sustained.

Design has been, to date, underestimated as a resource to implement the invaluable insights provided by positive psychology research. The impact such design solutions would have on people's well-being far surpasses the negligible effect of their potential material value; the true impact results from the effects it achieves by stimulating experiences of pleasure and meaning. This kind of design is positive design.

Acknowledgments The author wishes to thank Julia Mattaar, Lisa van de Merwe, Frank Stemerding, and Max Tak for permitting the use of their images, Sanne Kistemaker for her assistance in student supervision, and copyeditor Jianne Whelton.

References

Archor, S. (2010). *The happiness advantage*. London: Virgin Books.

Bergsma, A. (2008). Do self-help books help? *Journal of Happiness Studies, 9*(3), 341–360.

Boehm, J. K., & Lyubomirsky, S. (2009). The promise of sustainable happiness. In S. J. Lopez (Ed.), *Handbook of positive psychology* (2nd ed., pp. 667–677). Oxford, UK: Oxford University Press.

Bolier, L., & Abello, K. M. (2014). Online positive psychological interventions: State of the art and future directions. In A. C. Parks & M. S. Schueller (Eds.), *The Wiley Blackwell handbook of positive psychological interventions* (pp. 286–309). Hoboken: Wiley.

Bolier, L., Haverman, M., Westerhof, G. J., Riper, H., Smit, F., & Bohlmeijer, E. (2013). Positive psychology interventions: A meta-analysis of randomized controlled studies. *BMC Public Health, 13*, 119.

Boswell, W. R., Boudreau, J. W., & Tichy, J. (2005). The relationship between employee job change and job satisfaction: The honeymoon-hangover effect. *Journal of Applied Psychology, 90*(5), 882–892.

Brickman, P., & Campbell, D. T. (1971). Hedonic relativism and planning the good society. In M. H. Appley (Ed.), *Adaptation-level theory: A symposium* (pp. 287–302). New York, NY: Academic Press.

Brickman, P., Coates, D., & Janoff-Bulman, R. (1978). Lottery winners and accident victims: Is happiness relative? *Journal of Personality and Social Psychology, 36*(8), 917–927.

Bryant, F. B., & Veroff, J. (2007). *Savoring: A new model of positive experience*. Mahwah, NJ: Lawrence Erlbaum Associates Publishers.

Calvo, R., & Peters, D. (2014). *Positive computing: Technology for wellbeing and human potential*. Cambridge, MA: MIT Press.

Carter, T. J., & Gilovich, T. (2014). Getting the most for the money: The hedonic return on experiential and material purchases. In M. Tatzel (Ed.), *Consumption and well-being in the material world*. Dordrecht, Netherlands: Springer.

Casais, M., Mugge, R., & Desmet, P. M. A. (2015). Extending product life by introducing symbolic meaning: An exploration of design strategies to support subjective well-being. In *Proceedings of product lifetimes and the environment conference*, Nottingham, UK.

Christensen, H., Griffiths, K., Groves, C., & Korten, A. (2006). Free range users and one hit wonders: Community users of an internet-based cognitive behaviour therapy program. *Australian and New Zealand Journal of Psychiatry, 40*, 59–62.

Christensen, H., Griffiths, K. M., & Farrer, L. (2009). Adherence in internet interventions for anxiety and depression: Systematic review. *Journal of Medical Internet Research, 11*(2), e13.

Csikszentmihalyi, M., & Rochberg-Halton, E. (1981). *The meaning of things: Domestic symbols and the self*. New York, NY: Cambridge University Press.

Desmet, P. M. A., & Pohlmeyer, A. E. (2013). Positive design: An introduction to design for subjective well-being. *International Journal of Design, 7*(3), 5–19.

Di Tella, R., Haisken-De New, J., & MacCulloch, R. (2010). Happiness adaptation to income and to status in an individual panel. *Journal of Economic Behavior and Organization, 76*(3), 834–852.

Diener, E., Lucas, R. E., & Napa Scollon, C. (2006). Beyond the hedonic treadmill: Revising the adaptation theory of well-being. *American Psychologist, 61*(4), 305–314.

Dolan, P. (2014). *Happiness by design: Change what you do, not what you think*. London, UK: Hudson Street Press.

Emmons, R. A., & McCullough, M. E. (2003). Counting blessings versus burdens: An experimental investigation of gratitude and subjective well-being in daily life. *Journal of Personality and Social Psychology, 84*(2), 377–389.

Farvolden, P., Denisoff, E., Selby, P., Bagby, R. M., & Rudy, L. (2005). Usage and longitudinal effectiveness of a web-based self-help cognitive behavioral therapy program for panic disorder. *Journal of Medical Internet Research, 7*(1), e7.

Fogg, B. J. (2003). *Persuasive technology: Using computers for what we think and do*. San Francisco, CA: Morgan Kaufman Publishers.

Fournier, S., & Richins, M. L. (1991). Some theoretical and popular notions concerning materialism. *Journal of Social Behavior and Personality, 6*, 403–414.

Frederick, S., & Loewenstein, G. (1999). Hedonic adaptation. In D. Kahneman, E. Diener, & N. Schwartz (Eds.), *Well-being: The foundations of hedonic psychology* (pp. 302–329). New York, NY: Russel Sage Foundation.

Guevarra, D. A., & Howell, R. T. (2015). To have in order to do: Exploring the effects of consuming experiential products on well-being. *Journal of Consumer Psychology, 25*(1), 28–41.

Hassenzahl, M., Eckoldt, K., Diefenbach, S., Laschke, M., Lenz, E., & Kim, J. (2013). Designing moments of meaning and pleasure. Experience design and happiness. *International Journal of Design, 7*(3), 21–31.

Huppert, F. A., & So, T. T. C. (2013). Flourishing across Europe: Application of a new conceptual framework for defining well-being. *Social Indicators Research, 110*, 837–861.

ISO. (2010). *ISO 9241–210: Ergonomics of human-system interaction—Part 210: Human-centred design for interactive systems*. Geneva: International Organization for Standardization.

Jimenez, S., Pohlmeyer, A. E., & Desmet, P. M. A. (2015). *Positive design reference guide*. Delft: Delft University of Technology.

Kaplan, J. (2012). Gratitude survey. Conducted for the John Templeton Foundation.

Kasser, T. (2002). *The high price of materialism*. Cambridge, MA: MIT Press.

Kelders, S. M., Kok, R. N., Ossebaard, H. C., & Van Gemert-Pijnen, J. E. W. C. (2012). Persuasive system design does matter: A systematic review of adherence to web-based interventions. *Journal of Medical Internet Research, 14*, e152.

Linley, P. A., & Joseph, S. (2004). *Positive psychology in practice*. Hoboken, NJ: Wiley.

Lucas, R. E., Georgellis, Y., Clark, A. E., & Diener, E. (2003). Reexamining adaptation and the set point model of happiness: Reactions to changes in marital status. *Journal of Personality and Social Psychology, 84*(3), 527–539.

Ludden, G. D. S., van Rompay, T. J. L., Kelders, S. M., & van Gemert-Pijnen, J. E. W. C. (2015). How to increase reach and adherence of web-based interventions: A design research viewpoint. *Journal of Medical Internet Research, 17*(7), e172.

Lykken, D., & Tellegen, A. (1996). Happiness is a stochastic phenomenon. *Psychological Science, 7*(3), 186–189.

Lyubomirsky, S. (2007). *The how of happiness*. London: Piatkus.

Lyubomirsky, S. (2011). Hedonic adaptation to positive and negative experiences. In S. Folkman (Ed.), *The Oxford handbook of stress, health, and coping* (pp. 200–224). New York: Oxford University Press.

Lyubomirsky, S. (2013). *The myths of happiness*. New York: The Penguin Press.

Lyubomirsky, S., & Layous, K. (2013). How do simple positive activities increase well-being? *Current Directions in Psychological Science, 22*(1), 57–62.

Lyubomirsky, S., Sheldon, K. M., & Schkade, D. (2005). Pursuing happiness: The architecture of sustainable change. *Review of General Psychology, 9*(2), 111–131.

Lyubomirsky, S., Dickerhoof, R., Boehm, J. K., & Sheldon, K. M. (2011). Becoming happier takes both a will and a proper way: An experimental longitudinal intervention to boost well-being. *Emotion, 11*(2), 391–402.

Mohr, D. C., Burns, M. N., Schueller, S. M., Clarke, G., & Klinkman, M. (2013). Behavioral intervention technologies: Evidence review and recommendations for future research in mental health. *General Hospital Psychiatry, 35*(4), 332–338.

Morris, R. R., & Picard, R. (2014). Crowd-powered positive psychological interventions. *The Journal of Positive Psychology, 9*(6), 509–516.

Nicolao, L., Irwin, J. R., & Goodman, J. K. (2009). Happiness for sale: Do experiential purchases make consumers happier than material purchases? *Journal of Consumer Research, 36*(2), 188–198.

Parks, A. C., & Szanto, R. K. (2013). Assessing the efficacy and effectiveness of a positive psychology-based self-help book. *Terapia Psicologica, 31*(1), 141–149.

Parks, A. C., Della Porta, M. D., Pierce, R. S., Zilca, R., & Lyubomirsky, S. (2012). Pursuing happiness in everyday life: The characteristics and behaviors of online happiness seekers. *Emotion, 12*(6), 1222–1234.

Patterson, L., & Biswas-Diener, R. (2012). Consuming happiness. In P. Brey, A. Briggle, & E. Spence (Eds.), *The good life in a technological age* (pp. 147–156). New York, NY: Routledge.

Pohlmeyer, A. E. (2012). Design for happiness. *Interfaces, 92*, 8–11.

Pohlmeyer, A. E. (2014). Enjoying joy. A process-based approach to design for prolonged pleasure. In *Proceedings of the 8th Nordic conference on human-computer interaction, NordiCHI'14* (pp. 871–876). New York, NY: ACM Press.

Pohlmeyer, A. E., & Desmet, P. M. A. (2017). From good to the greater good. In J. Chapman (Ed.), *The Routledge handbook of sustainable product design* (pp. 469–486). London: Routledge.

Quoidbach, J., Berry, E. V., Hansenne, M., & Mikolajczak, M. (2010). Positive emotion regulation and well-being: Comparing the impact of eight savoring and dampening strategies. *Personality and Individual Differences, 49*(5), 368–373.

Riva, G., Banos, R. M., Botella, C., Wiederhold, B. K., & Gaggioli, A. (2012). Positive technology: Using interactive technologies to promote positive functioning. *Cyberpsychology, Behavior, and Social Networking, 15*(2), 69–77.

Ruitenberg, H. P., & Desmet, P. M. A. (2012). Design thinking in positive psychology: The development of a product-service combination that stimulates happiness-enhancing activities. In *Proceedings of the 8th international conference on design and emotion,* London, UK.

Ryan, R. M., & Deci, E. L. (2000). Self-determination theory and the facilitation of intrinsic motivation, social development and well-being. *American Psychologist, 55*(1), 68–78.

Sander, T. (2011). Positive computing. In R. Biswas-Diener (Ed.), *Positive psychology as social change* (pp. 309–326). New York, NY: Springer.

Schueller, M. S., & Parks, A. C. (2014). The science of self-help: Translating positive psychology research into increased individual happiness. *European Psychologist, 19*(2), 145–155.

Schueller, S. M., Muñoz, R. F., & Mohr, D. C. (2013). Realizing the potential of behavioral intervention technologies. *Current Directions in Psychological Science, 22*(6), 478–483.

Seligman, M. E. P. (2011). *Flourish*. New York, NY: Free Press.

Seligman, M. E. P., Steen, T. A., Park, N., & Peterson, C. (2005). Positive psychology progress: Empirical validation of interventions. *American Psychologist, 60*(5), 410–421.

Sheldon, K. M., & Elliot, A. J. (1999). Goal striving, need satisfaction, and longitudinal well-being: The self-concordance model. *Journal of Personality and Social Psychology, 76*(3), 482–497.

Sin, N. L., & Lyubomirsky, S. (2009). Enhancing well-being and alleviating depressive symptoms with positive psychology interventions: A practice-friendly meta-analysis. *Journal of Clinical Psychology: In Session, 65*(5), 467–487.

Sleeswijk Visser, F., Stappers, P. J., van der Lugt, R., & Sanders, E. B.-N. (2005). Contextmapping: Experiences from practice. *CoDesign, 1*(2), 119–149.

Van Boven, L. (2005). Experientialism, materialism, and the pursuit of happiness. *Review of General Psychology, 9*(2), 132–142.

Yang, Y. (2015). *Sentimental value and its influence on hedonic adaptation*. Ph.D. thesis, Carnegie Mellon University.

Chapter 15
How Can Positive Psychology Influence Public Policy and Practice?

Roger G. Tweed, Eric Mah, Madeline Dobrin, Rachel Van Poele, and Lucian Gideon Conway III

Abstract Positive psychologists who decline to involve themselves in government policy issues may be similar to medical doctors who refuse to work in hospitals or clinics. Both the positive psychologist and the doctor may greatly reduce their positive effect if they avoid involvement in these institutions that widely impact the population. This chapter explains what positive psychologists bring to policy discussions: An emphasis on measurable well-being, a desire to do more than just ameliorate pathology, and a broad knowledge of psychological findings. The chapter provides examples of policy relevant findings related to: (a) measurement of well-being, (b) identification of groups with particular needs, and (c) exploration of paths to the good life. The chapter also gives warnings about ways to fail in policy engagement, such as limiting efforts to legislative lobbying, ignoring lessons from policy-engaged academics, failing to consider costs, seeking to change fundamental belief systems of opponents, ignoring unintended consequences, expressing hubris, providing imbalanced emphasis on particular types of well-being, and failing to test policies incrementally. The chapter closes by proposing a strategy for policy engagement that not only promotes, but also embodies positive psychology.

Abbreviation

SWB Subjective well-being

R.G. Tweed (✉) • E. Mah • M. Dobrin • R. Van Poele
Department of Psychology, Kwantlen Polytechnic University,
12666 – 72nd Avenue, Surrey, BC, Canada, V3W 2M8
e-mail: roger.tweed@kpu.ca; eric0mah@hotmail.com; madelinedobrin@gmail.com; rachelvanpoele@hotmail.com

L.G. Conway III
Department of Psychology, University of Montana, Skaggs Bldg., Missoula, MT 59812, USA
e-mail: luke.conway@umontana.com

C. Proctor (ed.), *Positive Psychology Interventions in Practice*,
DOI 10.1007/978-3-319-51787-2_15

Can Positive Psychology Influence Public Policy and Practice?

Why Positive Psychology and Public Policy?

Imagine a brilliant doctor who can to accurately diagnose any disease and cure any ailment. This doctor, who has a wealth of knowledge and ability, chooses to stay away from clinics and hospitals, and instead lives night and day on a secluded mountain frequented only by the occasional hiker. This doctor treats the occasional passer-by on the mountain trails and once saved the life of a climber in extremis, but in the end the brilliant doctor's contributions to the greater good fall short of what they might have been had the doctor worked at a clinic or other location that attracts people in need. If the doctor spent workdays in a clinic or hospital, the doctor would encounter and help people in need many times every day rather than every few weeks or months.

Now imagine a positive psychologist who through rigorous research becomes a prodigy in the field. As a result of countless studies, the psychologist understands much about the good life, character strengths, positive emotions, and so forth. Naturally, this psychologist publishes extensively and the research becomes well-known in academia. Despite lifelong contributions to the field in the form of well-designed experiments and top-notch academic publications, the psychologist's valuable understanding of human flourishing—knowledge that has the potential to promote positive and widespread social and institutional change—remains of interest almost only to scholars and university students.

The analogy of the brilliant doctor may seem farfetched, but serves to highlight an important distinction between individual excellence—expertise, ability, and knowledge—and practical outcomes in the form of social and institutional change. Unfortunately, the fictional case of the positive psychologist may not be far from reality in some cases. Our objective here will be to examine ways in which the many robust, interesting, and significant findings of positive psychologists can be translated successfully into policies that can improve the lives of members of society. If positive psychologists are interested in creating effective interventions, possibly the most impact will be had by influencing the ways that governments intervene in people's lives.

Is There Reason to Believe that Positive Psychology Can Uniquely Contribute to Public Policy?

Perhaps we go too fast. We do not generally question the value of a good doctor; but some could ask what makes the application of positive psychology to policy uniquely useful to begin with? Here, we discuss three reasons. First, positive psychology, at least academic positive psychology, relies on empirical measures of psychological well-being. This may sound like an abstract or even practically irrelevant distinctive, but it is not. Many other policy perspectives will seek to maximise outcomes, such as income, education, or health, that are presumed to increase well-being. In contrast, positive psychologists seek to measure well-being more directly to assess which elements of these more usual foci (income, health, education, and other variables) contribute the most to well-being. For example, positive psychologists do not merely assume that wealth is a desirable policy outcome, but they actually study this empirically. In fact, recent research suggests that increased wealth does tend to produce greater psychological well-being, but only if certain other social factors accompany the increased wealth (Diener et al. 2013).

Second, positive psychologists are not satisfied with merely ameliorating problems. They want to help people build lifestyles enhancing positive well-being. As Gable and Haidt (2005) suggested, much of psychology has historically focused on healing, that is, bringing 'people from negative eight to zero', but positive psychologists seek to bring people from 'zero to positive eight' (p. 103). Most positive psychologists would argue that merely reducing depression, for example, is not a sufficient goal. People also deserve help in building a meaningful and fulfilling life.

Third, positive psychologists draw on a different literature than typical policy analysts. Academically trained positive psychologists will have familiarity with a broad range of psychological research that will not be familiar to and will less often be referenced by other decision makers in government bodies. Thus, positive psychologists can bring a fresh perspective to the discussion. According to Seligman et al. (2005), positive psychology involves the comprehensive study of three topics: (1) positive emotions, (2) positive character traits, and (3) institutions that enable the first two components. The third element, the study of institutions facilitating positive states and traits may be the most understudied of the three (Schueller 2009). Nonetheless, the importance of this third element is inestimable; after all, ideas cannot often effect widespread change without institutional forces to back them.

Other policy and practice analysts may bring one of these elements (i.e., focus on measures of well-being, focus on doing more than ameliorating problems, or broad familiarity with empirical findings from psychology), but fewer will bring all three of these elements. Thus, applying positive psychology to policy and practice decisions can break new ground.

The Rocky Road from Positive Psychology to Public Policy

Admittedly, the road from any clear-cut psychological finding to a public policy decision is often a rocky one, and thus the path from knowledge to societal benefit is not as straightforward as our opening analogy might imply. As a field, we may fully establish that factor X causes outcome Y at an individual level, but it does not always follow that attempting to manipulate X from a public policy standpoint will lead to widespread change in Y. Enacting public policy has many potential consequences outside of the specific effect of X➔Y. For example, overt pressures such as those implied in top-down public policy might: (a) cause reactance (e.g., Knowles and Linn 2004), (b) invoke backfiring based on informational contamination (e.g., Conway and Schaller 2005), or (c) involve other moral or psychological principles outside of the scope of the X→Y relationship.

Consider an example from aggression research. There is a lot of evidence that violent video games cause subsequent aggression; meta-analyses of a large body of research reveals that the effect of violent media on aggressive behaviour is larger than the effect of condoms on HIV, calcium intake on bone mass, homework on academic achievement, and a number of other commonly-accepted effects (Bushman and Anderson 2001). But that alone does not mean that, to create a better society, we should encourage a public policy banning violent video games. A ban might invoke culturally shared values about freedom of choice and possibly bring a backlash or create other reactions that could eventually do more harm than good. What we do with that knowledge of effects from violent games is itself a separate question that ought to be subject to empirical scrutiny. For example, we might think it more effective in the long run to use that knowledge to create a grass-roots, bottom-up campaign that aims for long-term cultural change and not for quick policy fixes (for the predictive power of bottom-up vs. top-down processes, see Conway et al. 2006).

Left alone, the above paragraph would support a proscription suggesting we ignore policy altogether. However, we think that would be a mistake because public policy will influence people's lives, and positive psychologists can help that influence be for the good.

There are at least three major questions when applying positive psychology to policy: (1) What can we infer from positive psychology research regarding public policies that will be helpful? (2) How does one effectively influence policy and practice in response to these findings? and (3) Does that policy when implemented have a positive impact on peoples' lives. All these questions are important. The third, policy impact, can only be researched after we engage and influence policy makers or at least policy implementers. The impact of the policy once implemented is exceedingly important and amenable to research, but we will assume, for the purposes of this chapter, that many positive psychologists need to take the first steps of developing policy positions and engaging policy-makers. Only then will the third question be feasible to address. Thus, this chapter focuses more on responding to the first two questions: implications of research findings and strategies for influencing policy.

Examples of Research Findings with Policy Implications

As a starting point, some policy implications of empirical findings will be discussed. This brief discussion can only begin to explore this topic. For further discussion of these types of issues, we recommend seeing: Mulgan (2013) and Diener et al. (2009).

Psychological Well-Being Can Be Measured

Positive psychology researchers have devoted much effort toward developing valid measures of psychological well-being (see Proctor et al. 2015) and there is evidence these can work well (e.g., Veenhoven 2015). According to Diener et al. (2009), however, current government policies are often built: (a) without awareness of which population groups have different levels of psychological needs, and (b) on erroneous assumptions regarding factors that promote well-being. Thus, they recommend that measures of subjective well-being (SWB) be regularly administered to populations and consulted when making policy decisions. These measures would help identify subgroups with elevated needs. The measures could also provide feedback on the effectiveness of the interventions. Governments currently gather information on many indicators of performance: Just as indicators of gross national product, current account deficits, and employment rates are regularly tracked by government bodies, likewise, psychological well-being could be regularly measured and tracked.

From a more technical perspective, it is worth noting that some measures of psychological well-being may place excessive emphasis on hedonic indicators of well-being (e.g., short-term happiness) and comparatively neglect eudaimonic indicators of well-being (e.g., life purpose, self-actualisation, sense that one is contributing to society, belief that one is living a good life). As a result, selecting the best set of psychological measures will require careful thinking (Diener and Diener 2011; Hone et al. 2014; Proctor et al. 2015).

Particular Subgroups Have Elevated Needs (e.g., Youth at Risk of Mental Illness and Caregivers)

The approaches from the prior section would serve to add psychological measures to the data that policy makers may use when making decisions, but these measures of course do not directly ensure other specific policy changes. As such, positive psychologists who stop there would be like doctors who provide data to patients but refuse to do surgery. Thus, it is useful to also look more deeply into some examples of additional policy changes that might be implemented based on positive psychology research. A few specific examples will be mentioned here.

One relevant finding relates to the decreased SWB scores evident among one subgroup of the population: People who have experienced ongoing issues with mental illness. In response to this finding, Diener et al. (2009) recommend preventive treatment targeting youth at risk of mental illness. In particular, they recommend school-wide screening to identify children with risk indicators and subsequent targeted preventive treatment with the identified children to reduce their likelihood of progression to full-scale mental illness. Just like a polio vaccine can inhibit the onset of disease, some research suggests that psychological training targeting kids in this situation can reduce the likelihood of future depression (Seligman et al. 2007). In this case, there is not only research on the X→Y relationship, but also research on the positive consequences of attempting to directly manipulate X from a top-down, policy level.

Measures of SWB also indicate that people who provide daily care for infirm significant others tend to experience particular SWB deficits. Thus, Diener et al. (2009) recommend policies to support caregivers through connection to support groups and counselling in order to reduce the negative effects brought upon by the burden of caregiving. These steps and others to support this subpopulation could potentially lower the chance of depression in relation to caregiving (Lin et al. 2013) and thereby the chance of institutionalisation for the person receiving care (Diener et al. 2009). More research is needed on the specific implications of policy change. Nonetheless, the current findings do suggest that efforts toward an ameliorative policy make sense.

Relationships Matter, but Pursuit of Wealth Can Be Problematic

Humans are inherently social beings. One of the largest lessons learned so far from SWB research is the importance of relationships in comparison to financial pursuits. While we need financial resources to live, some research suggests that pursuit of money at an intensity above the population average, tends to make people less happy (Kasser and Ryan 1993). More generally, life goals related to wealth, fame, and good looks are associated with poor psychological outcome, but life goals related to building relationships and contributing to the community are associated with well-being (Kasser and Ryan 1996). Further evidence comes from the fact that there has been a steady increase in wealth for developed nations following WWII, but this is associated with relatively static levels of well-being (Marks 2011; http://www.worlddatabaseofhappiness.eur.nl). This disconnect suggests reconsideration of the issues currently driving public policy. Nic Marks (2011) argued that once basic needs are met, chasing primarily material wealth is an unsustainable and ill-informed approach to achieving societal well-being. In response to this type of finding, Tim Kasser (2004) has suggested practical solutions to reduce the materialistic impulses induced by advertising. His suggestions include media literacy campaigns for children and their parents, new regulations for psychological research in advertising and marketing, reductions in the amount of advertising children are exposed to in the educational system, and more dissemination of information on the negative well-being effects of a society that equates wealth with happiness (2004).

Also, the UK's Foresight programme (Aked et al. 2008) has advocated for publicly sponsored campaigns teaching the populace about five reliable ways to well-being. They use the following terms to summarise the strategies: Connect, Be active, Take notice, Keep learning, and Give. Also, other relationship-sustaining policies such as provision of skill training for parents at-risk may help build positive relations within families (Mulgan 2013; Sanders et al. 2014), so are worthy of consideration.

Admittedly, healthy human social relationships are complex and hard to manufacture widely across society. For example, enforced social interaction through population-wide interventions such as cohousing and meal sharing could manufacture many relationships, but many of these relationships will be negative. Furthermore, clashing value systems regarding relationships can create resistance to government policy in this domain (Mulgan 2013). As a result, more research is specifically needed that directly ties policy change to relationship facilitation, and in turn to more SWB. Nonetheless, it would be foolish to ignore this research on the value of relationships when developing policy. It is a good goal to at least consider how policies might influence the success of people attempting to meet their social needs.

Physical Activity Promotes Well-Being

In quite a different domain, much research indicates that regular physical activity is associated with increased well-being (e.g., Marks 2011; Mutrie and Faulkner 2004). Some research suggests that regular physical activity may also reduce depression, with effects possibly as large as the impact of antidepressant medication (see Daley 2008 for a review). In some regions such as Canada, tax breaks have been provided for parents who enrol their children in regular programmes of physical fitness. Initially, the credit in Canada was especially problematic because families whose incomes were too low to pay income tax were not eligible for any benefit. The policy was later made more universal, but, then, after an election, the subsequent government completely removed the policy. Nonetheless, this is one example of a policy to increase well-being by inducing activity while still letting families choose the programme in which to enrol their children.

Many Other Findings Have Policy Implications

Many more topics could be discussed in terms of policy implications from positive psychology. Diener et al. (2009) argued that empirical findings linking commute time with reduced well-being justify policies aimed at reducing commute time. Mulgan (2013) has argued that because well-being is associated not only with actual victimhood, but also fear of crime, police agency benchmarks should measure not only actual crime rates, but also fear of crime; he argued that police agencies would then probably engage with citizens more and focus more on reducing antisocial behaviour that frightens citizens. Mulgan (2013) also argued that much of government spending on the arts, sports, and culture is focused on large, spectator events, but much research instead shows that participation is conducive to well-being (e.g., playing sports and producing music and art). Thus, he argues that governments should spend less on spectator activities and more on participation opportunities and incentives. Also, some evidence suggests that positive psychology character education in schools promotes well-being and improved relationships (Proctor et al. 2011; Quinlan et al. 2015). Many other studies also have implications for public policy.

Some Ways to Fail in Policy Engagement

As we have discussed, the road from psychological findings to policy recommendations is a rocky one. Premature implementation of policy can cause problems; however, an equally concerning mistake would be failure in persuading policy makers to successfully implement effective policies reflecting findings from positive psychology. If our hypothetical doctor cannot get patients to receive surgery when they need it, then she is of little value to society. As a cautionary note, here are some failure-inducing strategies that may be worth avoiding.

Ignore Lessons Shared by Others Who Have Succeeded (and as a Result, Bore Policymakers)

The instincts of academics may often guide them to ineffective strategies for engaging policy makers. Bogenschneider and Corbett (2010) wrote a helpful guide based on years of work facilitating relations between policy makers and academics. Based on surveys, interviews, and experience, they suggest the engagement with policy makers will be most effective when the academics: (1) provide brief oral (rather than only written) presentations summarising several studies and the policy implication; (2) describe comparative policy and practice from other jurisdictions; (3) conduct interactive seminars encouraging cross-talk between academics, policymakers, and policy implementers; (4) maintain an ongoing relationship with the policymaker; and (5) when speaking to an elected official, tell a story about a person in that electoral district who will be affected by the policy. This last point might not seem obvious to academics accustomed to discussing theory and data, but the relevance would be dangerous to ignore. Bogenschneider and Corbett (2010) quote one high-ranking politician who said, 'If you give legislators the research and facts, and I tell a heart-wrenching story, I will win every time' (p. 41; cf. Slovic 2007).

Limit Efforts to Legislative Lobbying

Though legislators often dictate formal written policy, the reality in practice is that operational managers at a variety of levels have much influence on how policies are implemented (Bogenschneider and Corbett 2010). As a result, positive psychologists interested in influencing policy may reasonably choose to work with officials lower down in the system that determine how policy is implemented and who feed information into the system. Focusing exclusively on legislative lobbying could be unnecessarily restrictive.

Ignore Unintended Consequences

Any step forward in new policy directions will inevitably have unintended consequences. For example, once well-being measures are implemented, any effect could be undermined by governments that could manipulate these statistics just as some have manipulated statistics on GNP, debt, and unemployment rates (Frey 2011). Alternatively, subgroups of the population could alter their responses on questionnaires to get more funding. Furthermore, tax policy changes intended to promote positive behaviour may cause people to game the system (e.g., creating false fitness programmes to get tax breaks), thereby defeating the intended purpose of the policy. Unintended consequences are hard to predict. Groups proposing new policies will need to carefully monitor effects to maximise the chance of success.

Fail to Consider Costs (and Be Perceived as Irrelevant or Unrealistic)

Positive psychologists are mostly untrained in economic analysis. However, to motivate those who ultimately enact policy change, positive psychologists will have to consider cost issues. An impressive model of this type of analysis has been provided by the Washington State Institute for Public Policy (e.g., 2014a). That group has assessed a variety of possible interventions including specific programmes for parent training, early prison release, nurse home visits, and many others. For each intervention, they calculated the overall cost to government, the financial benefit to society as a whole, and the return to government in cost savings or increases in tax revenue. These analyses are not easy; for example, some may require estimates of the reduced earnings due to substance abuse or even the monetary cost of pain and suffering resulting from victimisation (Washington State Institute for Public Policy 2014b). Nonetheless, cost-benefit analyses provide information that policy-makers value. Some positive psychologists could apply for grants to conduct exactly this type of analysis of the cost-benefit outcomes of implementing positive psychology components into government policy. This type of analysis could require much effort, but the information could potentially greatly extend the reach of positive psychology and provide information regarding which interventions should or should not be expanded.

Indeed, it is worth noting that if positive psychologists continually call for vastly increased government spending without simultaneously being open to, or even suggesting strategies for raising government revenue or reducing other government expenses, their missives might seem unrealistic and unworthy of attention. The kneejerk responses of saying governments can save money through reducing politicians' pay or expenses might seem tempting to policy neophytes, but these are often relatively small portions of government budgets. Big policy changes often require big budgets and big increases in tax or reductions in spending. Similarly, the idea of raising corporate taxes often seems to be popular among academics, and this may be appropriate, but academics should be aware that simple ideas like this often have unintended consequences. For example, some corporations may counteract the tax increase by booking their profit in other countries, by reducing the number of employees, or by raising prices charged to consumers rather than reducing profits. We are not recommending or countermanding particular tax directions here, but simply urging caution and awareness of budget limitations. Positive psychologists need to learn about budget limitations and consider these realistically given their proposals. Some possible positive psychology interventions can be successful at a relatively low cost. For example, online positive psychology interventions even without any face-to-face therapy have produced promising outcomes in randomized control trials (e.g., Boettcher et al. 2014; Bolier et al. 2014). Low cost interventions like these may deserve attention as first steps when advocating policy related to positive psychology.

Focus on Changing the Fundamental Belief System of Opponents

Positive psychologists also need to recognise that some disagreements will not be resolved in their lifetime, so they will need to find common ground amidst continued disagreement. Yuval Harari (2015), for example, pointed out the societal conflict between equality and individual freedom. He argued that enforced equality (e.g., seizing and redistributing tax dollars) reduces liberty, but utter liberty (freedom to run one's business as one pleases) can reduce equality. He argues that such conflicting values are normal in societies. Individuals will often differ in the extent to which they value each of two conflicting values, and empirical findings may not be able to override that conflict. At that point, the conversation might need to shift away from trying to change fundamental beliefs of others toward finding common ground and common goals (Fisher et al. 2011). Fighting against fundamental belief systems in others may be like fighting the rising of the sun, but seeking common ground may promote collaborative and synergistic efforts.

Express Hubris

Also, positive psychologists who enter policy discussions might find a temptation toward hubris. In our experience, policymakers often have a dichotomous response to social science evidence: They want to treat social science evidence as either indisputable or worthless. They often have difficulty remaining cognizant of the fact that much evidence from social science is valuable, justifiably convincing, but seldom equivalent to absolute proof (the same could be said about much of the evidence policymakers deal with every day, whether it be in the domain of health, economics, education, or other domains). When positive psychologists become the explicator of the evidence, it may be tempting to likewise treat your own evidence at one of these extremes.

In reality, however, some intellectual humility might be appropriate. Even well-researched interventions often show shrunken effect sizes when implemented on a larger scale (Welsh et al. 2010). Also, much of positive psychology is based on correlational studies, longitudinal studies, or small-scale experiments on nonrandom samples. As discussed earlier, often positive psychologists will not have evidence directly related to policy implementation (element #3), and will only have evidence concerning the X➔Y relationship at the individual level. Thus, positive psychologists would do well to proceed with humility and caution. They can, nonetheless, provide valuable perspective – especially because the alternative is often policy guided by gut feelings, party policy, or current practices. Bogenschneider and Corbett (2010), suggest that academics may be wise to sometimes refrain from using the term 'evidence-based policy', and instead discuss 'evidence-informed policy' or 'research-shaped decision making' (p. 4). Such a change may seem small, but this small change in terminology communicates intellectual humility by admitting that the research evidence will not always be able to give a definitive answer regarding policy, but can give some guidance about the types of policies most likely to produce desirable outcomes.

Provide Imbalanced Emphasis Regarding Well-Being

When positive psychologists refer to well-being, they often assume this means frequent positive emotion, infrequent negative emotion, and high life satisfaction (the 'Big Three' model of well-being). A recent analysis, however, suggests that this Big Three framework puts excessive emphasis on one type of well-being called hedonic well-being and neglects any indicator of pure eudaimonic well-being (Proctor et al. 2015). Measures of life satisfaction seem to assess a mix of hedonic and eudaimonic well-being, and the frequency of emotion measures assess hedonic well-being.

Here's a clarification of why a focus on eudaimonic well-being matters: Consider an example of a psychotherapist. The therapist might get short-term hedonic pleasure from daily life experiences such as food and entertainment. The therapist might also get deeper joy and stability from eudaimonic experiences such as using her strengths and serving others. If the therapist, when working with clients, seeks to facilitate only hedonic pleasure and avoidance of pain, then she will be failing to help them achieve the deeper joy and stability that she gets from eudaimonic experiences. When providing therapy, the clinician will ideally provide clients with strategies not only for finding hedonic short-term happiness and avoidance of pain, but also the longer term eudaimonic well-being that derives from finding meaning, using one's strengths, and serving a purpose beyond oneself. The same care to be balanced may be necessary for policymakers. Their policy work should also seek to facilitate both these types of experiences among citizens. Even people in extremely difficult circumstances often can find joy in eudaimonic experiences of helping others (Schwartz and Sendor 1999) and using their personal strengths (e.g., Tweed et al. 2012).

The value of eudaimonic experiences suggests that the inauguration speech of at least one politician, John F. Kennedy (United States and Library of Congress 1961), expressed wisdom from a positive psychology perspective. He suggested that the populace not ask what their country could do for them, but instead ask what they could do for their country. The research on eudaimonia suggests that policies helping people do exactly this, use their strengths to serve their neighbourhood, country, and even world, might promote a broader well-being, something to add to the short-term pleasure of hedonia. Also, this eudaimonic emphasis would support innovations such as public ministries devoted to facilitating volunteer work or facilitating time banks or other strategies promoting eudaimonia among the populace. It would also support monitoring of eudaimonic well-being in the population in order to assess needs and monitor the success of interventions. Thus, focusing exclusively on promoting hedonic well-being would be a failure in terms of promoting policy reflective of empirical findings from positive psychology.

Do Not Include Separate Sections on Policy in Texts, Conferences, and Courses

Many positive psychologists attend conferences, teach courses, or write text books. To the extent that policy-related issues are ignored in these domains, future positive psychologists will lack skills. Adding sections on public policy in conferences, texts, and courses could help overcome this deficit. Public policy could receive attention more broadly in positive psychology conferences, texts, and courses. In graduate programmes in particular, students may benefit from exposure to more general introductions to public policy analysis (e.g., Bardach 2012; Bogenschneider and Corbett 2010; Diener et al. 2009; Cartwright and Hardie 2012; Manski 2013; Mulgan 2013).

Fail to Test Policies Incrementally

Polices will have the greatest chance to succeed if the policy can be tested on a small scale in order to identify effect sizes, problems, and unintended effects prior to broad implementation. The Abdul Latif Jameel Poverty Action Lab provides a helpful model of such research (http://www.povertyactionlab.org). Pilot programmes testing policy changes on a small scale could save vast resources that would be spent on ineffective programmes and could protect the reputation of positive psychologists by enhancing the chance of success when large-scale positive psychology interventions are implemented.

Concluding Thoughts: A Positive Psychology of Facilitating Policy Changes

Social change of any kind is fraught with difficulties. Interestingly, in pursuing social change based on positive psychology, it may be that positive psychology can offer lessons to itself about how best to pursue that change. Scott Sherman (2011) argued for an approach that in some ways befits positive psychology. His quantitative analysis of social movements also suggests this method is particularly effective. In his model, a person will uncover injustice within society, recruit others to help demand change, and then not demonise those committing the injustice; but rather, seek to collaborate with others—including former enemies—to create the change. Working with people who disagree about fundamental values or who come from a different political orientation is difficult. The relation may break down without any malicious intent on either side. For example, each party may insult the other party through word choice, through negative assumptions about motives, or through other actions that are not consciously malicious (for a helpful framework for productive conversations amidst serious disagreements, see http://www.livingroomconversations.org).

As a historical example, consider Martin Luther King. According to Sherman (2011), a central motivating element of Martin Luther King's nonviolent methods was, in conjunction with his religious beliefs, the fact that King envisioned a better world for all, even his enemies. Bringing harm would be inconsistent with those values. According to King:

> A big danger for us is the temptation to follow the people we are opposing. They call us names, so we call them names…I remind you that in many people, in many people called segregationists, there are other things going on in their lives: this person or that person, standing here or there may also be other things—kind to neighbors and family, helpful and good-spirited at work…Let us not do to ourselves as others (as our opponents) do to us: try to put ourselves into one all-inclusive category—the virtuous ones as against the evil ones…there is the danger: the 'us' or 'them' mentality takes hold, and we do, actually, begin to run the risk of joining ranks with the very people we are opposing. I worry about this a lot these days. (Coles 1994, p. 32)

Sherman (2011) suggests this type of attitude need not be relegated to the past. He argues that this method of uncovering injustice, demanding change, but not demonizing and instead working with all people, including those committing the injustice, to enact a better future is still particularly effective in promoting positive social change. Sherman recognises that anger has great value for mobilising people, so they are ready to take action; however, Sherman (2011) suggests that subsequent action for positive psychologists will be more likely to produce lasting change if the anger that initiates motivation is transformed. The anger that helps motivate can subsequently be transformed into something that changes society while building relationships rather than destroying them. Sherman claims to have been surprised when his empirical analysis showed this approach to be more effective than alternative strategies for creating broad social change. If Sherman is right that this method is effective, we should pay attention. This would be a truly positive psychology approach to influencing policy. His findings suggest that if we ultimately want to avoid being like our hypothetical doctor who does not fulfil her potential to help society, we should not only recommend positive psychology to others, but also enact positive psychology in the way we pursue change.

References

Aked, J., Marks, N., Cordon, C., & Thompson, S. (2008). Five ways to wellbeing. *New Economics Foundation*. Retrieved from http://www.neweconomics.org/publications/entry/five-ways-to-well-being-the-evidence

Bardach, E. (2012). *A practical guide for policy analysis* (4th ed.). Thousand Oaks, CA: Sage.

Boettcher, J., Astrom, V., Pahlsson, D., Schenstrom, O., Andersson, G., & Carlbring, P. (2014). Internet-based mindfulness treatment for anxiety disorders: A randomized controlled trial. *Behavior Therapy, 45*(2), 241–253.

Bogenschneider, K., & Corbett, T. J. (2010). *Evidence-based policymaking: Insights from policy-minded researchers and research-minded policymakers*. New York: Routledge.

Bolier, L., Majo, C., Smit, F., Westerhof, G. J., Haverman, M., Walburg, J. A., Riper, H., & Bohlmeijer, E. (2014). Cost-effectiveness of online positive psychology: Randomized controlled trial. *The Journal of Positive Psychology, 9*(5), 460–471.

Bushman, B. J., & Anderson, C. A. (2001). Media violence and the American public: Scientific facts versus media misinformation. *American Psychologist, 56*(6/7), 477–489.

Cartwright, N., & Hardie, J. (2012). *Evidence-based policy: A practical guide to doing it better*. Oxford: Oxford University Press.

Coles, R. (1994). *The call of service*. New York: Houghton Mifflin Harcourt.

Conway III, L. G., & Schaller, M. (2005). When authority's commands backfire: Attributions about consensus and effects on deviant decision making. *Journal of Personality and Social Psychology, 89*(3), 311–326.

Conway III, L. G., Clements, S. M., & Tweed, R. G. (2006). Collectivism and governmentally initiated restrictions: A cross-sectional and longitudinal analysis across nations and within a nation. *Journal of Cross-Cultural Psychology, 37*(1), 1–23.

Daley, A. (2008). Exercise and depression: A review of reviews. *Journal of Clinical Psychology in Medical Settings, 15*(2), 140–147.

Diener, E., & Diener, C. (2011). Monitoring psychosocial prosperity for social change. In R. Biswas-Diener (Ed.), *Positive psychology as social change* (pp. 53–72). Dordrecht: Springer.

Diener, E., Lucas, R., Schimmak, U., & Helliwell, J. (2009). *Well-being for public policy*. Oxford: Oxford University Press.

Diener, E., Tay, L., & Oishi, S. (2013). Rising income and the subjective well-being of nations. *Journal of Personality and Social Psychology, 104*(2), 267–276.

Fisher, R., Ury, W., & Patton, B. (2011). *Getting to yes: Negotiating agreement without giving in*. New York: Penguin Books.

Frey, B. S. (2011). Tullock challenges: Happiness, revolutions, and democracy. *Public Choice, 148*(3/4), 269–281.

Gable, S. L., & Haidt, J. (2005). What (and why) is positive psychology? *Review of General Psychology, 9*(2), 103–110.

Harari, Y. (2015). *Sapiens: A brief history of humankind*. New York: HarperCollins.

Hone, L. C., Jarden, A., Schofield, G. M., & Duncan, S. (2014). Measuring flourishing: The impact of operational definitions on the prevalence of high levels of wellbeing. *International Journal of Wellbeing, 4*(1) Retrieved from http://internationaljournalofwellbeing.org/ijow/index.php/ijow/article/view/286.

Kasser, T. (2004). The good life or the goods life? Positive psychology and personal well-being in the culture of consumption. In P. A. Linley & S. Joseph (Eds.), *Positive psychology in practice* (pp. 55–67). Hoboken: Wiley.

Kasser, T., & Ryan, R. M. (1993). A dark side of the American dream: Correlates of financial success as a central life aspiration. *Journal of Personality and Social Psychology, 65*(2), 410–422.

Kasser, T., & Ryan, R. M. (1996). Further examining the American dream: Differential correlates of intrinsic and extrinsic goals. *Personality and Social Psychology Bulletin, 22*(3), 280–287.

Knowles, E. S., & Linn, J. A. (2004). The importance of resistance to persuasion. In E. S. Knowles & J. A. Linn (Eds.), *Resistance and persuasion* (pp. 3–9). Mahwah: Erlbaum.

Lin, W. F., Chen, L. H., & Li, T. (2013). Adult children's caregiver burden and depression: The moderating roles of parent-child relationship satisfaction and feedback from others. *Journal of Happiness Studies, 14*(2), 673–687. doi:10.1007/s10902-012-9348-0.

Manski, C. F. (2013). *Public policy in an uncertain world: Analysis and decisions*. Cambridge: Harvard University Press.

Marks, N. (2011). *The happiness manifesto: How nations and people can nurture well-being*. New York: TED Books.

Mulgan, G. (2013). Well-being and public policy. In S. A. David, I. Boniwell, & A. C. Ayers (Eds.), *The Oxford handbook of happiness* (pp. 517–532). Oxford: Oxford University Press.

Mutrie, N., & Faulkner, G. (2004). Physical activity. In P. A. Linley & S. Joseph (Eds.), *Positive psychology in practice* (pp. 146–164). Hoboken: Wiley.

Proctor, C., Tsukayama, E., Wood, A. M., Maltby, J., Fox Eades, J. M., & Linley, P. A. (2011). Strengths Gym: The impact of a character strengths-based intervention on the life satisfaction and well-being of adolescents. *The Journal of Positive Psychology, 6*(5), 377–388. doi:10.1080/17439760.2011.594079.

Proctor, C., Tweed, R., & Morris, D. (2015). The naturally emerging structure of well-being among young adults: "Big Two" or other framework? *Journal of Happiness Studies, 16*(1), 257–275.

Quinlan, D. M., Swain, N., Cameron, C., & Vella-Brodrick, D. A. (2015). How 'other people matter' in a classroom-based strengths intervention: Exploring interpersonal strategies and classroom outcomes. *The Journal of Positive Psychology, 10*(1), 77–89.

Sanders, M. R., Kirby, J. N., Tellegen, C. L., & Day, J. J. (2014). The Triple P-Positive Parenting Program: A systematic review and meta-analysis of a multi-level system of parenting support. *Clinical Psychology Review, 34*(4), 337–357. doi:10.1016/j.cpr.2014.04.003.

Schueller, S. M. (2009). Promoting wellness: Integrating community and positive psychology. *Journal of Community Psychology, 37*(7), 922–937. doi:10.1002/jcop.20334.

Schwartz, C. E., & Sendor, R. M. (1999). Helping others helps oneself: Response shift effects in peer support. *Social Science and Medicine, 48*(11), 1563–1575.

Seligman, M. E. P., Steen, T. A., Park, N., & Peterson, C. (2005). Positive psychology progress: Empirical validation of interventions. *American Psychologist, 60*(5), 410–421.

Seligman, M. E. P., Reivich, K., Jaycox, L., & Gillham, J. (2007). *The optimistic child*. New York: Houghton Mifflin.

Sherman, S. (2011). Changing the world: The science of transformative action. In R. Biswas-Diener (Ed.), *Positive psychology as social change* (pp. 329–345). London: Springer.

Slovic, P. (2007). "If I look at the mass I will never act": Psychic numbing and genocide. *Judgment and Decision Making, 2*(2), 79–95.

Tweed, R. G., Biswas-Diener, R., & Lehman, D. R. (2012). Self-perceived strengths among people who are homeless. *The Journal of Positive Psychology, 7*(6), 481–492.

United States., & Library of Congress. (1961). I*naugural addresses of the Presidents of the United States from George Washington, 1789, to John F. Kennedy, 1961*. Washington: United States Government Printing Office.

Veenhoven, R. (2015). Happiness as a priority in public policy. In S. Josephs (Ed.), *Positive psychology in practice* (2nd ed., pp. 731–750). Hoboken: Wiley.

Washington State Institute for Public Policy. (2014a). *Benefit-cost results*. Olympia: Author.

Washington State Institute for Public Policy. (2014b). *Benefit-cost technical documentation*. Olympia: Author.

Welsh, B. C., Sullivan, C. J., & Olds, D. L. (2010). When early crime prevention goes to scale: A new look at the evidence. *Prevention Science, 11*(2), 115–125. doi:10.1007/s11121-009-0159-4.

ERRATUM

Positive Psychology Interventions in Practice

Carmel Proctor

© Springer International Publishing AG 2017
C. Proctor (ed.), *Positive Psychology Interventions in Practice*,
DOI 10.1007/978-3-319-51787-2

DOI 10.1007/978-3-319-51787-2_16

Chapter 11 in: Suzy Green, Olivia Evans, and Belinda Williams, Positive Psychology at Work: Research and Practice, DOI 10.1007/978-3-319-51787-2_11.

The original version of this book was published with an additional affiliation for Dr. Suzy Green. It is removed and updated in the current version:

S. Green
The Positivity Institute, Level 57, MLC Centre, 19-29 Martin Place, Sydney, NSW 2000, Australia

---

The updated original online version for this book can be found at
DOI 10.1007/978-3-319-51787-2

© Springer International Publishing AG 2017
C. Proctor (ed.), *Positive Psychology Interventions in Practice*,
DOI 10.1007/978-3-319-51787-2_16

Lightning Source UK Ltd.
Milton Keynes UK
UKOW06n1438111217
314180UK00003BA/345/P

9 783319 517858